The Geography of Disease

**Also Available from
Bloomsbury Academic**

*Pandemics in American Popular Culture: Depicting Disease and
Confronting Contagion*
James Craig Holte

Endangered Places: Disappearing Sites around the World
Leslie A. Duram

Human Migration and the Refugee Crisis: Origins and Global Impact
Eliot Dickinson

The Geography of Disease

How Location and Culture Influence Health in Today's World

Jing Luo

BLOOMSBURY ACADEMIC
NEW YORK • LONDON • OXFORD • NEW DELHI • SYDNEY

BLOOMSBURY ACADEMIC

Bloomsbury Publishing Inc, 1359 Broadway New York NY 10018 USA
Bloomsbury Publishing Plc, 50 Bedford Square London WC1B 3DP UK
Bloomsbury Publishing Ireland 29 Earlsfort Terrace Dublin 2, D02 AY28 Ireland

BLOOMSBURY, BLOOMSBURY ACADEMIC and the Diana logo are
trademarks of Bloomsbury Publishing Plc

First published in the United States of America 2026

Copyright © Jing Luo, 2026

Cover image © MattLphotography/Alamy Stock Photo

All rights reserved. No part of this publication may be: i) reproduced or transmitted in
any form, electronic or mechanical, including photocopying, recording or by means of
any information storage or retrieval system without prior permission in writing from the
publishers; or ii) used or reproduced in any way for the training, development or operation
of artificial intelligence (AI) technologies, including generative AI technologies. The rights
holders expressly reserve this publication from the text and data mining exception
as per Article 4(3) of the Digital Single Market Directive (EU) 2019/790.

Bloomsbury Publishing Inc does not have any control over, or responsibility for,
any third-party websites referred to or in this book. All internet addresses given
in this book were correct at the time of going to press. The author and publisher
regret any inconvenience caused if addresses have changed or sites have ceased
to exist, but can accept no responsibility for any such changes.

Library of Congress Cataloging-in-Publication Data
Names: Luo, Jing, 1900- author.
Title: The geography of disease : how location and culture influence
health in today's world / Jing Luo.
Description: New York, NY : Bloomsbury Academic, 2026. |
Includes bibliographical references and index.
Identifiers: LCCN 2025013787 (print) | LCCN 2025013788 (ebook) |
ISBN 9781440875595 hardback | ISBN 9798765114520 epub | ISBN 9781440875601 pdf
Subjects: LCSH: Medical geography | Environmental health | World health
Classification: LCC RA792 .L86 2026 (print) | LCC RA792 (ebook)
LC record available at https://lccn.loc.gov/2025013787
LC ebook record available at https://lccn.loc.gov/2025013788

ISBN: HB: 978-1-4408-7559-5
ePDF: 978-1-4408-7560-1
eBook: 979-8-7651-1452-0

Typeset by Integra Software Services Pvt. Ltd.

For product safety related questions contact productsafety@bloomsbury.com.

To find out more about our authors and books visit www.bloomsbury.com
and sign up for our newsletters.

Contents

Preface ix
Acknowledgments xiii

Introduction 1

1 Ecology and Disease 7
   Climate Change and the Spread of Zoonotic Disease 8
      Hantavirus and Babesiosis—A Red Flag of Climate Change and Environmental Stress 8
      Marburg Virus Disease Outbreaks—Lessons Learned 12
      Middle East Respiratory Syndrome (MERS) 16
      Severe Acute Respiratory Syndrome (SARS) and the Importance of Information Transparency 19
      Yellow Fever—A Continuing Challenge under Climate Change and Globalization 24
      Zika—A Virus with Impacts on Societies' Value Systems 28
   Geographic Factors and Natural Hazards 32
      Cancer and Geographical Environment 32
      Chemical Releases in Natech Events 37
      Health Impacts of the Chernobyl and Fukushima Daiichi Accidents 40
      Epidemics after Natural Disasters 44
      Malaria Control—Progress and Challenges 48
      Systemic Lupus Erythematosus and the Socioeconomic Environment 52
   Impact of Environmental Damages on Health 55
      Alberta Struggles to Contain Health Risks from Oil Sands 55
      Could Lab Leaks Pose Serious Threats to Public Health? 59
      Deforestation and Increasing Risks of Lyme Disease 66
      Dengue Fever and Runaway Urbanization in Asian Cities 69
      Radioactive Contamination due to Mining—What Can Be Learned? 72

2	Population Health and Well-Being	77
	Aging and Health Challenges	80
	Cultural Perspectives on Aging	80
	Combatting Dementia—What Japan and the United States Can Share to Improve Care and Innovation	83
	Global Aging—Exploring the Role of Geography, Genetics, and Socioeconomic Factors	88
	Environmental Triggers of Parkinson's Disease—Insights for Prevention and Management	92
	Why Societies Must Be Prepared for Population Aging	96
	Education and Public Health	100
	The Revival of TCM: Heritage, Health, and the Role of the State	100
	Comprehensive Sexuality Education in China, Japan, and Korea—Cultural Challenges and Reforms	104
	The Power of Words and the Stigma of Contagion	109
	Nutrition Education in Japan	112
	Promoting Health Education in Africa through Artistic Forms	117
	Health Care Systems and Public Health	120
	China's Health Care System—Challenges and Opportunities	120
	Health Care in Africa—Challenges and Opportunities	124
	Japan's Health Care System	129
	How Health Care Systems in the United States and Canada Address Their Challenges Differently	132
	What Can the United States Learn from Other Industrialized Countries in Controlling Drug Prices?	138
	Lifestyle and Health Issues	142
	China's Struggle with Mental Health Challenges	142
	E-Cigarettes and Their Associated Health Risks	149
	China's Struggle with Fatty Liver Disease and Gout	153
	Could GLP-1 Drugs End Obesity?	158
	Japanese Tips for a Healthy Diet—Insights and Practices	162
	Overwork-Related Health Consequences in Japan and Korea	166
	Traditional Chinese Medicine and Its Contribution to Treatment and Prevention of Disease	170
3	Social Determinants of and Policy Impacts on Health	175
	Public Policies' Impact on Public Health	178
	China's Zero-Covid Policy and Its Abrupt Ending	178

Covid-19 and Politics in the United States—It's More Than Fighting the Virus	184
Eradication of Smallpox—The First Major Milestone of Modern Vaccination	189
Resurgence of Syphilis in China	192
The Healing Power of Belief: Worship as a Societal Antibiotic	199
Socioeconomic Divide and Health	203
China's Blueprint for Hepatitis B Control—An Extraordinary Public Health Success Story	203
Depression and Anxiety in College Population in the United States	207
Preventable Diseases in an Unequal World—Addressing Diphtheria, Tetanus, and Pertussis	211
Malnutrition in the United States—A Socioeconomic Challenge	214
Beyond Outbreaks: The Global Rise of *Salmonella* and *E. coli* Infections	218
Synthetic Opioids and Methamphetamine Addiction: Escalating Crises in American Public Health	224
War and Forced Migration	227
Control and Prevention of Polio in Africa	227
Impact of Migration on the Spread of HIV/AIDS	231
Resurgence of Louse-Borne Diseases due to Migration	236
The 1918 Flu—How War Promotes Pandemics	240
Forced to Flee, Left Behind: Health Consequences of the Syrian Refugee Crisis	244
The Surge of Covid, TB, and HIV in War-Torn Ukraine	247
Addressing the Health Needs of Migrant Populations	250
4 Globalization and Public Health	**255**
Mpox: Understanding Its Origins, Global Spread, and Strategies for Control	256
Prion Diseases—Navigating Global Health Risks in an Era of Zoonotic Threats and Globalization	260
Influenza in a Globalized World—Swine Flu and Bird Flu	264
Globalization, Forced Migration, and the Growing Threat of Tuberculosis Outbreaks	268
Ebola in West Africa—The Clash of Globalization and Tradition	272

5 Spatial Technology and Public Health 277
   John Snow's Legacy in Modern Disease Control and Prevention 279
   Enhancing Public Health through Geographic Information
      Systems (GIS) 282
   How China and the United States Used Spatial Technology
      to Fight the Covid-19 Pandemic 285
   How Spatial Tools Empower Global Health Organizations 290
   Mapping the Future—How Spatial Technology Is Revolutionizing
      Chronic Disease Prevention and Management 294

Index 298
About the Author 307

Preface

The Geography of Disease: How Location and Culture Influence Health in Today's World explores the relationships between diseases and their social, economic, and geographical contexts—the contextual determinants of health. The book presents a collection of case studies, each typically providing a detailed description of a disease and its associations with social, cultural, and geographical determinants, based on published research. It is organized into five chapters: ecology and disease, population health and well-being, social determinants and policy impacts on health, globalization and public health, and spatial technology and public health. Sidebars throughout the book provide additional information related to each set of cases.

The contents of each chapter are presented as follows.

Ecology and Disease

Ecological impacts on public health are a major challenge of the twenty-first century, with environmental degradation, climate change, and human activities profoundly influencing disease spread and management. This chapter examines pollution from Alberta's oil sands raising cancer risks for Indigenous communities and climate shifts driving diseases such as Lyme and dengue fever. It explores the long-term health effects of radioactive contamination, industrial pollution, and disasters like Chernobyl and Fukushima, highlighting the vulnerabilities of marginalized populations. The rise of zoonotic diseases, fueled by deforestation, habitat changes, and wildlife trade, including outbreaks of MERS, SARS, yellow fever, and Zika, stresses the need for global collaboration, surveillance, and equitable health care. Preventable diseases such as malaria and the socioeconomic burdens of conditions like lupus further reveal the intersection of environmental and societal factors.

Population Health and Well-being

Global aging, lifestyle-related health challenges, health care efficiency, and education are pivotal factors shaping public health and well-being globally. Aging populations in countries such as Japan, the United States, and other developed nations place significant pressure on health care systems, particularly with the increasing prevalence of dementia and Parkinson's disease. Socioeconomic disparities, environmental issues, and genetic predispositions further influence health outcomes, disproportionately affecting vulnerable populations. Education plays a vital role in fostering health literacy, encouraging healthier behaviors, and addressing issues such as sexually transmitted infections and xenophobia. Lifestyle-related conditions, including obesity and metabolic disorders, highlight the need for preventive measures, public awareness, and systemic reforms. Efficient health care systems, as seen in countries such as Japan and Canada, offer valuable insights into achieving a balance between equity, affordability, and innovation. The integration of traditional practices, such as Traditional Chinese Medicine, with modern approaches also presents opportunities to address chronic diseases and global health challenges effectively.

Social Determinants and Policy Impacts on Health

Poorly designed public health policies, socioeconomic disparities, and conflicts are significant obstacles to public health, often intertwining to hinder disease control and prevention while exacerbating existing crises. Cases such as China's Zero-Covid policy and the U.S. fragmented Covid-19 response illustrate how governance and political divides can influence health outcomes. Socioeconomic disparities further magnify health challenges, as seen in the rising mental health issues among U.S. college students, malnutrition in low-income communities, and the opioid crisis fueled by poverty. Meanwhile, conflicts such as the Syrian war and the crisis in Ukraine have devastated health care infrastructure, driving disease outbreaks and worsening non-communicable conditions. Migration, whether caused by war or economic hardship, deepens vulnerabilities, exposing displaced populations to infectious diseases and inadequate health care access. Historical examples, including the eradication of smallpox and the 1918 flu pandemic, showcase the potential of coordinated global action while underscoring the importance of equitable policies and preparedness.

Globalization and Public Health

The modern era of globalization has fostered interconnectedness and collaboration, raising global living standards while also introducing significant health challenges. Increased trade, travel, migration, conflict, climate change, and zoonotic diseases have amplified the risk of infectious disease outbreaks, requiring coordinated global responses. The 2013–16 Ebola outbreak in West Africa, exacerbated by weak health care systems and cultural practices, and the spread of prion diseases such as vCJD from industrial farming, demonstrate the dangers of zoonotic transmission. Influenza pandemics like H1N1 and H5N1 reveal the speed with which zoonotic viruses can spread globally, emphasizing the importance of a One Health approach and improved biosecurity. Tuberculosis, worsened by overcrowding, migration, and health care disruptions, remains a persistent threat, especially in developing regions. These examples reveal the transboundary nature of infectious diseases and the urgent need for international collaboration in prevention, early detection, equitable health care access, and the strengthening of health systems to mitigate future pandemic risks.

Spatial Technology and Public Health

Spatial technologies, such as Geographic Information Systems (GIS), have become essential in modern public health, providing tools for tracking, analyzing, and responding to health challenges in a world increasingly affected by climate change, migration, conflict, and zoonotic diseases. Building on John Snow's 1854 cholera mapping, GIS now enables advanced data visualization and integration, supporting efforts to manage both infectious and chronic diseases. During the Covid-19 pandemic, countries such as China and the United States used GIS to monitor infection hotspots, allocate resources, and address health care disparities, showcasing its value in real-time crisis management. Beyond infectious diseases, GIS plays a key role in tackling chronic health conditions by identifying environmental and social determinants, such as access to nutritious food and health care. It also enhances global cooperation through frameworks such as the United Nations' One Health initiative, which integrates human, animal, and environmental health. Although challenges such as data privacy and interoperability persist, the proven effectiveness of spatial technologies has them indispensable for early detection, prevention, and equitable health responses in the future.

The cases in this book are carefully selected to effectively illustrate key themes while addressing current public health concerns. For example, the management of Covid-19, the emergence and resurgence of infectious diseases such as mpox and syphilis, global aging and its associated health care challenges, and the application of spatial technologies are each analyzed in relation to their socio-environmental contexts. These include factors such as cultural influences, global economic shifts, conflict and war, and disease prevention within the One Health framework.

The case analyses are grounded in findings from up-to-date and reputable studies. It is important to emphasize that this book is not intended to serve as a clinical guide. Rather, its purpose is to explore the intricate relationship between health and the environment, promoting the idea that improving the contextual determinants of health can lead to healthier lives and better preparedness for future pandemics.

Acknowledgments

This book explores the critical relationship between environmental and sociocultural factors in shaping public health outcomes. As the Covid-19 pandemic demonstrated, disease control extends beyond medical interventions; it is deeply influenced by governance, economic conditions, and cultural values. The contrasting responses to the Covid-19 pandemic highlighted how social structures and policy choices shape health outcomes, sometimes with unintended consequences. By understanding these contextual determinants, we can foster more effective and equitable public health strategies for the future.

I extend my deep appreciation to ABC-CLIO, now part of Bloomsbury Publishing, for its foresight in supporting this project. By recognizing the importance of this topic, the publisher has provided a valuable platform for examining the intersections of geography, culture, and health.

My sincere gratitude goes to Mr. Kevin Downing, the editorial director, for his leadership and unwavering support in facilitating this project to completion. I also thank Ms. Kaitlin Ciarmiello, former senior acquisition editor, for her editorial guidance on the book's structure and her thoughtful approach to shaping the layout of case studies. Finally, I am grateful to Ms. Maxine Taylor, senior acquisition editor, for her dedication in ensuring the manuscript successfully moved through the final stages of publication. This book could not have been realized without their dedicated support.

Introduction

Diseases are not solely biological processes; their spread, morbidity, and mortality are deeply influenced by social, cultural, geographic, and other contextual determinants. A notable example is the contrasting approaches taken by the United States and China to control the spread of Covid-19, each shaped by its unique sociocultural context. Neither country could have effectively implemented the other's strategy.

Science and technology were instrumental in the US rapid development of Covid-19 vaccines, saving tens of millions of lives. Federalism and individual rights are foundational aspects of the U.S. social system, often giving the states considerable autonomy in crafting their control policies. This resulted in a diverse array of strategies, ranging from personal protective measures to vaccine mandates. Although individual rights were strongly protected, studies showed that many decisions were heavily shaped by partisan politics, turning public health measures into highly polarizing issues.

China, by contrast, adopted a centralized, top-down approach to managing the pandemic. Its strategy focused on extensive quarantines, including policies such as "Zero-Covid" and "Dynamic Zero," alongside mandatory antigen testing. From January 2020 to December 2022, dozens of megacities, each with populations in the millions or tens of millions, endured prolonged lockdowns. Wuhan, a city of 11 million, was locked down for 76 days, while many other large cities faced weeks-long lockdowns. During these periods, citizens were confined to their apartments and their movements were strictly monitored through a Health Code system that tracked infection status and exposure. Compliance was enforced through strict media censorship, which promoted pro-government narratives—referred to as "positive energy"—while suppressing dissenting opinions. Adherence to the measures was framed as an act of loyalty and patriotism.

Centralized response versus decentralized response, tech-driven monitoring versus a focus on vaccine development, strict restrictions on individual mobility versus substantial resistance to measures, tight media control versus mixed messaging from various sources, and proactive prevention versus reactive management—these are some of the differences between the United States and China in systemic approaches that contributed to varying mortality and morbidity outcomes.

In 2022, the Johns Hopkins Coronavirus Resource Center reported that the U.S. Covid-19 death toll had exceeded one million, while China's official death toll remained at approximately 5,000, though some experts raised concerns about potential underreporting. China's Zero-Covid policy successfully minimized infections and deaths in the early stages of the pandemic but came at significant mental, political, and economic costs. Prolonged lockdowns sparked widespread frustration, culminating in public protests and growing economic pressures by late 2022. In response, the government abruptly abandoned its lockdown strategy in December 2022. This sudden policy reversal left citizens unprepared for a surge of Omicron-induced infections, overwhelming health care systems and exposing vulnerabilities after years of stringent containment measures.

The true mortality rate in China during this period remains uncertain. A study by Du et al. (2023) estimated the death toll at 1.4 million following the relaxation of the Zero-Covid policy. The researchers attributed the high fatality rate to several factors, including a lack of infection-acquired immunity, the moderate effectiveness of commonly used vaccines, low vaccination coverage among the elderly, and limited access to effective antiviral drugs. Similarly, a study published in Lancet Regional Health estimated that China's Covid-19 death toll exceeded one million (Lancet 2023). However, questions have been raised about the accuracy of China's official figures, highlighting potential gaps in data reporting.

In comparison, Covid-19 deaths in the United States were estimated to have reached approximately 1.13 million by April 2023 (Statista.com 2025). Unlike China, the United States faced significant challenges related to public trust, vaccine hesitancy, and political polarization, which hindered the consistent implementation of public health measures.

Both countries might have reduced their Covid-19 death tolls by addressing key social and cultural determinants, such as improving access to health care, increasing vaccination rates among vulnerable populations, and fostering greater public trust in scientific evidence and policies backed by science. These systemic barriers significantly influenced the outcomes of their pandemic responses.

Contextual Determinants of Disease

The Covid-19 pandemic brought wider recognition to an important truth: the success of disease control and prevention is shaped not only by medical interventions but also by contextual factors, such as social, cultural, and environmental conditions. According to the World Health Organization (WHO), these determinants account for 30–55 percent of health outcomes, highlighting their significant impact on a community's capacity to manage and recover from diseases. Therefore, addressing these non-medical determinants is crucial for creating effective public health strategies.

Socioeconomic disparities, for example, directly impact access to health care. Studies show that health follows a social gradient—individuals in lower socioeconomic positions consistently experience poorer health outcomes. These disparities, although unjust and avoidable, persist and contribute to a greater and more widespread burden of disease.

Governance policies play a critical role in shaping public health by influencing the prioritization of health needs, determining resource allocation for social welfare, and guiding crisis response and prevention efforts. Cultural values can both support and hinder health care. On one hand, they promote health by encouraging preventive practices, fostering strong family support, embracing holistic approaches, driving community initiatives, and building trust in health care providers. On the other hand, they can impede health care through factors such as stigma surrounding certain conditions, reliance on traditional medicine, mistrust of scientific systems, language barriers, restrictive gender roles, unhealthy dietary habits, and fatalistic beliefs.

Geographical conditions significantly impact public health by influencing disease prevalence, resource availability, and access to health care. Climate and terrain shape risks such as vector-borne diseases in tropical regions, water scarcity in arid areas, and limited health care access in remote locations. Urbanization can exacerbate issues like overcrowding, pollution, and the rapid spread of diseases, while natural disasters often disrupt health care systems and infrastructure. To be effective, public health strategies must address these location-specific challenges.

Conflict and war can lead to a breakdown of sanitation, overcrowding in refugee settings, and a lack of access to clean water, all of which facilitate the rapid spread of infectious diseases such as cholera, malaria, and respiratory infections. Additionally, immunization programs are often halted, increasing the population's vulnerability to outbreaks.

Climate change, driven by human activities such as deforestation and fossil fuel consumption, has a profound impact on health care and the spread of diseases. Events like the 2025 Los Angeles wildfires, intensified by rising temperatures and drought, increase respiratory illnesses and disrupt communities, heightening the risk of disease outbreaks in crowded shelters. Rising temperatures also expand the habitats of disease vectors such as mosquitoes, leading to increased cases of malaria and dengue. Additionally, extreme weather events like floods disrupt sanitation and water systems, causing waterborne illnesses. These challenges place significant strain on health care systems, underscoring the need for climate-resilient strategies and proactive efforts to address the root causes of climate change.

Global aging poses significant challenges to health care systems by increasing demand for services, driving up costs, and creating strain on resources. Older populations are more prone to chronic diseases, require specialized geriatric care, and often face mental health conditions such as dementia and depression. To address these challenges, health care systems must adapt by tackling workforce shortages, emphasizing targeted fiscal policies, preventive care, and prioritizing effective management of chronic diseases. These measures are essential to meet the needs of aging populations and ensure the sustainability of health care delivery.

Lifestyles play a crucial role in public health by shaping behaviors and habits. Healthy practices, such as maintaining a balanced diet, engaging in regular exercise, seeking preventive care, and avoiding harmful substances, support physical and mental well-being while reducing the risk of chronic diseases. In contrast, unhealthy diets, sedentary lifestyles, risky behaviors such as smoking or excessive alcohol consumption, and neglect of preventive care contribute to a higher prevalence of diseases and place additional strain on health care systems. Stressful, overworked lifestyles further exacerbate both mental and physical health challenges. Promoting positive lifestyle changes through education, supportive policies, and enabling environments is essential for improving public health outcomes.

Racism and xenophobia undermine disease control by eroding trust in health care, limiting access to care, and fueling stigma that discourages treatment and cooperation. These biases deepen health disparities, strain social cohesion, and divert attention from effective, evidence-based strategies. On both local and global scales, they obstruct equitable health care and hinder collective efforts, making inclusive and culturally sensitive approaches essential for improving public health outcomes.

These factors, contextual to the biological mechanisms of disease, are key determinants that influence how diseases are managed, experienced, and prevented across populations. Addressing them is essential, as they impact not only individual health outcomes but also the effectiveness of public health strategies. Ignoring these determinants can deepen health disparities, perpetuate unequal care, and weaken disease prevention efforts. By prioritizing them, policymakers and health systems can foster more equitable and sustainable health outcomes for entire communities.

Further Reading

Bridgeland, John, Elizabeth Cameron, J. Stephen Morrison, Jennifer B. Nuzzo, and Aquielle Person. 2024. "Strengthening Democracy and Pandemic Preparedness Go Hand in Hand." *Bulletin of the Atomic Scientists*. https://thebulletin.org/2024/09/strengthening-democracy-and-pandemic-preparedness-go-hand-in-hand/.

Du, Zhanwei, Yuchen Wang, Yuan Bai, Lin Wang, Benjamin John Cowling, and Lauren Ancel Meyers. 2023. "Estimate of COVID-19 Deaths, China, December 2022–February 2023." *Emerging Infectious Diseases*. https://wwwnc.cdc.gov/eid/article/29/10/23-0585.

Ellwanger, Joel Henrique, and José Arur Bogo Chies. 2021. "Zoonotic Spillover: Understanding Basic Aspects for Better Prevention." *Genetics and Molecular Biology*, 44(1) (Suppl 1). https://doi.org/10.1590/1678-4685-GMB-2020-0355.

Lancet Regional Health—Western Pacific (Lancet). 2023. "The End of Zero-Covid-19 Policy Is Not End of COVID-19 for China." https://www.thelancet.com/journals/lanwpc/article/PIIS2666-6065(23)00020-2/fulltext.

Statista.com. 2025. "Total Number of Cases and Deaths from COVID-19 in the United States as of April 26, 2023." https://www.statista.com/statistics/1101932/coronavirus-covid19-cases-and-deaths-number-us-americans/.

The World Health Organization (WHO). "Social Determinants of Health." https://www.who.int/health-topics/social-determinants-of-health#tab=tab_1.

1

Ecology and Disease

Ecological impacts on public health are a defining feature of the twenty-first century. The degradation of natural environments, unfavorable geo-environmental changes, and climate shifts have profoundly affected disease control and prevention. This chapter examines these dynamics through seventeen articles, each exploring how human activities, environmental disruption, and climate change contribute to the spread and management of diseases, shaping global health outcomes.

Canada's reliance on Alberta's oil sands reflects the tension between economic development and environmental costs, where pollution has heightened cancer risks for nearby Indigenous communities. Lab leaks, whether from human error or advanced bioengineering experiments, underscore the global risks of inadequate biosafety measures. Lyme disease, linked to deforestation and warming climates, continues to spread as ecosystems shift, while dengue fever persists in urban regions with poor waste management and thriving Aedes mosquito populations. The legacy of radioactive contamination from uranium mining, such as the Church Rock spill, reveals long-term health and ecological consequences that demand stronger oversight and community engagement.

Geographic and environmental conditions amplify health challenges worldwide. Environmental exposures, from industrial pollutants to lifestyle factors, contribute to cancer rates, with marginalized populations often bearing the greatest burden. Natech disasters, where natural hazards trigger chemical spills, illustrate the vulnerabilities of industrial systems to environmental hazards, emphasizing the need for disaster preparedness. The nuclear accidents at Chernobyl and Fukushima revealed the immense human and environmental toll of nuclear energy mishaps, calling for transparency and collaboration to mitigate future risks. Natural disasters frequently lead to outbreaks of diseases such as cholera and malaria, exacerbated by inadequate sanitation and health care in affected regions. Malaria, though preventable and treatable, remains a significant global health challenge, requiring innovative approaches to vaccines and genetic solutions. Diseases like systemic lupus erythematosus (SLE) highlight how socioeconomic disparities and environmental exposures disproportionately affect women and minorities.

The growing prevalence of zoonotic diseases further manifests the consequences of ecological disruption. Warming climates and habitat changes drive the spread of diseases such as babesiosis and hantavirus, while deforestation and wildlife trade fuel outbreaks of Marburg Virus Disease. The emergence of Middle East respiratory syndrome (MERS) and severe acute respiratory syndrome (SARS) demonstrates the need for global cooperation, early surveillance, and robust public health systems to combat zoonotic threats. Yellow fever and Zika, both exacerbated by climate-driven mosquito proliferation, stress the importance of vaccination and public health interventions. The Zika outbreak, in particular, highlighted social challenges, sparking debates over reproductive rights and ethical considerations during health crises.

These interconnected issues demand urgent, coordinated action to safeguard public health. Strategies that integrate environmental conservation, equitable health care, climate resilience, and scientific innovation are essential to address these challenges. By confronting the ecological factors driving disease emergence and spread, the global community can work toward a healthier, more sustainable future.

Climate Change and the Spread of Zoonotic Disease

Hantavirus and Babesiosis—A Red Flag of Climate Change and Environmental Stress

Babesiosis and hantavirus infections are serious diseases transmitted by rodents that can result in hemorrhagic fever, organ failure, and death in humans. These diseases are increasingly prevalent worldwide, primarily due to three key factors: climate change, human intervention of eco-environment, and specific human activities.

Babesiosis is a tick-borne illness, caused by a protozoan parasite that feeds on red blood cells. The babesia species that infects people is known as *Babesia microti* (*B. microti*). The primary reservoir of this parasite is the white-footed mice which have high populations in Northeastern and Upper Midwestern regions of the United States, particularly in parts of New England, New York,

New Jersey, Wisconsin, and Minnesota. The transmission occurs through the bite of an infected blacklegged tick known as *Ixodes scapularis* or "deer ticks" that have fed on an infected carrier mouse. In rare cases, blood transfusion can be a pathway of transmission. As a result, the inclusion of babesia contamination testing is part of the standard blood screening procedure. Because black-legged ticks can also spread Lyme disease, co-infection of babesiosis and Lyme disease can occur in a same individual, according to the Centers for Disease Control and Prevention (CDC).

Compared to infections of Lyme disease, the number of reported cases of babesiosis in the United States is relatively low, with approximately 1,000 cases per year, while Lyme disease accounts for approximately 30,000 cases. However, the rate of occurrences of babesiosis between 2011 and 2019 in Vermont, Maine, and New Hampshire experienced the highest increase, according to the CDC. Scientists believe that the warmer climate in the northern United States may have been an important factor responsible for the rise in babesiosis cases. Warmer winters contribute to increased vegetation that sustains larger deer populations, which in turn lead to an abundance of ticks that feed on deer (Anthes 2023).

Symptoms of babesiosis can range from asymptomatic to mild, resembling flu-like symptoms that typically resolve in two to three weeks. However, approximately one-fourth of individuals who become infected, especially those who are over the age of fifty or younger than three months, may develop severe infections that can prove fatal. In the advanced stage, anemia, unstable blood pressure, blood clotting, and malfunction of vital organs such as the kidneys, lungs, and liver can occur and even lead to death. According to the CDC, the fatality rate can range from 10 percent to 30 percent in certain high-risk groups—such as the elderly, those without a spleen, people with weakened immune systems, and those with other severe health conditions. Treatment for babesiosis involves the use of antibiotics; prevention measures include wearing appropriate clothing and using insect repellent. Unfortunately, a vaccine for babesiosis is not yet available.

Globally, babesiosis infects many parts of the world. In Europe, the tick-borne subspecies *B. divergens* is prevalent, while in Asia *B. venatorum* is commonly found. Both sub-species are transmitted by tick bites. In Asia, the reservoirs for these subspecies have been reported to be domestic animals such as cattle and roe deer, which shows the remarkable adaptability of babesia to human-influenced environment. In China, *B. miroti and B. Venatorum* both have a high prevalence which can be attributed to significant modification to the natural environment and the increasing production of beef and dairy products (Hussein et al. 2022; He 2021).

Hantaviruses are transmitted from rodents to people through aerosolized dust particles infested with mouse urine, feces, and saliva. Occasionally, transmission can also occur through a bite from an infected host. Hantavirus can be carried by various rodents commonly found in the United States, including Cotton rat, white-footed mice, and deer mice. While the primary mode of transmission is through inhalation of dust with viral particles, in rare cases blood transfusion can also lead to infection. Individuals who engage in vacuuming infested areas, such as cabins, sheds, and barns, as well as construction workers, campers, and soldiers, are at higher risk of contracting hantavirus. Research shows that many outbreaks of symptoms documented during the Korean War are now attributed to hantavirus infections (Mohammed 2010).

Hantavirus infections pose a significant global health risk, attracting widespread attention. These infections can manifest in two distinct forms, depending on geographic locations and the associated host rodents. The "New World" hantaviruses are found mostly in the Americas and may cause "hantavirus pulmonary syndrome" (HPS). Conversely, the "Old World" hantaviruses are predominantly found in Europe and Asia, and are capable of causing "hemorrhagic fever with renal syndrome" (HFRS). Both HPS and HFRS can result in internal bleeding, fever, and organ failure and, in severe cases, death. However, HPS is particularly severe due to symptoms such as cardiogenic shock and pulmonary edema (fluid buildup). Fatality of HPS ranges between 30 percent and 50 percent, while HFRS has a fatality rate of 12 to 40 percent, studies show (Avšič-Županc et al. 2015; CDC). In the United States and Canada, the primary hantavirus responsible for HPS is the *Sin Nombre* virus which is typically transmitted by the deer mouse (CDC).

The spread of zoonotic diseases is often influenced by both climate change and environmental deterioration. One outbreak associated with climate change is the Four Corner outbreak. In 1993, a hantavirus outbreak occurred in the Four Corners area where Colorado, Utah, New Mexico, and Arizona meet in the southwestern United States. This outbreak resulted in cases of HPS and caused approximately twenty deaths. The outbreak was attributed to an unusually moist winter in 1993, following several years of drought. Scientists observed that warmer winter temperatures and increased rainfall resulted in abundant vegetation in subsequent spring. This abundance of vegetation allowed deer mice to reproduce rapidly, with their population reaching ten times larger than the previous year. The larger mouse population increased the likelihood of contact between mice and humans, facilitating the transmission of the hantavirus carried by the mice to humans (Van Hook 2018).

Encroachment into forest areas can contribute to the emergence of hantavirus infections. For example, when cropland or urban expansion encroaches on forests and pastures, it can lead to shifts in rodent species diversity (Garcia-Peña 2021). This phenomenon was observed in China during the early stages of its economic boom in the late 1970s and early 1980s, a period marked by rapid urbanization. Reports of rodents infiltrating cities became a major concern and widely reported in local media. The winter season saw the highest incidence of infections, particularly with the Hantaan virus and Seoul virus, two subspecies of hantaviruses carried by a range of rodents, including wild mice and urban rats. The most severe outbreak occurred in 1985, with 115,804 cases of hemorrhagic fever with renal syndrome (HFRS), representing over 90 percent of global cases at the time and a fatality rate of 12.98 percent. In response, China implemented a series of rodent control measures, resulting in subsequent outbreaks in 1994 and early 2001 with fewer than 40,000 cases and a reduced fatality rate of approximately 2 percent (Zhang 2004).

Globally, rodent-transmitted diseases have been major concerns for public health due to their ability to spread rapidly and widely. Research suggests that in addition to advancement in medical treatment, mitigating impact of climate change and environment deterioration are key to prevention.

Further Reading

Anthes, Emily. 2023. "Lyme Isn't the Only Tick Disease to Worry about in the Northeast, CDC Says." *The New York Times.* https://www.nytimes.com/2023/03/16/health/babesiosis-tick-disease-northeast.html.

Avšič-Županc, Tatjana, Ana Saksida, and Miša Korva. 2015. "Hantavirus Infections." *Clinical Microbiological Infections, 21S*(2019): e6–e16. doi: 10.1111/1469-0691.12291.

CDC. "Parasites -Babesiosis." https://www.cdc.gov/parasites/babesiosis/epi.html.

Eby, Peggy, Alison J. Peel, Andrew Hoegh, et al. 2023. "Pathogen Spillover Driven by Rapid Changes in Bat Ecology." *Nature, 613*: 340–44. doi: 10.1038/s41586-022-05506-2.

García-Peña, Gabriel E., André V. Rubio, Hugo Mendoza, Miguel Fernandez, Matthew T. Milholland, A. Alonso Aguirre, Gerardo Suzan, and Carlos Sambrana-Torrelio. 2021. "Land-Use Change and Rodent-Borne Diseases: Hazards on the Shared Socioeconomic Pathways." *The Royal Society*. https://doi.org/10.1098/rstb.2020.0362.

Gibb, Rory, David W. Redding, Kai Qing Chin, Christl A. Donnelly, Tim M. Blackburn, Tim Newbold, and Kate E. Jones. 2020. "Zoonotic Host Diversity Increases in Human-dominated Ecosystems." *Nature*. https://doi.org/10.1038/s41586-020-2562-8.

He, Lan, Reginaldo G. Bastos, Yali Sun, Guohua Hua, Guiquan Guan, Junlong Zhao, and Carlos E. Suarez. 2021. "Babesiosis as a Potential Threat for Bovine Production in China." *Parasites & Vectors*. https://doi.org/10.1186/s13071-021-04948-3.

Hussain, Sabir, Abrar Hussain, Muhammad Umair Aziz, Baolin Song, Jehan Zeb, David George, Jun Li, and Oliver Sparagano. 2022. "A Review of Zoonotic Babesiosis as an Emerging Public Health Threat in Asia." *Pathogens, 11*(1): 23. https://doi.org/10.3390/pathogens11010023.

Krause, Peter. 2018. "Babesiosis." *Youtube*. https://www.youtube.com/watch?v=vMWHW2w19pE.

Mir, Mohammed. 2010. "Hantaviruses." *Clin Lab Med*. doi: 10.1016/j.cll.2010.01.004.

Schmaljohn, Connie and Brian Hjelle. 1997. "Hantaviruses: A Global Disease Problem." *Emerging Infectious Disease, 3*(2) (April–June): 95–104. doi: 10.3201/eid0302.970202.

Swanson, Megan, Amy Pickrel, John Williamson, Susan Montgomery. 2023. "Trends in Reported Babesiosis Cases—United States, 2011–2019." *MMWR Morb Mortal Wkly Rep, 72*(11): 273–77. doi: http://dx.doi.org/10.15585/mmwr.mm7211a1.

Towner, Jonathan S., Marina L. Khristova, Tara K. Sealy, Martin J. Vincent, Bobbie R. Erickson, Darcy A. Bawiec, Amy L. Hartman, James A. Comer, Sherif R. Zaki, Ute Ströher, Filomena Gomes da Silva, Fernando del Castillo, Pierre E. Rollin, Thomas G. Ksiazek, and Stuart T. Nichol. 2006. "Marburgvirus Genomics and Association with a Large Hemorrhagic Fever Outbreak in Angola." *Journal of virology, 80*(13): 6497–516. doi:10.1128/JVI.00069-06.

Van Hook, and J. Charles. 2018. "Hantavirus Pulmonary Syndrome—The 25th Anniversary of the Four Corners Outbreak." *Emerging Infectious Diseases, 24*(11): 2056–60. https://doi.org/10.3201/eid2411.180381.

Zhang, Yong-zhen, Xiao dong-lou, Wang Yu, Wang Hong-xia, Sun Li, Tao Xiao-xia, Qu yong-gang. 2004. "The Epidemic Characteristics and Preventive Measures of Hemorrhagic Fever with Syndromes in China." *China Journal of Epidemiology, 25*(6): 466–9. https://pubmed.ncbi.nlm.nih.gov/15231118/.

Marburg Virus Disease Outbreaks—Lessons Learned

Marburg virus disease (MVD) is a highly virulent hemorrhagic fever caused by two filoviruses, Marburg and Ravn, both closely related to Ebola and presenting clinically similar symptoms. The virus was first identified in 1967 after simultaneous outbreaks occurred in Frankfurt and Marburg, Germany, and in Belgrade, Yugoslavia (now Serbia). These outbreaks were linked to laboratory work involving African green monkeys (*Cercopithecus aethiops*) imported from Uganda. Lab workers in Marburg—after which the disease was later named—were the first to be infected while handling these monkeys (Towner et al. 2006).

Researchers have identified the Egyptian rousette bat (*Rousettus aegyptiacus*) as the natural reservoir of the Marburg virus. Transmission to humans can occur through direct contact with infected bats—the virus is present in the saliva, urine, and feces of infected bats—or through intermediate hosts, such as infected nonhuman primates, as well as contact with body fluids from infected humans (WHO 2024).

According to the Centers for Disease Control and Prevention (CDC), symptoms of MVD typically include sudden onset of fever, chills, headache, and muscle aches. As the disease progresses, patients may experience nausea, vomiting, chest pain, sore throat, abdominal pain, and diarrhea. In more severe cases, symptoms can include jaundice, pancreatitis, liver failure, and severe hemorrhaging (bleeding), which may occur from multiple body sites. The case fatality rate for MVD ranges from 24 percent to 88 percent, depending on the virus strain and level of care provided. Currently, there are no specific vaccines or antiviral treatments for MVD, though supportive care—such as rehydration and symptom management—can improve survival rates. Because human-to-human transmission is the primary mode of spread, medical personnel and research scientists face direct risks of infection.

In September 2024, Rwanda experienced its first significant outbreak, with thirty-six confirmed cases and eleven reported deaths (Correal et al. 2024). Historical data shows that larger and deadlier outbreaks began emerging in the late twentieth century, such as the Democratic Republic of the Congo outbreak from 1998 to 2000 (154 cases, 128 deaths) and the 2005 Angola outbreak, the largest to date, with 374 cases and 329 deaths. More recent outbreaks, including those in Equatorial Guinea in 2023 (40 cases, 35 deaths) and Tanzania (9 cases, 6 deaths), demonstrate an increase in frequency. Smaller outbreaks in Guinea (2021), Ghana (2022), and Uganda (2007, 2012, 2014, 2017) indicate ongoing spillovers, with a rising trend from approximately once a decade to nearly once a year, particularly since the early 2000s (Sidik 2024).

Bat-borne diseases are a primary focus of research because bats are unique mammals capable of carrying over a thousand viruses without becoming ill. Some of these viruses have been linked to severe pandemics (Calisher et al. 2006), including Ebola, SARS, and MERS. Whether SARS-CoV-2, the virus responsible for Covid-19, originated from bats—and if so, how the spillover occurred—remains under investigation. Research suggests that key factors, such as deforestation (which disrupts bat habitats and increases human-bat contact), climate change (which alters bat behavior and migration patterns), wildlife trade (which brings humans into close contact with infected animals), and mining in bat roosting sites, may contribute to the increased frequency of outbreaks.

There is evidence that a warming climate can alter bat behavior, bringing them closer to human communities. A study by Australian scientists showed that El Niño events are linked to spillovers of the Hendra virus, which has a 50 percent fatality rate in humans. The mechanism works like this: flying fox bats, potential hosts of the Hendra virus, typically hibernate in forests during the winter season. However, due to climate change, winter zones are shrinking, and fewer forests remain for bats to hibernate in. As a result, bats experience food shortages, driving them to forage near farms with domestic animals, leading to virus transmission. Researchers suggest that restoring tree habitats could help reduce the risk of future spillovers (Eby et al. 2023).

Another study using climate models suggests that climate change will drive many mammal species toward colder regions, where they will encounter each other for the first time and potentially exchange viruses. If Earth's temperature rises by 2°C, this scenario is expected to unfold in biodiversity-rich regions like India and Indonesia, studies show. These areas may become hotspots for viral transmission, as species from different habitats interact due to shifting climates. This increased contact could elevate the risk of new zoonotic diseases emerging (Gilberg 2022).

Deforestation due to urbanization and the expansion of pastures and agricultural lands can also create spillover opportunities. A 2020 study examined the impact of human-driven land use changes, such as deforestation and urbanization, on the emergence of zoonotic diseases. Host species, such as rodents and bats, often persist or even increase in these disturbed ecosystems due to their ability to adapt to human-altered environments. In contrast, non-host species, such as large carnivores and primates—which often help regulate rodent populations—tend to decline in disturbed habitats. As a result, increased contact between humans and host species facilitates the transmission of pathogens from wildlife to humans, as these adaptable hosts thrive in fragmented landscapes (Tollefson 2020).

Mining activities in bat habitats are known to have triggered zoonotic outbreaks. Several Marburg virus outbreaks have been linked to human activity in caves where Egyptian fruit bats roost. For instance, during a 1998 outbreak in the Democratic Republic of the Congo, over half of the cases involved gold miners working in the Goroumbwa Mine. Similarly, in 2007, four miners in Uganda contracted the virus, and in 2008, two tourists became infected after visiting Python Cave in Uganda, resulting in one death. Given the frequency of such activities and the wide range of Egyptian fruit bats across sub-Saharan Africa and parts of the Middle East, there is a high potential for further zoonotic spillovers (UNMC 2023).

Among all commercial activities, wildlife trade is likely the most significant trigger for zoonotic diseases. Animals involved in the trade are often kept in cramped, unsanitary conditions, which facilitates the mixing of viruses across species. Examples include SARS, Ebola, and possibly Covid-19, which have been linked to wildlife species like pangolins and civets in market settings. The risk is heightened when wildlife is traded for food, medicine, or exotic pets (Mallapty 2020).

Outbreaks of Marburg virus disease (MVD) and other zoonotic diseases highlight the urgent need for global efforts in habitat conservation, reduction of wildlife trade, improved wildlife population surveillance, and stricter regulation of land use. More broadly, addressing climate change—which intensifies shifts in wildlife and human behavior—has never been more crucial.

Further Reading

Barron, Madeline. 2024. "How Studying Bat Viruses Can Help Prevent Zoonotic Disease." *American Society for Microbiology*. https://asm.org/Articles/2024/July/How-Studying-Bat-Viruses-Prevent-Zoonotic-Disease.

Calisher, Charles H., James E. Childs, Hume E. Field, Kathryn V. Holmes, and Tony Schountz. 2006. "Bats: Important Reservoir Hosts of Emerging Viruses." *Clinical Microbiology Reviews*, *19*(3): 531–45. doi: 10.1128/CMR.00017-06.

CDC. 2024. "Marburg." https://www.cdc.gov/marburg/about/index.html.

Correal, Annie, and April Rubin. 2024. "What to Know about the Marburg Virus Disease Outbreak." *The New York Times*. October 3. https://www.nytimes.com/2024/10/03/health/marburg-virus-disease.html.

Gilberg, Natasha 2022. "Climate Change Will Force New Animal Encounters—And Boost Viral Outbreaks." *Nature, 605*(20). doi: https://doi.org/10.1038/d41586-022-01198-w.

Mallapaty, Smriti. 2020. "Scientists Call for Pandemic Investigations to Focus on Wildlife Trade." *Nature, 583*. doi: https://doi.org/10.1038/d41586-020-02052-7.

Mallapaty, Smriti. 2022. "Why Do Bat Viruses Keep Infecting People?" *Nature*. doi: https://doi.org/10.1038/d41586-022-03682-9.

Okesanya, O. J., E. Manirambona, N. O. Olaleke, H. A. Osumanu, A. A. Faniyi, O. Bouaddi, O. Gbolahan, J. J. Lasala, and Lucero-Prisno DE 3rd. 2023. "Rise of Marburg Virus in Africa: A Call for Global Preparedness." *Ann Med Surg (Lond)*, *85*(10): 5285–90. doi: 10.1097/MS9.0000000000001257. PMID: 37811021; PMCID: PMC10553126.

Sidik, Saima. 2024. "Lethal Margurg Virus Is on the Rise in Rwanda: Why Scientists Are Worried." *Nature*. doi: https://doi.org/10.1038/d41586-024-03275-8.

Tollefson, Jeff. 2020. "Why Deforestation and Extinctions Make Pandemics More Likely." *Nature, 634*: 522–3. doi: https://doi.org/10.1038/s41586-020-2562-8.

UNMC. 2023. "Marburg Virus Outbreaks Are Increasing in Frequency and Geographic Spread – Three Virologists Explain." *Nebraska Medicine*. https://www.unmc.edu/healthsecurity/transmission/2023/03/14/marburg-virus-outbreaks-are-increasing-in-frequency-and-geographic-spread-three-virologists-explain/.

World Health Organization. 2024. "Marburg Virus Disease." https://www.who.int/news-room/fact-sheets/detail/marburg-virus-disease.

Middle East Respiratory Syndrome (MERS)

First isolated in 2012 in Saudi Arabia (WHO 2019), MERS-CoV is a coronavirus responsible for Middle East Respiratory Syndrome (MERS). There is currently no vaccine or antiviral treatment for this infection. MERS-CoV, along with SARS-CoV and SARS-CoV-2, belongs to the same family of coronaviruses with zoonotic origins, each having triggered deadly outbreaks. While the precise mechanisms of transmission among animals and from animals to humans are still under investigation, several transmission pathways have been confirmed. Evidence shows the virus can be present in aerosols and can spread through direct contact with infected bats and camels (Killerby et al. 2020; CDC).

A study on the influence of climate on MERS-CoV spread found that MERS-CoV infection is closely linked to specific climate conditions. Higher temperatures and increased ultraviolet (UV) index were associated with a rise in MERS-CoV cases, while lower relative humidity and reduced wind speeds correlated with fewer cases. Notably, MERS cases peaked between April and August, coinciding with the hotter months in Saudi Arabia. The study further identified that a one-degree Celsius increase in temperature could elevate the monthly incidence of MERS cases by 5.4 percent (Altamimi et al. 2020).

Strains of MERS-CoV were identified in camels in several Eastern Mediterranean countries such as Saudi Arabia, the UAE, Jordan, Oman, Qatar, Kuwait, Iran, and Lebanon have a higher rate of infection of MERS-CoV than in other countries. As a respiratory syndrome, MERS has been found to be transmissible from person to person through airborne droplets produced by sneezing and coughing. MERS infection rate is rather low compared to SARS and Covid-19. As of 2019, 2,494 cases had been reported. However, the fatality rate of MERS is the highest among Corona virus infections: MERS has been reported to have a fatality rate of 34.4 percent, compared to 9.5 percent for SARS and 2.13 percent for Covid-19 (Pustake et al. 2022).

Coronavirus infections present a range of symptoms, from asymptomatic cases to severe respiratory distress and even death. Common symptoms include fever, cough, and shortness of breath, with patients who have underlying health conditions at a higher risk for severe or fatal outcomes. Conversely, some patients may experience mild flu-like symptoms or remain asymptomatic, allowing for the possibility of asymptomatic transmission. MERS infections, however, are often marked by severe complications, and the rate of renal dysfunction is notably higher than in both SARS and Covid-19 cases. For instance, a study shows that in a case series of seventy MERS patients, thirty (or 42.9 percent) developed acute renal failure. Among chronically ill MERS patients, this rate was even higher; in one study, seven out of twelve patients (or 58 percent) required renal replacement therapy. Researchers noted heightened renal risks, as MERS-CoV has been detected in the urine of infected individuals (Pustake et al. 2022).

Origin of MERS-CoV

In a study by Memish and colleagues on viruses in bats, the researchers identified in one bat sample 100 percent nucleotide match to the virus found in the human index case (the first documented patient). This suggests that bats likely play a significant role in human infection (Memish 2013). Meanwhile, El-Kafrawy and colleagues (2019) found MERS-CoV present in 22.8 percent of camels sampled in Saudi Arabia, indicating a high prevalence in camels and potential health risks for individuals who work closely with them.

Seroepidemiologic studies, which assess virus prevalence through antibody presence in blood, have shown a high rate of seropositivity among camel herders who lack proper hygienic practices (El-Kafrawy 2019). Research by Killerby and colleagues (2020) further supports that direct contact with camels is a plausible infection source. In a study of individuals in Saudi Arabia with occupational exposure to camels, a higher seroprevalence of MERS-CoV-specific antibodies was observed: 2.3 percent among camel herders and 3.6 percent among slaughterhouse workers, compared to only 0.2 percent among those without such exposure.

Additionally, 54.9 percent of primary cases (suspected animal-to-human transmissions) involved direct contact with dromedary camels, supporting the hypothesis that dromedary camels are a reservoir host, with bats as a likely original reservoir. Studies also suggest that, beyond direct contact, handling contaminated equipment could lead to indirect transmission. In another investigation in Abu Dhabi, 17 percent of 235 market and slaughterhouse workers were found to be seropositive (Killerby et al. 2020).

MERS Spread Worldwide

MERS appears to be less easily spread among humans than the viruses associated with SARS and Covid-19. Almost all cases have been linked to countries in and near the Arabian Peninsula. The largest known outbreak of MERS outside the area occurred in the Republic of Korea in 2015 associated with a traveler returning to Seoul from a visit to Middle Eastern countries. The pattern of spread in South Korea suggested that MERS is narrower in scope, likely limited within health care environment, and could be relatively easily contained (Butler 2015).

Isolation of MERS-CoV

The process of isolating MERS-CoV involved resolving multiple obstacles. Virologist Dr. Ali Mohamed Zaki is accredited for isolating MERS-CoV. He was invited to examine a case of a sixty-year-old Saudi man admitted to a private hospital in Jeddah, Saudi Arabia, on June 13, 2012. The patient had a seven-day history of fever, cough, expectoration, and shortness of breath at the time. Despite anti-viral treatment, the patient died of respiratory and renal failure eleven days after admission. Collected samples tested negative for common respiratory viral pathogens at the researcher's lab and the lab of Saudi Ministry of Health to which the sample was submitted. Unconvinced by the negative results, Dr. Ali Mohamed Zaki pursued further testing weeks after the patient's death. Eventually, using pan-coronavirus primers designed by Erasmus Medical Center (EMC) in the Netherlands and with EMC's direct testing of a sample, he was able to confirmed that the pathogen was a novel coronavirus which was different from the previously identified SARS-CoV. The finding was published in the *New England Journal of Medicine* in November 2012 (Zaki 2012).

An intriguing twist accompanied the publication of Dr. Ali Mohamed Zaki's findings. Before publication, Dr. Zaki submitted an alert to ProMED in September 2012, which immediately drew criticism from the Saudi Ministry of Health for failing to obtain permission before sending samples to a Dutch lab. This led to suspicion of his involvement in the virus's spread, the closure of his lab, and his return to Cairo. In his defense, Dr. Zaki cited his professional training, experience in virology research, and BSL-2+ lab conditions meeting the biosafety standards. He stated that he was prepared to face the political "storm," including the potential loss of his job, "My job is worth nothing compared to saving lives" (Islam Hussein 2014).

Further Reading

Altamimi, Asmaa, and Anwar E. Ahmed. 2020. "Climate Factors and Incidence of Middle East Respiratory Syndrome Coronavirus." *Journal of Infection and Public Health, 13*(5): 704–8. doi: https://doi.org/10.1016/j.jiph.2019.11.011.

Butler, Declan. 2015. "South Korean MERS Outbreak Is Not a Global Thread." *Nature*. doi: 10.1038/nature.2015.17709.

Centers for Disease Controls and Prevention (CDC). 2024. "About Middle East Respiratory Syndrome (MERS)." *Cdc.gov*. https://www.cdc.gov/mers/about/index.html.

El-Kafrawy, Sherif A., Victor M. Corman, Ahmed M. Tolah, Saad B. Al Masaudi, Ahmed M. Hassan, Marcel A. Müller, Tobias Bleickere, Steve M. Harakeh, Abdulrahman A. Alzahrani, Ghaleb A. Alsaaidi, Abdulaziz N. Alagili, Anwar M. Hashem, Alimuddin Zumla, and Christian Drosten. 2019. "Enzootic Patterns of Middle East Respiratory Syndrome Coronavirus in Imported African and Local Arabian Dromedary Camels: A Prospectivegenomic Study." *Lancet Planet Health, 3*(12): e521–28.

Houssein, Islam. 2004. "The Story of the First MERS Patient." *Nature Middle East*. doi: 10.1038/nmiddleeast.2014.134.

Johns Hopkins University. 2020. Coronavirus Resource Center. https://coronavirus.jhu.edu/.

Killerby, Marie E., Holly M. Biggs, Claire M. Midgley, Susan I. Gerber, and John T. Watson. 2020. "Middle East Respiratory Syndrome Coronavirus Transmission." *Emerging Infectious Diseases, 26*(2): 191–8. doi: https://dx.doi.org/10.3201/eid2602.190697.

Memish, Ziad A., Nischay Mishra, Kevin J. Olival, Shamsudeen F. Fagbo, et al. 2013. "Middle East Respiratory Syndrome Coronavirus in Bats, Saudi Arabia." *Emerging Infectious Diseases, 19*(11): 1819–23. doi: https://dx.doi.org/10.3201/eid1911.131172.

Pustake, Manas, Isha Tambolkar, Purushottam Giri, and Charmi Gandhi. 2022. "SARS, MERS and Covid-19: An Overview and Comparison of Clinical, Laboratory and Radiological Features." *Journal of Family Medicine and Primary Care, 11*(1): 10–17. doi: 10.4103/jfmpc.jfmpc_839_21.

WHO. 2019. "Middle East Respiratory Syndrome Coronavirus (MERS-COV)." https://www.who.int/emergencies/mers-cov/en/.

Zaki, Ali M., Sander van Boheemen, Theo M. Bestebroer, Albert D. M. E. Osterhaus, and Ron A. M. Fouchier. 2012. "Isolation of a Novel Coronavirus from a Man with Pneumonia in Saudi Arabia." *New England Journal of Medicine, 367*(19): 1814–20. doi: 10.1056/NEJMoa1211721.

Severe Acute Respiratory Syndrome (SARS) and the Importance of Information Transparency

SARS-CoV is a coronavirus identified as the cause of Severe Acute Respiratory Syndrome (SARS). The virus spreads from person to person, primarily through respiratory droplets in the air. The outbreak was traced to Foshan City in

Guangdong Province, China, in November 2002. Five nearby cities within the initial spread zone, including the densely populated Guangzhou, were affected (WHO 2003). Studies suggest that multiple lab leaks and a lack of transparency may also have contributed to the virus's spread (Senio 2003; Walgate 2004; Congressional-Executive Commission on China 2003; WHO 2003).

Clinically, SARS presents with flu-like symptoms, including fever, cough, chills, fatigue, shortness of breath, headache, and diarrhea. The infection can progress rapidly, often requiring hospitalization and isolation to prevent further spread, particularly among health care workers. During the 2003 outbreak, SARS led to over 8,000 cases across 29 countries, including 29 cases in the United States, and resulted in 774 deaths globally, though none occurred in the United States. The virus was fatal for approximately one in ten patients, with mortality risk rising significantly for those over sixty—nearly half of whom did not survive. While most patients fully recovered, a small percentage experienced lasting effects such as depression, anxiety, chronic lung or kidney disease, or persistent respiratory symptoms like cough and shortness of breath, according to the Centers for Disease Control and Prevention (CDC).

SARS, MERS, and Covid-19, all caused by coronaviruses, share notable similarities in clinical characteristics, transmission routes, and demographic patterns. Clinically, these diseases present with symptoms such as fever, cough, fatigue, and shortness of breath, which can progress to severe respiratory complications like acute respiratory distress syndrome (ARDS). Transmission primarily occurs through respiratory droplets and close human contact, with possible fomite transmission, especially in health care settings. Demographically, these infections primarily affect adults, with older adults and those with comorbidities at higher risk for severe outcomes and higher case fatality rates. While SARS and MERS exhibit higher case fatality rates, Covid-19 has a notably broader and faster transmission rate, resulting in significant global spread (Zhu et al. 2020).

There are varied accounts of the first SARS cases. According to one report, the earliest known case may have been a 46-year-old man from Foshan who experienced fever and respiratory distress for nine days. He was hospitalized, treated in intensive care, and eventually recovered. However, his wife, aunt, and his aunt's daughter fell ill shortly afterward. Subsequently, multiple independent clusters of cases were reported across seven municipalities in Southern China. Between November 10, 2002, and February 9, 2003, hundreds of SARS cases were identified in Guangdong Province, many involving health care workers. The first known spread of SARS to Hong Kong occurred on February 21, 2003, involving a 64-year-old physician from Zhongshan University in Guangdong Province who traveled to Hong Kong for a wedding. Before being hospitalized, he stayed one night at the Metropole Hotel, where ten secondary cases emerged among other guests. These secondary cases directly led to tertiary cases in two Hong Kong hospitals and outbreaks in Singapore, Toronto, and Hanoi. SARS eventually spread to twenty-nine countries or regions (Cherry 2004).

The main phase of SARS transmission was brought under control by July 2003. However, a secondary wave occurred in spring 2004 in Beijing, likely originating from the Diarrhea Virus Laboratory at the National Institute of Virology. Although the WHO declared the outbreak contained in May, the exact source of the infection was never confirmed. In its "Update 7," the WHO issued a strong warning on biosafety procedures for the research and storage of SARS coronavirus samples (WHO 2004). The outbreak was ultimately contained through quarantines implemented in multiple international cities.

Zoonotic Transmission

The process by which a virus transfers from animal hosts to humans is known as zoonotic transmission. In the case of SARS, civet cats—a raccoon-like animal unrelated to domestic cats—were widely believed to be the original carriers. In southern China, civet cats are sometimes sold live in food markets as a delicacy. Consuming wild animals as exotic foods or for medicinal purposes is not uncommon in China. In 2004, experts discovered evidence of the virus in civet cages at a restaurant where a patient had consumed civet dishes. This finding prompted Guangdong provincial authorities to cull thousands of civets and ban their consumption that same year. However, since these cages were also used to house other wild animals, some of which carry similar virus strains, there remains uncertainty about the findings. A joint study by the Chinese CDC and Hong Kong University in 2007 confirmed that the SARS coronavirus found in human patients was identical to the strain found in civet cats, demonstrating that civet cats are indeed capable of transmitting the SARS virus to humans (Reuters 2007; Cherry 2004).

Later studies found that the precursor virus exists in certain wild bats. A SARS-like CoV strain was isolated from Chinese horseshoe bats, sharing 88–92 percent genomic similarity with viruses found in humans and civet cats, suggesting that bats may be the natural hosts for SARS-CoV (Zhu et al. 2020). These findings indicate that civets and other mammals could have served as intermediate hosts, where the virus mutated into a form transmissible to humans (Li et al. 2005; Zhu et al. 2020).

What Lessons Could Be Learned?

Several lessons can be drawn from the handling of the SARS pandemic. First, transparent and prompt reporting is crucial. The initial cover-up by the Guangdong government and the delayed response by the central government—understandably due to concerns about socioeconomic impacts (U.S. Congress 2003; Pomfret 2003)—are believed to have hindered timely actions that could have saved lives. Coincidentally, a power transition from Jiang Zemin to Hu Jintao was taking place in Beijing during the month of March. The central government eventually openly made its move to contain the infection toward mid-April 2003 under the new leadership (Eckholm 2023). However, by this time the virus was already spreading in Beijing and had even sickened a number of party and government leaders (Pomfret 2003). The WHO issued a global warning on March 15, 2003, which circulated via mobile phones, email, and the internet despite China's media restrictions. On March 25, after WHO experts arrived, the Chinese government finally acknowledged that SARS had spread beyond Guangdong (Huang 2004).

The most important lesson learned is perhaps that leaders worldwide must recognize that suppressing information on infectious diseases carries a high cost: such actions lead to loss of life, suffering, and damage to the government's credibility. Second, biosafety protocols in laboratories must be strictly enforced and diligently followed, as multiple lab leaks in Beijing, Taiwan, and Singapore resulted in employees being infected. This suggests that scientific labs can be sources of outbreaks. Third, weaknesses in health care systems may exacerbate virus transmission. One significant weakness is the lack of adequate protection for health care workers, exposing them to infection risks—in the 2003 SARS outbreak, health care workers accounted for 24 percent of early cases (Xu et al. 2004). Finally, virus infections can cross countries' borders; global collaboration is essential to developing strong monitoring systems to prevent future outbreaks.

Further Reading

Centers for Disease Control and Prevention (CDC). 2017. "SARS Basics Fact Sheet." https://archive.cdc.gov/www_cdc_gov/sars/about/fs-sars.html.

Congressional-Executive Commission on China. 2003. "Freedom of the Press and the 2002–2003 SARS Outbreak." https://www.cecc.gov/freedom-of-the-press-and-the-2002-2003-sars-outbreak.

Eckholm, Erik. 2003. "The Sars Epidemic: Epidemic; China Admits Underreporting Its SARS Cases." *The New York Times*. https://www.nytimes.com/2003/04/21/world/the-sars-epidemic-epidemic-china-admits-underreporting-its-sars-cases.html.

Cherry, James D. 2004. "The Chronology of the 2002–2003 SARS Mini Pandemic." *Pediatric Respiratory Reviews*, 5(4): 262–9. doi: 10.1016/j.prrv.2004.07.009.

Huang, Yanzhong. 2004. "The SARS Epidemic and Its Aftermath in China: A Political Perspective." In Institute of Medicine (US) Forum on Microbial Threats; Knobler, S., Mahmoud, A., Lemon, S., et al., (eds.), *Learning from SARS: Preparing for the Next Disease Outbreak: Workshop Summary*. Washington, DC: National Academies Press (US), pp. 116–36. https://www.ncbi.nlm.nih.gov/books/NBK92479/.

Li, Wendong, Zhengli Shi, Yu Meng, Wuze Ren, Craig Smith, Jonathan H. Epstein, Hanzhong Wang, Gary Crameri, Zhihong Hu, Huajun Zhang, Jianhong Zhang, Jennifer McEachern, Hume Field, Peter Daszak, Bryan T. Eaton, Shuyi Zhang, and Lin-Fa Wang. 2005. "Bats Are Natural Reservoirs of SARS-Like Coronaviruses." *Sciencemag.org*. https://zenodo.org/records/3949088.

Pomfret, John. 2003. "Outbreak Gave China's Hu an Opening." *The Washington Post*. May 13. https://www.washingtonpost.com/archive/politics/2003/05/13/outbreak-gave-chinas-hu-an-opening/6e7ebf75-9689-48bb-81a9-3e28e7f25b56/.

Reuters. 2007. "China Scientists Say SARS-Civet Cat Link Proved." *Science News*. https://www.reuters.com/article/world/china-scientists-say-sars-civet-cat-link-proved-idUSPEK109397/.

Senio, Kathryn. 2003. "Recent Singapore SARS Case a Laboratory Accident." *Lancet Infectious Diseases*, 3(11): 679. https://pmc.ncbi.nlm.nih.gov/articles/PMC7128757/.

U.S. Congress. 2003. "Dangerous Secrets--Sars and China's Healthcare System." https://www.congress.gov/event/108th-congress/house-event/LC74062/text.

Walgate, Robert. 2004. "SARS Escaped Beijing Lab Twice." *Genome Biol*. doi: 10.1186/gb-spotlight-20040427-03.

World Health Organization (WHO). 2004. "China's Latest SARS Outbreak Has Been Contained, But Biosafety Concerns Remain—Update 7." https://www.who.int/emergencies/disease-outbreak-news/item/2004_05_18a-en.

World Health Organization (WHO). 2003. "Consensus Document on the Epidemiology of Severe Acute Respiratory Syndrome (SARS)." https://iris.who.int/bitstream/handle/10665/70863/WHO_CDS_CSR_GAR_2003.11_eng.pdf?sequence=1.

World Health Organization (WHO). 2003. "SARS Case in Laboratory Worker in Taiwan, China." https://www.who.int/news/item/17-12-2003-sars-case-in-laboratory-worker-in-taiwan-china.

Xu, Rui-Heng, Jian-Feng He, Meirion R. Evans, et al. 2004. "Epidemiologic Clues to SARS Origin in China." *Emerging Infectious Diseases*, 10(6): 1031–7. https://doi.org/10.3201/eid1006.030852.

Zhu, Zhixing, Xihua Lian, Xiaoshan Su, Weijing Wu, Giuseppe A. Marraro, and Yiming Zeng. 2020. "From SARS and MERS to Covid-19: A Brief Summary and Comparison of Severe Acute Respiratory Infections Caused by Three Highly Pathogenic Human Coronaviruses." *Respiratory Research*, *21*(1): 224. doi: https://doi.org/10.1186/s12931-020-01479-w.

Yellow Fever—A Continuing Challenge under Climate Change and Globalization

Yellow fever (YF) is a zoonotic disease caused by the yellow fever virus, a member of the *Flaviviridae* family. The virus originated in Africa, with non-human primates identified as the primary reservoir. Transmission occurs mainly through mosquito bites, particularly from *Aedes aegypti* mosquito. Although native to Africa, this mosquito species has expanded its range to Asia, tropical islands, and the Americas. People in these regions can contract the infection and, in some cases, become carriers themselves. Genetic studies suggest that the virus may have been introduced to the Americas as early as during the transatlantic slave trade (Gianchecci et al. 2022).

The clinical symptoms of YF infection can vary widely. About half of cases are asymptomatic, around 33 percent present with flu-like symptoms that typically resolve on their own, and approximately 12 percent progress to severe symptoms. Severe YF infection is marked by jaundice, body aches, fever, liver and kidney failure, bleeding from the mouth and nose, and internal bleeding. Nearly 50 percent of severe cases result in fatalities (Gianchecchi et al. 2022; CDC).

Currently, there is still no specific antiviral cure for yellow fever. Treatment focuses on easing symptoms such as fever, muscle pain, and dehydration (CDC). The good news is, it can be effectively prevented through vaccination. The YF vaccine is both highly effective and safe, with a single dose providing lifetime protection for most people without the need for booster shots. The World Health Organization (WHO) recommends vaccination for children aged nine months and older and strongly advises all international travelers visiting regions where the disease is endemic to receive the vaccine.

YF outbreaks in the Western Hemisphere are extremely rare, aside from a limited outbreak in Brazil in 2017–18. However, the disease remains endemic in Africa and South America, causing approximately 200,000 cases and 30,000 deaths annually, with over 90 percent of cases occurring in Africa. The spread of the disease is believed to be influenced by three key factors: (a) low population immunity, (b) increased migration, and (c) climate and environmental factors that have boosted mosquito populations (WHO 2023).

The United States has a long and memorable history of grappling with YF, dating back to the late 1600s. Two major outbreaks earned the disease the nickname "American Plague." One occurred in New York City in 1702, claiming the lives of 10 percent of the city's population; another notable outbreak struck Philadelphia in 1793, resulting in 5,000 deaths and causing widespread panic and migration. Both cities had large, densely populated areas that facilitated the spread of the disease. Smaller outbreaks continued throughout the nineteenth century, especially in southern states.

The disease was finally contained thanks to findings by U.S. Army surgeon Major Walter Reed, who was sent to Cuba to investigate widespread illness among American soldiers during the Spanish-American War (1898). His research confirmed that mosquitoes, rather than poor sanitation, were the disease's vectors, leading to mosquito control campaigns that significantly reduced YF cases. The last U.S. outbreak occurred in 1905, claiming 900 lives in Louisiana (PBS).

It's essential to recognize Dr. Carlos Finlay, a Cuban physician and scientist who, in 1881, hypothesized the role of the mosquito *Culex cubensis* (now known as *Aedes aegypti*) in transmitting the disease. Reed and his team proved Finlay's pivotal insight (Bryan et al. 2004).

In the 1930s, the development of a YF vaccine took a major leap forward. Max Theiler, a Harvard scientist and member of the Rockefeller Foundation's International Health Division, conducted experiments using mouse brains and developed an attenuated vaccine known as "17-D." This vaccine was first administered in large-scale immunizations in 1937 and remains the standard YF vaccine today, playing a crucial role in the global fight against YF (CDC). Theiler was awarded the Nobel Prize in 1951 for his groundbreaking work.

The successful elimination of YF in Africa and South America will depend on increasing population immunity through large-scale vaccination efforts. According to the World Health Organization (WHO), African countries need to improve their relatively low vaccination rates. For example, vaccination coverage in Cameroon is 54 percent, in the Central African Republic 41 percent, and in Chad 45 percent. Overall, the childhood vaccination rate across the continent is below 50 percent. To achieve the goal of eliminating YF epidemics, the WHO developed the Eliminate Yellow Fever Epidemics (EYE) strategy, which aims to raise childhood vaccination rates above 80 percent. The EYE strategy focuses on protecting at-risk populations, preventing international spread, and containing outbreaks swiftly (WHO 2024).

Walter Reed and the Control of Yellow Fever

Walter Reed (1851–1902), a U.S. Army physician, is widely celebrated for his groundbreaking work in identifying the transmission route and controlling the spread of yellow fever a disease that plagued regions in the Americas and Africa. The yellow fever virus is a mosquito-borne virus belonging to the *Flaviviridae* family, which includes other viruses like dengue, Zika, and West Nile viruses. During the Spanish-American War (1898), more soldiers died from yellow fever and malaria than from combats. In 1900, Reed led the Yellow Fever Commission, a team of scientists, to investigate the transmission of yellow fever. At the time, many believed the disease spread was due to poor sanitation conditions, but Cuban physician Dr. Carlos Finlay believed that mosquitoes were responsible for transmission.

Reed's team conducted experiments in Cuba to test Finlay's hypothesis. Several researchers volunteered to expose themselves to mosquito bites and lost their lives due to infection. Thanks to their dedicated work, the experiments confirmed that the *Aedes aegypti* mosquito was the primary vector for yellow fever. This knowledge shifted focus from treating symptoms to controlling mosquitoes. Eradication of mosquitoes through fumigation and elimination of mosquito breeding sites later proved effective in reducing the disease, and remains standard control today.

Reed's findings would soon prove life-saving for American soldiers and civilians alike. The implementation of mosquito control during the Panama Canal construction protected workers and assured the project's completion in 1914.

In the late 1930s, Dr. Max Theiler, a South African virologist, developed the first effective yellow fever vaccine. Theiler's breakthrough, known as the 17D strain, was a weakened version of the virus that provided immunity. For this accomplishment, he was awarded the Nobel Prize in Physiology or Medicine in 1951. The vaccine remains globally used for controlling yellow fever.

Today, organizations like the World Health Organization (WHO) and the Centers for Disease Control and Prevention (CDC) monitor outbreaks, promote vaccination campaigns, and support rapid response teams in yellow fever-endemic areas in Africa and South America. Walter Reed and his contributions to the control of yellow fever is considered one of the most important contributions to public health in modern history.

Further Reading

Centers for Disease Control and Prevention. 2020. "Yellow Fever Vaccine: A Brief History." Last modified February 26, 2020. https://www.cdc.gov/yellowfever/history.

Crosby, Molly Caldwell 2006. *The American Plague: The Untold Story of Yellow Fever, the Epidemic That Shaped Our History*. New York: Berkley Books.

Feng, Patrick. "Major Walter Reed and the Eradication of Yellow Fever." *The Army Historical Foundation*. https://armyhistory.org/major-walter-reed-and-the-eradication-of-yellow-fever/.

World Health Organization. 2023. "Yellow Fever." https://www.who.int/news-room/fact-sheets/detail/yellow-fever. Accessed October 28, 2023.

It is important to recognize two major continuing challenges: climate change and globalization. Climate change has led to warmer and more humid conditions in many parts of the world, creating environments where mosquito populations can thrive, which increases the risk of spreading mosquito-borne diseases like Zika virus, West Nile virus, and Chikungunya virus. Globalization has also become a significant factor in the spread of infectious diseases. A notable example is the YF outbreak in China in 2016. That year, approximately 200,000 Chinese workers were in Angola during a YF outbreak. Some returned to China carrying the virus, leading to a local outbreak in Guangdong province (Li et al. 2020).

Global travel and climate change present complex challenges for controlling vector-borne diseases in today's world. It could be said that no place is truly safe. However, global health can improve if countries are willing to proactively address and reduce these contributing factors.

Further Reading

Bryan, Charles S., Sandra W. Moss, and Richard J. Khan. 2004. "Yellow Fever in the Americas." *Infectious Disease Clinics of North America, 18*: 275–92. https://www.sciencedirect.com/sdfe/pdf/download/eid/1-s2.0-S0891552004000224/first-page-pdf.

Centers for Disease Control and Prevention (CDC). "Yellow Fever." https://www.cdc.gov/yellow-fever/index.html.

Centers for Disease Control and Prevention (CDC). 2025. "Yellow Fever Vaccine information for Healthcare Providers." https://www.cdc.gov/yellow-fever/hcp/vaccine/?CDC_AAref_Val=https://www.cdc.gov/yellowfever/healthcareproviders/vaccine-info.html.

Gianchecchi, Elena, Virginia Cianchi, Alessandro Torelli, and Emanuele Montomoli. 2022. "Yellow Fever: Origin, Epidemiology, Preventive Strategies and Future Prospects." *Vaccine (Basel), 10*(3): 372. doi: 10.3390/vaccines10030372.

Li, Chao, Dan Li, Shirley JoAnn Smart, Lei Zhou, Peng Yang, Jianming Ou, Yi He, Ruiqi Ren, Tao Ma, Nijuan Xiang, Haitian Sui, Yali Want, Jian Zhao, Chaonan Wang, Yeping Wang, Daxin Ni, Isaac Chun-Hai Fung, Dexin Li, Yangmu Huang, and Qun Li. 2020. "Evaluating the Importation of Yellow Fever Cases into China in 2016 and Strategies Used to Prevent and Control the Spread of the Disease." *WHO WPSAR*, *11*(2). doi: https://doi.org/10.5365/wpsar.2018.9.1.007.

PBS. "Yellow Fever in America." https://www.pbs.org/wgbh/americanexperience/features/fever-timeline-yellow-fever-america/.

Prinzi, Andrea. 2021. "History of Yellow Fever in the U.S." *American Society for Microbiology*. https://asm.org/Articles/2021/May/History-of-Yellow-Fever-in-the-U-S.

World Health Organization. "Eliminate Yellow Fever Epidemics by 2026." https://www.who.int/initiatives/eye-strategy.

World Health Organization (WHO). 2024. "Yellow Fever—African Region." https://www.who.int/emergencies/disease-outbreak-news/item/2024-DON510.

Zika—A Virus with Impacts on Societies' Value Systems

In the course of human history, there have been occasions during which epidemics or pandemics have prompted societies to reconsider their long-standing rules and moral ethics, and sometimes resulting in a change of direction. The Zika pandemic was one of such diseases.

Zika virus is a member of *Flaviviridae* family of viruses that also include Dengue, West Nile virus, yellow fever, Japanese encephalitis, and tick-borne encephalitis. Flaviviruses are typically transmitted through arthropod vectors, including mosquitoes and ticks. Flaviviruses have been known to affect the central nervous system in humans and can result in severe injuries.

In 2015, Zika outbreaks were reported in Brazil and several countries in Latin America and Central America. The disease was associated with an increasing number of microcephaly (a condition where children were born with smaller brain), Guillain-Barre syndromes (a paralyzing disease due to damages to nerve cells), and myelitis (inflammation of the spine cord). In January 2016 the World Health Organization (WHO) Emergency Committee declared Public Health Emergency of International Concern (PHEIC) after receiving case reports from Brazil, France, the United States, and El Salvador which highlighted a potential association between Zika virus and microcephaly as well as other neurological disorders (WHO 2016). According to WHO and Pan American Health Organization (PAHO), Zika had resulted in half a million infections and nearly 4,000 congenital birth defects in 86 countries and territories, predominantly in Central and Latin America (PAHO 2018).

Clinically, the majority of individuals infected with Zika experience no symptoms or very mild symptoms, such as red eye, rash, headache, fever, and joint/muscle pain. These symptoms typically subside within a week. The primary concern, however, lies in the potential for Zika to cause birth defects, specifically microcephaly, when pregnant women became infected. Scientists believe that the virus in pregnant women's blood during a state known as viremia can be transmitted to fetus and affect fetus' neural cells, leading to its proliferation in the brains and central nervous system where Zika virus exert neurovirulence like other flaviviruses (CDC).

As of present moment, there are no available antiviral treatments or vaccines targeting Zika. The concern that Zika can potentially result in fetal abnormalities had a significant moral and social impact in affected countries, including Brazil, El Salvador, and Colombia, leading to increased calls for legalization of abortion. Zika outbreaks became a major public health concern in 2015 and peaked in 2016 with 522,720 cases, when infections started to drop which scientists attribute to the development of herd immunity. Since 2016, the number of cases reported in Latin America and the Caribbean has stabilized in the range of 20,000 to 55,000 cases per year (Nebehay et al. 2016; Mendoza 2024).

Research shows that the original reservoir of Zika virus was nonhuman primates. Zika virus was first isolated in 1947 in the Zika forest in Uganda from a rhesus macaque. Subsequent serum samplings among residents in Uganda showed the presence of neutralizing antibodies against the virus, which was evidence that the virus had infected humans. The vector that effected the transmission was identified to be *Aedes Aegypti* mosquitoes. However, infested individuals could pass on the virus through sex and blood transfusion. By 2007 outbreaks had already been reported in Pacific Islands and south America and association suspected with nervous abnormalities in newborns, per CDC data. The widespread outbreaks in 2015–16 were likely related to accelerated climate-induced ecological changes. Warmer temperature and more rainfalls encourage mosquito populations to thrive, leading to an increasing number of outbreaks, such as dengue, Zika, and chikungunya around the world (Schlein 2023).

The Zika virus outbreak in Latin America led to a significant increase in the demand for abortion which is forbidden in many countries. Advocates argued that abortion should be treated as a medical decision rather than a moral issue during the years of the pandemic. Reproductive rights and reproductive justice emerged as the central theme in the social and political arena. In countries like

Brazil the law prohibits abortion except in cases of incest or when the woman's life is at risk. Opponents cite moral grounds, with arguments framed abound eugenics and religious beliefs, asserting that microcephaly does not justify abortion as the condition is compatible with life (Gressick et al. 2019). In El Salvador, the law criminalizes abortion under all circumstances. Abortion control has led to instances where women were imprisoned following miscarriages, and some faced lengthy sentence on abortion charges (Wenham et al. 2019; Grant 2022).

Abortion activists pointed out the biases in Zika policies, for instance, that while governments urged women to avoid or delay pregnancy through contraceptive use, they made little effort to ensure affordable and available contraceptive devices. Furthermore, government policies unjustly shifted responsibilities to women for not properly following medical advice when their child is born with brain defects, despite the fact that many of these women lacked access to necessary material support and education. Additionally, activists argued that these policies failed to address the governments' own failures in ensuring effective sanitation facilities to reduce mosquito infestation. In Brazil and El Salvador, activists demand the governments to adopt a rights-based approach to the Zika outbreak by implementing legislative reforms. Essentially, these requests emphasize a breach in the social contract between the state and individuals, one that required a renegotiation (Valente 2017).

During the Zika pandemic, the World Health Organization (WHO) and the United Nations (UN) supported the demands of the activists and called on countries that restrict comprehensive sexual and reproductive services including contraception, emergency contraception, maternal health care, and safe abortion services to reassess their policies and align them with human rights obligations in order to ensure the right to health for all individuals (UN 2016). Furthermore, these international organizations encouraged the governments to adopt policies that empower women and girls to make their own decisions regarding pregnancy and childbirth. However, countries such as Brazil and El Salvador have made minimal efforts to ease restrictions citing the protection of rights of children with disability, and arguing that restriction of abortion serves a broader societal benefit (Wenham et al. 2019).

A concerning trend in the handling of the Zika pandemic is that in countries where abortion is not accessible through formal health care channels, there tends to be a surge of unsafe abortions. According to a 2016 study, requests for abortion medication through Women on Web (WOW), a nonprofit organization that provides access to abortion medications (mifepristone and misoprostol) through online telemedicine in countries such as in Brazil, Costa Rica, El Salvador, Ecuador, Honduras, and Venezuela, witnessed an increase ranging from 36 percent to 108 percent during 2015–16 (Aiken et al. 2016). These findings strongly indicate that the prohibition of abortion can increase health risks to women. Consequently, for nearly a decade, Zika infection, particularly with its association with birth defects like microcephaly, has spurred debates across Latin America about relaxing legal and moral restrictions on abortion.

Further Reading

Aiken, Abigail R. A., James G. Scott, Rebecca Gomperts, James Trussell, Marc Worrell, and Catherine E. Aiken. 2016. "Requests for Abortion in Latin America Related to Concern about Zika Virus Exposure." *New England Journal of Medicine*. doi: 10.1056/NEJMc1605389.

CDC. "Zika Virus." https://www.cdc.gov/zika/index.html.

Grant, Will. 2022. "El Salvador's Abortion Ban: 'I Was Sent to Prison for Suffering a Miscarriage.'" *BBC News*.

Gressick, Kimberly, Adriane Gelpi, and Toni Chanroo. 2019. "Zika and Abortion in Brazilian Newspapers: How a New Outbreak Revived an Old Debate on Reproductive Rights." *Sex Reprod Health Matters, 27*(2): 1586818. doi: 10.1080/26410397.2019.1586818.

Mendoza, Jennifer. 2024. "Zika Virus Cases in Latin America 2015–2023." *Statista.com*. https://www.statista.com/statistics/1006814/latin-america-zika-virus-cases/.

Nebehay, Stephanie, and Julie Steenhuysen. 2016. "WHO Declares End of Zika Emergency But Says Virus Remains a Threat." *Reuters*. Https://www.reuters.com/article/us-health-zika-who/who-declares-end-of-zika-emergency-but-says-virus-remains-a-threat-idUSKBN13D2G2.

Noorbakhsh, Farshid, K. Abdolmohammadi, Y. Fatahi, H. Dalili, M. Rasoolinejad, F. Rezaei, M. Salehi-Vaziri, N. Z. Shafiei-Jandaghi, E. S. Gooshki, M. Zaim, M. H. Nicknam, et al. 2019. "Zika Virus Infection, Basic and Clinical Aspects: A Review Article." *Iranian Journal of Public Health, 48*(1): 20–31. https://www.ncbi.nlm.nih.gov/pmc/articles/PMC6401583/.

Pan American Health Organization and World Health Organization. 2018. "Zika Cases and Congenital Syndrome Associated with Zika Virus Reported by Countries and Territories in the Americas, 2015–2018 Cumulative Cases." https://www3.paho.org/hq/index.php?option=com_docman&view=download&category_slug=cumulative-cases-pdf-8865&alias=43296-zika-cumulative-cases-4-january-2018-296&Itemid=270&lang=en.

Schlein, Lisa. 2023. "Who Warns Climate Change Causing Surge in Mosquito-Borne Diseases." *Science & Health*. https://www.voanews.com/a/who-warns-climate-change-causing-surge-in-mosquito-borne-diseases/7043700.html.

Sedgh, Gilda, Jonathan Bearak, Susheela Singh, Akinrinola Bankole, Anna Popinchalk, Bela Ganatra, Clémentine Rossier, Caitlin Gerdts, Özge Tunçalp, Brooke Ronald Johnson Jr, Heidi Bart Johnston, and Leontine Alkema. 2016. "Abortion Incidence between 1990 and 2014: Global, Regional, and Subregional Levels and Trends." *Lancet.* https://doi.org/10.1016/S2468-2667(19)30204-X.

United Nations. 2016. "Upholding Women's Human Rights Essential to Zika Response—UN Rights Chief." *UN News.* https://news.un.org/en/story/2016/02/521662.

Valente, Pablo K. 2017. "Zika and Reproductive Rights in Brazil: Challenge to the Right to Health." *AJPH.* https://doi.org/10.2105/AJPH.2017.303924.

Wenham, Clare, Amaral Arevalo, Ernestina Coast, Sonia Corrêa, Katherine Cuellar, Tiziana Leone, and Sandra Valongueiro. 2019. "Zika, Abortion and Health Emergencies: A Review of Contemporary Debates." *Global Health, 15*: 49. doi: 10.1186/s12992-019-0489-3.

World Health Organization. 2016. "The History of Zika Virus." https://www.who.int/news-room/feature-stories/detail/the-history-of-zika-virus.

World Health Organization. 2016. "WHO Statement on the First Meeting of International Health Regulations (2005) (IHR2005) Emergency Committee on Zika Virus And Observed Increase in Neurological Disorders And Neonatal Malformation." https://www.who.int/en/news-room/detail/01-02-2016-who-statement-on-the-first-meeting-of-the-international-health-regulations-(2005)-(ihr-2005)-emergency-committee-on-zika-virus-and-observed-increase-in-neurological-disorders-and-neonatal-malformations.

World Health Organization. 2022. "Zika Virus." https://www.who.int/news-room/fact-sheets/detail/zika-virus.

Geographic Factors and Natural Hazards

Cancer and Geographical Environment

Cancer research has revealed that environmental factors play a far greater role in the development of cancer than commonly thought. The conventional view, which largely attributes cancer to genetic inheritance or random chance, is increasingly being challenged. Studies suggest that up to two-thirds of cancer cases could be linked to environmental substances and lifestyle factors. Although inherited cancer genes are a factor, they often require environmental triggers to mutate and lead to somatic mutations. This indicates that while cancer risk is universal, it is not uniformly distributed across the population. For instance, inherited mutations in genes such as *BRCA1* and *BRCA2* notably increase the risk of breast and ovarian cancers. Yet, these hereditary factors represent only a minor proportion of total cancer cases. The degree of susceptibility to cancer can significantly vary among different individuals and populations (Terry 2023). These findings suggest that, as we identify more cancer risks, our prevention strategies are becoming progressively more effective. The U.S. Department of Health and Human Services (HHS) compiles and updates a list of substances, both biological and chemical, known or suspected to cause cancer in humans. This information is crucial, guiding policymakers in their decisions and individuals in their daily lifestyle choices.

An essential component of cancer research is understanding the mechanisms by which carcinogens become integrated into our daily environment. For instance, extensive research has confirmed that exposure to tobacco smoke, radiation, and specific chemicals significantly elevates cancer risk. Notably, since the 1960s, the chronic use of tobacco has been identified as a primary contributor to lung cancer incidence (Hirayama 1981).

The impact of socioeconomic status (SES) on cancer risks and outcomes is equally critical. Individuals in lower SES brackets are often disproportionately exposed to cancer risk factors and face barriers in accessing health care, which critically hampers timely cancer detection and treatment (James et al. 2012).

Lifestyle factors, including dietary habits, physical activity levels, and alcohol consumption, also play a significant role in modulating cancer risks. For example, diets rich in processed and red meats have been associated with an increased risk of prostate cancer, while regular physical activity has been shown to mitigate the risk of various cancer types.

Age emerges as another vital factor in cancer risk assessment, with most cancer types demonstrating an increased prevalence with advancing age. This trend is attributed to the cumulative impact of various risk factors over time, coupled with the natural senescence of cellular mechanisms (Klassen et al. 2006).

Ethnicity and race exert a notable influence on cancer prevalence, with certain types of cancers showing higher incidence in specific racial or ethnic groups. Such patterns are typically the result of an intricate interplay of genetic predispositions, environmental exposures, and sociocultural factors (Bruning 2023).

Furthermore, geographical variations play an instrumental role in determining exposure levels to different risk factors. Studies on the influence of geographical environments on cancer epidemiology have contributed to the understanding of the diverse and complex factors contributing to cancer risk. They shed light on the complex interplay between genetics, environment, and lifestyle in the pathogenesis of cancer (Klassen et al. 2006). A few outstanding studies are introduced below.

Hirayama's Study on Passive Smoking

In 1981, by the time Takeshi Hirayama published his groundbreaking research on passive smoking, it had not been widely recognized that air polluted by nearby smokers posed risks comparable to those of direct cigarette smoking. Hirayama noted that although only 15 percent of women in Japan were smokers, the mortality rate from lung cancer among women increased in tandem with the trend observed in men, 73 percent of whom were smokers.

Hirayama conducted a longitudinal study over fourteen years (1966–79) involving 91,540 non-smoking women married to smokers. He discovered that these non-smoking wives faced up to twice the risk of developing lung cancer compared to women not exposed to passive smoking. Significantly, the study also found that the risk for these non-smoking wives increased in proportion to the number of cigarettes their husbands smoked. Thus, Hirayama's research provided compelling evidence of the carcinogenic effects of passive smoking.

Additionally, Hirayama's study revealed that the wives of agricultural workers in rural areas had a higher risk of lung cancer compared to smokers in urban environments. He attributed this to rural residents spending more time at home, thus increasing their exposure to passive smoke. This important finding highlighted the crucial role of the living environment in determining levels of exposure to carcinogens embedded as part of many people's daily routine.

Studies on Geography and Prostate Cancer

Prostate cancer is highly prevalent both in the United States and globally. Statistics indicate that about one in eight men in the United States will receive a prostate cancer diagnosis in their lifetime. According to the American Cancer Society, prostate cancer is the second leading cause of death among American men, trailing only lung cancer. Although a single triggering agent has yet to be identified, geographical research has provided valuable insights into understanding the disease's causative factors and progression. In a review of several geographical studies on prostate cancer, Klassen and colleagues (Klassen et al. 2006) indicated that geographical disparity appears to be a significant characteristic of prostate cancer. This disparity exists alongside other known risk factors such as age, African heritage, and family history. The incidence rates vary widely; for example, men in China have the lowest incidence rate at 2.9 per 100,000, compared to 107.8 among white Americans and 185.4 among Black Americans in the United States.

Multiple studies have suggested that dietary differences, such as the high consumption of soy and tea products in Asian diets versus the high intake of red meat in Western diets, may contribute to the lower prostate cancer risk observed in Asian men. This hypothesis is supported by additional geographical observations. For instance, research has shown that Japanese men who migrated to Hawaii, where a Western diet and lifestyle predominate, tend to have higher rates of prostate cancer. On a global scale, studies indicate a positive correlation between prostate cancer risk and a country's GDP, as well as its population's expenditure on sugar, meat, milk, animal protein, and overall energy intake. Conversely, an inverse relationship has been identified as well. Research involving the Dutch population, who experienced severe famine during the Second World War, demonstrated that famine and physical stature were not significant risk factors. However, dietary abundance in the post-war period, leading to a rapid increase in BMI, appeared to be a greater risk factor. Thanks to geographical observations, researchers were able to highlight a potential link between protein consumption and prostate cancer (Klassen et al. 2006).

Geo-economic Disparity and Cancer Risk in Vulnerable Groups

The case of Cancer Alley in Louisiana reflects how environmental mismanagement can disproportionally expose people of lower socioeconomic status (SES), particularly African Americans, to higher cancer risks (James et al. 2012).

Cancer Alley is an industrial corridor spanning approximately 100 miles from Baton Rouge to New Orleans in Louisiana. This area is home to over 130 industrial facilities, including plants, refineries, landfills, and factories, and contributes to a quarter of the petrochemical production in the United States. The communities within Cancer Alley have a notably high proportion of African Americans, accounting for 40 percent, compared to Louisiana's average of 32 percent and the national average of 12 percent in the United States (James et al. 2012).

A 2012 study by James and colleagues revealed that the average cumulative cancer risk in Cancer Alley was 45.8 per million. This means that up to forty-six individuals out of every million could potentially develop cancer over their lifetime due to exposure to carcinogenic air toxins in the ambient air. This risk level is statistically higher than the national average of 30.3 per million, the Delta Region Authority's average of 35.3 per million, and Louisiana State's average of 37.1 per million. Key contributors to the total cancer risks in this region include emissions of formaldehyde, acetaldehyde, carbon tetrachloride, ethylene oxide, benzene, 1,3-butadiene, and naphthalene, all of which were found to exceed benchmark levels. The study also found that the highest cancer risks were concentrated in the lowest-income areas, particularly in East Baton Rouge and Orleans Parishes. In East Baton Rouge Parish, most communities had a Black population of at least 75 percent, with some areas exceeding 90 percent.

In a recent 2022 investigation, the U.S. Environmental Protection Agency identified chloroprene emissions from the Denka Performance Elastomer plant in LaPlace, a predominantly Black parish, as a significant source of pollution. The EPA classifies chloroprene as a probable human carcinogen, known to potentially cause damage to the brain, lungs, heart, stomach, skin, and eyes. Moreover, the investigation discovered that schools near Denka and other similar polluting facilities exposed children to heightened cancer risks. In a letter to the Louisiana Department of Health, the EPA criticized both the Louisiana Department of Health (LDH) and the Louisiana Department of Environmental Quality (LDEQ) for their "actions/inactions" that have led to "an adverse disparate impact on the basis of race" (EPA 2022).

These findings illustrate the pivotal role of geographical studies in identifying carcinogenic factors around us, and bring the hope that cancer risks can be reduced and prevented.

Further Reading

American Cancer Society. "Key Statistics for Prostate Cancer." https://www.cancer.org/cancer/types/prostate-cancer/about/key-statistics.html#:~:text=Prostate%20cancer%20is%20the%20second,do%20not%20die%20from%20it.

Bruning, Madeline. 2023. "EPA Finds Evidence of Racial Discrimination in Cancer Alley." *The Regulatory Review*. https://www.theregreview.org/2023/03/21/bruning-epa-finds-evidence-of-racial-discrimination-in-cancer-alley/.

Department of Health and Human Services and updated regularly (HHS). 2021. "15th Report on Carcinogens." https://ntp.niehs.nih.gov/whatwestudy/assessments/cancer/roc.

Hirayama, Takeshi. (1981). "Non-Smoking Wives of Heavy Smokers have a Higher Risk of Lung Cancer: A study from Japan." *British Medical Journal* (Clinical research ed.), *282*(6259): 183–5. doi: https://doi.org/10.1136/bmj.282.6259.183

James, Wesley, Chunrong Jia, and Satish Kedia. 2012. "Uneven Magnitude of Disparities in Cancer Risks from Air Toxics." *Environmental Research and Public Health, 9*(12). https://doi.org/10.3390/ijerph9124365.

Klassen, Ann C., and Elizabeth A. Platz. 2006. "What Can Geography Tell Us about Prostate Cancer?" *American Journal of Preventive Medicine, 30*(2 Suppl): S7–15. doi: 10.1016/j.amepre.2005.09.004.

Terry, Mary Beth. 2023. "Cancer Susceptibility across the Life Course." Columbia University and Weill Cornell Medicine Meyer Cancer Center Conference. https://www.youtube.com/watch?v=bpuIORyIrDA.

United States Environmental Protection Agency (EPA). 2022. "In Reply refer to: EPA Complaint Nos. 01R-22-R6, 02R-22-R6, and 04R-22-R6." *EPA.gov*. https://www.epa.gov/system/files/documents/2022-10/2022%2010%2012%20Final%20Letter%20LDEQ%20LDH%2001R-22-R6%2C%2002R-22-R6%2C%2004R-22-R6.pdf.

Chemical Releases in Natech Events

Modern life is increasingly reliant on chemically manufactured products. However, uncontrolled release of chemicals into the food chain and drinking water has also become a major source of health risks. Natural disasters such as earthquakes, floods, and cyclones can trigger chemical spills, resulting in what's known as natech (natural-hazard-triggered-technological) events. An illustrative instance would be an event that happened in Santa Cruz, California in 2020, where a dry lightning storm sparked a forest fire leading to the leakage of benzene, a known carcinogen, from overheated plastic piping, into water supply (Sever 2020). These events can exacerbate the impact of natural disasters, rendering contaminated areas uninhabitable and causing economic losses and mental distress for displaced populations.

The occurrence of natech events has been steadily increasing worldwide, particularly over the past two decades. Scientists have identified two factors that contribute significantly to natech disasters. First, the expanding construction of urban and rural communities into wilderness areas, where natural disasters are more likely to happen. Second, climate change has resulted in more frequent occurrences of extreme weather patterns. According to National Oceanic and Atmospheric Administration (NOAA), the number of weeks in a year with weather conditions that pose risks of very large wildfires will exceed sixfold in the United States alone by 2070 (Kennedy 2015). Rising temperature and frequent hurricanes have the potential to devastate power grids and facilities for storing chemicals. Hurricane Katrina and a cyanide spill in Romania are two events that stand out in notable natech disasters.

Hurricane Katrina 2005

Hurricane Katrina, a Category 5 hurricane, caused widespread devastation in the coastal region, particularly in the vicinity of New Orleans, in 2005. The powerful winds and extensive flooding led to 1,392 fatalities and staggering economic damages amounting to nearly $150 billion. However, Hurricane Katrina's extended damages are even more consequential, as researchers gradually uncovered in the subsequent years (Picou 2009). The following are notable findings that later emerged.

Air pollution in the city of New Orleans was primarily attributed to the practice of waste burning during the cleanup work, which was authorized by the Environmental Protection Agency (EPA) and state regulatory agencies. This operation led to the release of harmful toxins in the atmosphere. Numerous open burning sites were scattered across the city, exacerbating the problem of air pollution.

As waters receded, homes that had been inundated became susceptible to mold infestation. The presence of airborne mold spores and endotoxins in both the indoor and outdoor environment exposed restoration workers and returning residents to contaminated air, resulting in respiratory infestations.

The flooding washed up arsenic compounds that had either accumulated in the soil naturally or due to the past use of pesticides, resulting in areas with elevated concentration of arsenic on the land surface. Analysis of collected sediment samples revealed that 95 percent of the samples exceeded the screening levels set by the Environmental Protection Agency (EPA), and some 30 percent samples indicated necessity of cleanup operations. Arsenic poisoning can have fatal consequences, and children are particularly susceptible to its harmful effects.

The powerful winds and extensive flooding resulted in fuel spills from abandoned vehicles and fuel storage facilities. Analysis of sediment samples collected in New Orleans revealed widespread diesel contamination, requiring urgent and systematic cleanup. Petroleum fuel products contained carcinogenic compounds, including one of the most hazardous chemical of Benzo(a)pyrene which poses a grave threat to both the ecosystem and human health.

In addition to the pollutions, Hurricane Katrina imposed a high psychological burden on the affected populations. The aftermath of Katrina has reportedly led to a range of mental distress and emotional challenges to individuals who suffered from the contamination of the environment, from anxiety, depression to other psychological ailments.

Romania's Cyanide Spill 2020

In January 2020, a combination of heavy wintry rain and snowfall caused a reservoir at the Aurul gold mine to overflow. The reservoir was built to contain hundreds of thousands of cubic meters of water with high concentration of cyanide from the mining operations. Cyanide was being used at the Aurul mine to extract gold, instead of safer methods. Cyanide is a dangerous toxin to the human body, and can cause breathing difficulties, cardiac problems, and thyroid disease. In addition to the weather event causing the overflow, the gold mine was found to lack in monitoring capabilities and its emergency response readiness was rudimentary.

When approximately 100,000 cubic meters of the wastewater flowed into the Somes and Szamos rivers, the two largest tributaries of the River Tisza that merges with the Danube River, the resulting contamination had far-reaching impacts on neighboring countries, including Hungary, Yugoslavia, Bulgaria, and Ukraine (Encyclopedia.com 2023; UNEP 2000).

The environmental damages were acute, as stated in the assessment conducted by UNEP in 2000. The plume of contaminated water caused the decimation of various types of plankton along its path. Thousands of tons of fish were killed, according to Hungarian authorities' estimates. Dead fish were washed into the Danube River, affecting the fishing industry and tourism along multiple river systems.

In the vicinity of the dam where the overflow took place, the level of heavy metal contamination surpassed the standards set by neighboring countries. Additionally, investigations revealed that even the upstream areas unaffected by this specific spill exhibited elevated levels of heavy metal contamination, primarily due to shoddy mining operations. These problems also highlighted the region's history of contamination, which had been neglected and disregarded for an extended period under the influence of the former Soviet regime.

The chemical spills caused by natech events prompt us to revisit our understanding of natural disasters. They indicate that mitigating the effects of natural disasters extends beyond constructing stronger levees or infrastructure. It requires industries to embed natech-readiness as an integral part of their planning, due to the worsening climate change.

Further Reading

Encyclopedia.com. 2023. "Romania's Cyanide Spill." https://www.encyclopedia.com/history/energy-government-and-defense-magazines/romanias-cyanide-spill.

Kennedy, Caitlyn. 2015. "Risk of Very Large Fires Could Increase Sixfold by Mid-century in the US." *Climate.gov*. https://www.climate.gov/news-features/featured-images/risk-very-large-fires-could-increase-sixfold-mid-century-us.

Knabb, Richard D., Jamie R. Rhonme, and Daniel P. Brown. 2023. "Tropical Cyclone Report Hurricane Katrina 23-August 30, 2005." https://www.nhc.noaa.gov/data/tcr/AL122005_Katrina.pdf.

Picou, Steven J. 2009. "Katrina as a Natech Disaster: Toxic Contamination and Long-Term Risks for Residents of New Orleans." *Journal of Applied Social Science*, 3(2): 39–55. https://www.jstor.org/stable/23548914.

Sever, Megan. 2020. "Plastic Drinking Water Pipes Exposed to High Heat Can Leak Hazardous Chemicals." *ScienceNews*. https://www.sciencenews.org/article/plastic-drinking-water-pipes-high-heat-wildfire-hazardous-chemicals.

United Nations Economic Commission for Europe (UNECE). "The Industrial Accidents Convention and Natural Disasters: Natech." https://unece.org/industrial-accidents-convention-and-natural-disasters-natech.

United Nations Environment Programme (UNEP). 2000. "Cyanide Spill at Baia Mare—Assessment Mission Report." https://www.environmental-expert.com/articles/cyanide-spill-at-baia-mare-assessment-mission-report-unep-ocha-1324.

World Health Organization. "Chemical Incidents." www.who.int/health-topics/chemical-incidents/#tab=tab_1.

Health Impacts of the Chernobyl and Fukushima Daiichi Accidents

Harvesting energy through nuclear fission has become a cornerstone of electricity generation today. In a typical process, uranium fuel is shaped into ceramic pellets and stacked to form fuel rods. Each pellet produces as much energy as 150 gallons of oil. The nuclear reaction generates heat, which turns water into steam to drive turbines and produce electricity. When safety is ensured, this method is not only cleaner but also more versatile than traditional systems relying on fossil fuels or hydropower.

As of 2022, nuclear power accounts for over 10 percent of the world's electricity, with thirty-three countries operating commercial nuclear facilities.

France stands out, generating nearly 70 percent of its annual electricity from nuclear power, while the United States and Russia each produce over 20 percent of their electricity through nuclear energy. In the United States alone, there are fifty-four nuclear power plants and ninety-two nuclear reactors operating across twenty-eight states (EIA 2022).

However, safety concerns remain widespread, and not without justification. Two of the most infamous nuclear disasters—Chernobyl and Fukushima Daiichi—serve as stark reminders that reactor malfunctions can lead to devastating and long-lasting consequences.

On April 26, 1986, a nuclear accident at the Chernobyl Nuclear Power Plant located in Pripyat, Ukraine, administered under the Soviet Union at the time, caused severe damages to human health and the environment. The cause of the accident was attributed to human error and the faulty design of the Soviet-era nuclear reactor. The Soviet government initially attempted to cover up the disaster, until radiation levels were detected in Sweden and other European countries. Subsequently, radioactive fallouts were detected in countries as far as England and China.

Economic, environmental, and health-related consequences were staggering, according to reports. About 70 percent of the radioactive fallout rained down on Belarus, contaminating one-fourth of the country and one-fifth of its agricultural land. Lives of 7 million people were affected as a result of relocation, loss of jobs, and psychological depression. The Belarusian government still had to spend 22 percent of the total budget on response efforts five years after the accident (Hjelmgaard 2016; IAEA 2003–2005). Additionally, radioactive contamination affected even more people residing in nearby Russia and Ukraine; many suffered long-term health-related and psychological impacts.

The worst health impacts were experienced at the epicenter of the disaster. Of the more than 600 workers present at the site, 134 developed acute radiation sickness. Additionally, 530,000 recovery operation workers were exposed to high levels of radiation.

Children were particularly affected due to their smaller thyroid glands and faster metabolisms, which made them more vulnerable to radiation exposure. Their dietary habits further compounded this vulnerability. It is estimated that approximately 6,000 children and adolescents developed thyroid cancer at the time, with many more people expected to develop cancer in subsequent years (UNSCEAR 2000 Report).

Since 2016, the radioactive remains of Chernobyl have been contained within the New Safe Confinement (NSC), a structure designed to prevent further leaks for the next 100 years (Dubchak 2018). However, scientists estimate that due to the slow decay of the released isotopes, Chernobyl may remain uninhabitable for at least 3,000 years (Hinckley 2016).

The consequences continued into the early phase of the ongoing Russia-Ukraine war. During this time, Russian troops entered Chernobyl and disturbed previously treated radioactive soil, releasing additional radioactive materials into the environment (Kramer 2022).

Despite the safety design improvements and lessons learned from Chernobyl, another radioactive leak occurred at the Fukushima Daiichi nuclear power plant. This incident demonstrated that even with advanced safety measures, the plant's designers were unprepared to fully protect it from earthquakes and tsunamis—natural hazards that Japan routinely faces.

On March 11, 2011, a 9.0-magnitude earthquake triggered a tsunami that overwhelmed the seawall protecting the Fukushima Daiichi nuclear plant. This led to failures in cooling systems, meltdowns in three reactor cores, and the release of radioactive materials into the water and surrounding environment. Unlike the Chernobyl disaster, where explosions destroyed a reactor and sent a radioactive plume as far as Europe, the reactors at Fukushima retained partial containment, limiting the extent of radiation release. While the earthquake itself caused minimal damage to the reactors, the tsunami-induced cooling failures were catastrophic. According to the World Nuclear Association (2024), there have been no deaths directly attributed to radiation exposure from the incident, though significant environmental and societal impacts ensued.

Studies conducted over the following decade revealed significant secondary impacts on people's livelihoods. A report by the United Nations Scientific Committee highlighted the profound psychological and social toll caused by the disaster. Anxiety over potential radiation exposure, coupled with disruptions to daily life and medical care, led to widespread psychological distress, including post-traumatic stress disorder (PTSD).

Residents from the affected area faced stigmatization, often referred to as "radiation stigma" and "self-stigma," further exacerbating their challenges. Many evacuees suffered loss of jobs, severed social connections, and deteriorating mental health. According to one study, the severity of these impacts among the evacuees was of great severity, even when compared to other types of natural disasters (Maeda et al. 2017).

The world has learned many lessons from the Chernobyl and Fukushima disasters. From a technological perspective, even with enhanced safety precautions, unforeseen incidents can still occur. This underscores the need to remain vigilant and avoid complacency at all times.

The primary responsibility for ensuring the safety of nuclear energy lies with governments. When governments attempt to conceal nuclear accidents, the resulting devastation can be far more severe. Transparency is, therefore, a critical obligation for governments in managing nuclear energy safely.

Most importantly, nuclear risks are not confined by national borders—they pose a threat to humanity as a whole. This makes international cooperation essential for global safety. Countries involved in nuclear energy production must collaborate by sharing experiences, enhancing capabilities to manage hazards, preventing accidents, responding effectively to emergencies, and mitigating harmful consequences. These principles are emphasized in the International Atomic Energy Agency's (IAEA) "Safety Standards."

Further Reading

Centers for Disease Control and Prevention (CDC). 2023. "Fukushima Radiation Emergency: Lessons Learned." https://www.cdc.gov/nceh/features/fukushima-radiation/index.html.

Dubchak, Andriy. 2018. "Under the Shield: Inside Chernobyl's New Safe Confinement." https://www.rferl.org/a/inside-chernobyl-nuclear-power-plant-conferment-shelter-photo/29583945.html.

EIA.gov. 2022. "Nuclear Explained." https://www.eia.gov/energyexplained/nuclear/nuclear-power-plants.php.

Hinkley, Story. 2016. "Chernobyl Will Be Unhabitable for at Least 3,000 Years, Say Nuclear Experts." https://www.csmonitor.com/World/Global-News/2016/0424/Chernobyl-will-be-unhabitable-for-at-least-3-000-years-say-nuclear-experts.

Hjelmgaard, Kim. 2016. "In Secretive Belarus, Chernobyl's Impact is Breathtakingly Grim." *USA Today*. https://www.usatoday.com/story/news/world/2016/04/17/belarus-border-town-chernobyl-30th-anniversary/82888796/.

IAEA. 2003–5. "Chernobyl's Legacy: Health, Environmental and Socio-economic Impacts and Recommendations to the Governments of Belarus, the Russian Federation and Ukraine." https://www.iaea.org/sites/default/files/chernobyl.pdf.

International Atomic Energy Agency (IAEA). "Safety Standards." https://www.iaea.org/resources/safety-standards.

Kramer, Andrew. 2022. "Russian Blunders in Chernobyl: 'They Came and Did Whatever They Wanted.'" *The New York Times*. https://www.nytimes.com/2022/04/08/world/europe/ukraine-chernobyl.html.

Maeda, Msaharu and Misari Oe. 2017. "Mental Health Consequences and Social Issues after the Fukushima Disaster." *Asia-Pacific Journal of Public Health*, 29(2_suppl): 36S–46S. doi: 10.1177/1010539516689695.

United Nations. 2022. Sources, Effects and Risks of Ionizing Radiation—UNSCEAR 2020/2021 Report. Levels and effects of radiation exposure due to the accident at the Fukushima ... (unscear.org).

UNSCEARS. 2000. Assessments of the Radiation Effects from the Chernobyl Nuclear Reactor Accident. The Chernobyl Accident (unscear.org).

WHO. 2011. "Radiation: The Chernobyl Accident." https://www.who.int/news-room/questions-and-answers/item/radiation-the-chernobyl-accident.

World Nuclear Association. 2024. "Fukushima Daiichi Accident." https://world-nuclear.org/information-library/safety-and-security/safety-of-plants/fukushima-daiichi-accident.

Epidemics after Natural Disasters

Natural disasters such as earthquakes, volcanic eruptions, landslides, tsunamis, floods, and droughts can trigger severe disease outbreaks due to disruptions in sanitation systems and medical services. Furthermore, population displacement and overcrowding are also significant risk factors contributing to the spread of diseases.

Water-related diseases are among the most common health issues in the aftermath of disasters. Diarrheal outbreaks are frequently linked to the contamination of drinking water following floods. For instance, in 2004, flooding in Bangladesh resulted in 17,000 cases of diarrhea caused by *Vibrio cholerae* (associated with cholera) and *Escherichia coli* (*E. coli*). Both bacteria are known to cause severe acute watery diarrhea, leading to high morbidity and mortality rates. Cholera, in particular, is infamous for its potential to cause widespread infection and high death tolls.

Cholera outbreaks have been linked to significant mortality in past disasters, such as the floods in West Bengal in 1998 and Mozambique in 2000. However, the largest post-disaster cholera outbreak occurred in Haiti a decade later. In 2010, after a 7.0 magnitude earthquake killed 200,000 people and displaced one million, a cholera epidemic claimed an additional 4,500 lives (MacLachlan 2011). Due to the slow restoration of sanitation and drinking water systems in Haiti, cholera has remained a recurring issue, with a resurgence reported a decade later in 2022.

In addition to cholera, *E. coli* and *Salmonella* are frequently found in contaminated food and water, causing severe diarrhea. In the United States, outbreaks of *Salmonella* and norovirus—a virus that inflames the stomach and intestines—have been reported following hurricanes, such as Allison and Katrina in 2001 and 2005 respectively. However, these outbreaks did not result in fatalities.

What We Learn through Studying Health Geography

Health geography examines how place and space influence health outcomes and disease distribution. It studies patterns of health and illness, health care access, environmental impacts, and socioeconomic factors. By integrating geographic analysis, it identifies disparities and informs strategies to improve health care delivery tailored to specific locations.

This field adopts a holistic perspective, recognizing the interconnectedness of human and animal health within ecosystems. The One Health approach initiated by the United Nations, addresses complex health issues by considering ecological and human factors together.

Key areas include accessibility, environmental injustice, and the interaction between individual and social health determinants. Geographic location often affects access to care, with rural and underserved areas facing service gaps. Environmental injustice highlights how marginalized communities face greater exposure to hazards, leading to disparities. Studies also examine how personal factors like genetics and lifestyle interact with social determinants such as income, education, and policy.

For instance, Arcury et al. (2005) studied health care access in rural Appalachian North Carolina. Using Geographic Information Systems (GIS) and surveys from 1,059 adults, they found that long distances to providers and limited transportation reduced access to routine checkups and chronic care. Individuals without a driver's license faced added barriers to preventive and ongoing care.

Health geography provides spatial insights that help policymakers address health inequities, improve interventions, and promote better outcomes, contributing to a more equitable health care system.

Further Reading

Arcury, Thomas A., Wilbert M. Gesler, John S. Preisser, Jill Sherman, John Spencer, and Jamie Perin. 2005. "The Effects of Geography and Spatial Behavior on Health Care Utilization among the Residents of a Rural Region." *HSR: Health Services Research*, 40(1): 135–56. doi: 10.1111/j.1475-6773.2005.00346.x.

Vine, Michelle M., Kate Mulligan, Rachel Harris, and Jennifer L. Dean. 2023. "Health Geography on Public Health Research, Policy, and Practice in Canada." *International Journal of Environmental Research and Public Health*, 20(18): 6735. https://doi.org/10.3390/ijerph20186735.

The spread of communicable diseases can worsen under deteriorated sanitary conditions, such as limited access to clean water and compromised sewage systems. These conditions increase human exposure to pathogens that transmit via the fecal-oral route. Among the viruses capable of causing widespread disease are hepatitis A and E.

Hepatitis A is a highly contagious virus that affects the liver, causing symptoms such as jaundice, vomiting, abdominal pain, and dark urine. Infection occurs through the consumption of contaminated food or water or through direct contact with an infected individual. While hepatitis A is not typically associated with high mortality, its symptoms can be debilitating. In most cases, the infection resolves within weeks with adequate rest and proper nutrition.

In contrast, hepatitis E, which shares similar symptoms with hepatitis A, poses greater risks and can be life-threatening, particularly for pregnant women. The virus exploits immunological changes during pregnancy, which suppress the mother's immune system to support the fetus. Studies indicate that the mortality rate among pregnant women infected with hepatitis E can reach up to 25 percent, especially during the third trimester (Chaudhry 2015).

Both hepatitis A and E are prevalent in impoverished regions prone to frequent flooding and heavy rainfall. Research indicates that globally, one in eight individuals has experienced a viral hepatitis infection at some point (Li et al. 2020). Vaccines are available for hepatitis A, however; vaccines against hepatitis E are under development and with limited use in China, according to the World Health Organization (WHO).

Malaria and leptospirosis are diseases commonly associated with flooding, according to the CDC. Malaria is a mosquito-borne illness caused by *Plasmodium* parasites transmitted by mosquitoes in regions where the disease is endemic. Flooding often creates stagnant water, which serves as an ideal breeding ground for mosquitoes. Symptoms of malaria include nausea, vomiting, and recurring fever. While malaria vaccines have been developed, their availability is limited, and their effectiveness varies.

Leptospirosis, on the other hand, is a bacterial infection caused by *Leptospira*, a bacterium found in the urine of rodents, particularly mice. Symptoms include nausea, vomiting, diarrhea, and abdominal pain. In severe cases, patients may develop conjunctival suffusion (reddening of the eyes) and jaundice due to liver damage. Transmission occurs through direct contact with contaminated water. Flooding often forces rodents to higher ground, where humans seeking refuge are at increased risk of exposure. A vaccine for leptospirosis is still under development.

Natural disasters can force people into overcrowded shelters and camps, creating ideal conditions for the rapid spread of airborne infectious diseases. Diseases transmitted through respiratory droplets, such as the common flu, measles, meningitis, acute respiratory infections, and tuberculosis, thrive in such environments.

Take measles for example, a virus that is closely monitored globally due to its high transmission rate and severe symptoms. In addition to fever, cough, and skin rash, measles can lead to secondary complications such as pneumonia and encephalitis. Remarkably, the measles virus can remain active in the air for up to two hours after being released, and nine out of ten unimmunized individuals exposed to an infected person will contract the disease (Holt 2023). Vaccination against measles is highly effective and is part of the standard measles-mumps-rubella (MMR) vaccine. In Western countries, the MMR vaccine is typically administered to children at ages four to five and again around age fifteen. In the United States, most states require students to be vaccinated before attending school. However, the availability of the MMR vaccine remains limited in some parts of the world, particularly in regions of Africa and the Middle East, according to the CDC. For instance, between 2021 and 2023, measles claimed 182 lives in Ethiopia. Factors such as low population immunity, concurrent epidemics, conflict, forced displacement, and disruptions to childhood vaccination programs were cited as contributing causes of these outbreaks (WHO 2023). This has raised concerns about the resurgence of measles in vulnerable areas.

Beyond natural disasters, manmade crises such as wars and conflicts also significantly disrupt vaccination efforts, leading to outbreaks. For example, the Russia-Ukraine war has been linked to reported measles outbreaks in Ukraine due to interruptions in vaccination programs (Holt 2023).

In summary, natural disasters can exacerbate the spread of communicable diseases through factors such as displacement, overcrowding, water contamination, disrupted sanitation systems, and limited health care access. Similarly, wars and conflicts have comparable impacts. To mitigate post-disaster disease outbreaks, global health organizations emphasize the importance of routine surveillance, urgent supply readiness, access to clean water, and health care support.

Further Reading

CDC. 2025. "About Leptospirosis." https://www.cdc.gov/leptospirosis/about/index.html.
CDC. "Global Measles." https://wwwnc.cdc.gov/travel/notices/watch/measles-globe.
CDC. "Malaria." https://www.cdc.gov/malaria/index.html.
Chaudhry, Shahnaz. 2015. "Hepatitis E Infection during Pregnancy." *Can Fam Physician*. https://www.ncbi.nlm.nih.gov/pmc/articles/PMC4501603/.
Holt, Ed. 2023. "Experts Warn Over Potential for Measles in Ukraine." *The Lancet*. https://www.sciencedirect.com/science/article/pii/S0140673623004361?via%3Dihub.
Li, Pengfei, Jiaye Liu, Yang Li, Junhong Su, Zhongren Ma, Wichor M. Bramer, Wanlu Cao, Robert A de Man, Maikel P Peppelenbosch, Qiuwei Pan. 2020. "The Global Epidemiology of Hepatitis E Virus Infection: A Systematic Review and Meta-Analysis." *Liver International*, 40(7): 1516–28. doi: 10.1111/liv.14468.
MacLachlan, Allison. 2011. "The Quake That Brought Back Cholera." *Livescience.com*. https://www.livescience.com/15480-haiti-earthquake-cholera-outbreak.html.
Watson, John T., Michelle Gayer, and Maire A. Connolly. 2007. "Epidemics after Natural Disasters." *Emerging Infectious Diseases*, 13(1): 1–5. doi: 10.3201/eid1301.060779.
World Health Organization (WHO). 2023. "Measles—Ethiopia." www.who.int/emergencies/disease-outbreak-news/item/2023-DON460.
World Health Organization (WHO). 2024. "Safety of Hepatitis E Vaccines." https://www.who.int/groups/global-advisory-committee-on-vaccine-safety/topics/hepatitis-e-vaccines.

Malaria Control—Progress and Challenges

Malaria, one of humanity's oldest diseases, remains a major public health challenge worldwide. Transmitted to humans through the bites of infected female *Anopheles* mosquitoes, it is caused by *Plasmodium* parasites. Symptoms include fever, chills, muscle aches, diarrhea, and respiratory issues. In severe cases, malaria can result in anemia, organ failure, or death.

The disease predominantly affects tropical and subtropical regions, with a significant burden in parts of Africa and Asia. According to the World Health Organization (WHO) 2022 report, malaria caused approximately 619,000 deaths globally in 2021, making it one of the leading causes of death among young children, particularly in Africa. The report also notes that there were around 247 million cases of malaria across eighty-four endemic countries. Notably, Nigeria, the Democratic Republic of the Congo, and the United Republic of Tanzania accounted for 50 percent of global malaria-related deaths.

Research has indicated that socio-geographic determinants of transmission, such as high population density and poor hygiene conditions commonly found in impoverished neighborhoods, are among the most significant factors contributing to the spread of the disease. Additionally, irrigated agriculture and climate change, which lead to warmer temperatures and increased rainfall, have been linked to the growth of mosquito populations.

Historically, malaria parasites, which originated from the protozoan lineage, evolved into an organism that inhabits humans. This significant transition coincided with the development of agriculture and human settlements, approximately 100,000 years ago. Over time, four species of malaria *Plasmodium* have come to rely almost exclusively on humans as their natural intermediate hosts: *P. falciparum, P. vivax, P. ovale,* and *P. malariae*. Among these, *P. falciparum* is known to cause the most severe form of the disease (Noston 2022).

Documentation of malaria dates back to ancient times. The symptoms and various ways of treatment are found in archives of ancient civilizations of Egypt, China, and Europe. An herbal medicine known as "qinghao" (*Artemisia annua*) from which a critical anti-malarial compound, artemisinin, was later extracted was recorded in a Chinese medical handbook in a tomb of the Han dynasty circa the second century AD. In the West, scientists extracted quinine and chinchonine from cinchona tree bark to treat fevers in the 1800s.

It wasn't until the nineteenth century that scientific breakthroughs led to effective control measures against malaria. The malaria parasite, *Plasmodium*, was identified in red blood cells by French army surgeon Charles Louis Alphonse Laveran in 1880, an achievement for which he was awarded the Nobel Prize in 1907. Later, Ronald Ross, a British medical doctor, discovered the transmission of malaria parasites by *Anopheles* mosquitoes in 1897, earning him the Nobel Prize in 1902. These discoveries paved the way for twentieth-century strategies focused on controlling the vector mosquito by eliminating breeding sites. During this period, DDT (dichloro-diphenyl-trichloroethane) became the pesticide of choice, and its developer, Swiss chemist Paul Hermann Müller, was awarded the Nobel Prize for it in 1948. However, DDT was banned in 1978 due to its negative impact on wildlife and the development of resistance in the mosquitoes it was intended to control.

Notable progress has been made in the development of drugs to combat malaria. In the 1940s, the U.S. Army developed a drug named chloroquine, which became a preferred treatment until the emergence and rapid spread of chloroquine-resistant *P. falciparum* malaria. In the 1970s, Chinese scientists developed artemisinin, extracted from the plant "qinghao," which was used to treat soldiers infected with malaria during the Vietnam War. For her significant contributions to this drug discovery, Tu Youyou was awarded the Nobel Prize in 2015. In the 1990s, several Artemisinin Combination Therapies (ACTs) were developed to address drug resistance. However, the emergence of insecticide resistance in *Anopheles* mosquitoes and drug resistance in various species of *Plasmodium* has also increased alarmingly (Nosten 2022).

Currently, the most practical preventive measures in malaria-endemic regions of Africa remain rudimentary. These include the use of insecticide-treated nets (ITNs) and chemical sprays, accounting for 39 percent and 11 percent of prevention efforts, respectively. Other strategies involve modifying clothing and dwellings. However, these simple measures also face challenges. Despite only 54–47 percent of the at-risk population adopting ITNs, their use has reportedly led to insecticide resistance, evidenced by mosquitoes altering their feeding behavior, potentially increasing transmission risks. Another concern is that an increasing proportion of *P. falciparum* parasites no longer express the Pfhrp2/3 proteins, which are crucial for detecting malaria, posing a significant obstacle to reliable diagnosis, as reported by the WHO in 2022.

Faced with these challenges, scientists are increasingly turning to genetic approaches. Among the most promising strategies for malaria control and prevention are the development of vaccines and the genetic biocontrol of *Anopheles* mosquitoes. Efforts to create malaria vaccines began in the 1960s, but progress has been slow due to the *Plasmodium* parasite's complex and mutating genetic structure throughout its transmission cycle.

Additionally, socioeconomic challenges in endemic countries have often relegated malaria control to a lower priority. These efforts are further hampered by inadequate health care infrastructure and limited financial resources. Bureaucratic hurdles in vaccine licensing add another layer of difficulty, as highlighted by El-Moamly et al. in 2023.

Despite these challenges, the first-generation vaccine, RTS,S/AS01, was approved by the WHO in 2021. It offers about 56 percent protection over one year and 36 percent protection over four years. However, its protection is limited to *P. falciparum*, the deadliest malaria parasite globally and the most prevalent in Africa. The vaccine offers no protection against *P. vivax*, which predominates in many countries outside Africa. The WHO cautioned that RTS,S/AS01 is not sufficient as a stand-alone preventive measure. The WHO advocates that malaria control and prevention should continue to rely on a comprehensive approach, as emphasized (WHO 2020).

Genetic biocontrol technologies, such as gene-drive-modified mosquitoes (GDMMs), aim to control mosquito populations with objectives like replacing, suppressing, limiting, or localizing vector mosquitoes. One technology under experimentation is the Incompatible Insect Technique (IIT). This method involves releasing male mosquitoes treated with Wolbachia bacteria into the wild. The release is not harmful to humans, as male mosquitoes do not feed on human blood. However, when these males mate with female mosquitoes, the result is non-viable embryos. Another area of exploration in gene-drive technology focuses on skewing the sex ratio of mosquito progeny toward males, thereby reducing the population. These technologies, as noted by James et al. in 2023, are still in the preliminary stages.

A major benefit of genetic biocontrol is that modified mosquitoes, exhibiting the same natural behaviors as their target species, can access breeding sites that are often unreachable using traditional methods. Nevertheless, this approach faces challenges such as ensuring the sustainable delivery of genetically modified mosquitoes, as well as securing regulatory approval and public acceptance (James et al. 2023).

Further Reading

Centers for Disease Control and Prevention (CDC). 2004. "About Malaria." https://www.cdc.gov/malaria/about/.

El-Moamly, Amal A. and Mohamed A. El-Sweify. 2023. "Malaria Vaccines: The 60-Year Journey of Hope and Final Success—Lessons Learned and Future Prospects." *Tropical Medicine and Health, 51*: 29. doi: https://doi.org/10.1186/s41182-023-00516-w.

Geddes, Linda. 2021. "The Groundbreaking History of the World' First Malaria Vaccine." *VaccinesWork*. https://www.gavi.org/vaccineswork/groundbreaking-history-worlds-first-malaria-vaccine.

James, Stephanie and Michael Santos. 2023. "The Promise and Challenge of Genetic Biocontrol Approaches for Malaria Elimination." *Tropical Medicine and Infectious Disease, 8*(4): 201. doi:10.3390/tropicalmed8040201.

Nosten, François. 2022. "A Brief History of Malaria." *Sciencedirect.com, 51*(3): 104130. https://www.sciencedirect.com/science/article/pii/S0755498222000239?via%3Dihub.

The World Health Organization (WHO). 2020. "Malaria: The Malaria Vaccine Implementation Programme (MVIP)." https://www.who.int/news-room/questions-and-answers/item/malaria-vaccine-implementation-programme#:~:text=RTS%2CS%20is%20being%20evaluated,many%20countries%20outside%20of%20Africa.

The World Health Organization (WHO). 2022. "The 2022 World Malaria Report." https://www.who.int/publications/i/item/9789240064898.

Systemic Lupus Erythematosus and the Socioeconomic Environment

Systemic lupus erythematosus (SLE), commonly known as lupus, is an autoimmune disorder that affects millions of people worldwide each year. Common symptoms include muscle pain, joint swelling, and, in severe cases, inflammation impacting the lungs, kidneys, and cardiovascular system. This inflammation can cause long-term damage to these organs, as noted by the Centers for Disease Control and Prevention (CDC). Cardiovascular disease has become a leading cause of death among lupus patients, with mortality rates two to three times higher than those of the general population (Barber et al. 2023; CDC).

A notable characteristic of lupus is its considerable complexity, involving genetic factors, hormonal changes, gender, race, environmental influences, and socioeconomic status. Research indicates that lupus disproportionately impacts women of reproductive age, with a female-to-male ratio of approximately nine to one (Tian et al. 2022). The highest incidence rates per 100,000 people have been observed in American Indian/Alaskan women (270.6), Black women (230.9), Hispanic women (120.7), white women (84.7), and Asian/Pacific Islander women (84.4). Furthermore, lupus is among the leading causes of death for Black and Hispanic women between the ages of fifteen and twenty-five (Barber et al. 2023).

As a severe chronic disease, lupus affects individuals worldwide, though its geographic distribution varies significantly. It is estimated that around 400,000 new cases of lupus are diagnosed annually across the globe. The countries with the highest estimated rates of new cases per 100,000 individuals each year include Poland (83.51), Barbados (36.46), the United States (12.35), and China (8.77), research shows (Tian et al. 2022). The Lupus Foundation of the United States reports that about 1.5 million Americans and at least 5 million people globally are living with some form of this disease.

As a severe chronic condition, lupus has significant economic consequences. Among individuals diagnosed with lupus, 76 percent find themselves needing to reduce their participation in social activities due to fatigue, and 89 percent are unable to maintain full-time employment because of complications associated with the disease. Consequently, the Lupus Foundation reports that the average annual total cost for managing lupus per patient can reach as much as $50,000.

Like many autoimmune diseases, the exact cause of lupus remains unknown. Research centers worldwide are dedicating significant efforts to uncover the origins of this complex condition. In the United States, the Centers for Disease

Control and Prevention (CDC) manages five population-based registries across various regions to collect data on lupus.

Data from lupus programs in Georgia, Michigan, and the Indian Health Service reveal that lupus is more prevalent among non-Hispanic Asian women and Hispanic women of any race compared to non-Hispanic white women in the United States. These programs have provided valuable insights into various aspects of lupus. Here are some key findings:

According to the Johns Hopkins Lupus Center (JHLC), the development of lupus involves a complex interaction of genetics, hormones, and environmental factors. However, the direct trigger for the disease remains unidentified. It is believed that certain genes are associated with an increased risk of lupus, including the MHC class II and III genes, which are involved in the immune response and can vary by ethnicity. Additionally, multiple genes responsible for coding cell receptors and proteins, which function in identifying antigens, are also implicated. Mutations in these genes are thought to contribute to a general autoimmune reaction, where the immune system mistakenly attacks the body's own tissues instead of targeting foreign antigens.

However, genetic predisposition is just one of several contributing factors. The fact that women are nearly nine times more likely than men to develop lupus points to the role of sex hormones, notably estrogen, which is more abundant in females, in the disease's development, as noted by the Johns Hopkins Lupus Center. Environmental factors such as exposure to cigarette smoke, silica, and mercury are also under investigation. Certain viruses, including the herpes zoster virus, which causes shingles, and the Epstein-Barr virus, have been linked to lupus. Furthermore, exposure to ultraviolet light and stress have been implicated as potential triggers. Yet, none of these factors has been definitively identified as a direct cause of lupus, rendering the disease "overwhelming and mysterious at times," according to the Johns Hopkins Lupus Center.

Lupus research has explored the disease within socioeconomic and geographical frameworks. A notable study investigating differences between rural and urban environments found that individuals raised exclusively in urban areas are diagnosed with lupus approximately five years earlier than those from rural settings. Additionally, long-term residence in urban environments is associated with almost a two-fold increased risk of developing lupus compared to living in rural areas. Associated factors may include the level of education, exposure to sunlight and pesticides, and certain lifestyles. These observations imply that living environments may influence risk levels and manifestation of lupus (Gergianaski et al. 2019).

The geographical distribution has garnered considerable research. An analysis of forty-one studies highlighted a correlation between geographical latitudes and lupus nephritis (LN), a form of kidney disorder, in China. The research showed that the proportion of biopsy-confirmed LN among all biopsy-confirmed kidney diseases and among secondary glomerular diseases, which affect kidney's filtering functions, significantly increases from the northern to the southern regions of China as latitude decreases. However, no significant correlation was found with changes alongside geographic longitudes. This suggests that the lower latitudinal zones in China, which are associated with higher population densities and rapid economic development, may have a stronger connection with the incidence of LN (Pan et al. 2014).

Research into the connections between lupus, race, and socioeconomic status (SES) has provided important insights. In the United States, rates of lupus nephritis are notably higher among Hispanic and Black patients compared to white patients. This racial disparity also extends to hematological complications. Black, Asian/Pacific Islander, and Hispanic patients are at a heightened risk of developing severe hematological manifestations of lupus, such as thrombocytopenia (low platelet count) and anti-phospholipid antibody syndrome (APS), a condition associated with abnormal blood clotting, compared to their white counterparts.

Mortality studies reveal further disparities, showing that Black patients, whether newly diagnosed or with long-standing lupus, have a higher mortality rate and die on average 6.8 years earlier than white patients. These findings underscore the critical role of SES in lupus treatment and management. Individuals living in poverty, particularly Black women, often face significant barriers to accessing adequate health care. Likewise, on a global scale, data suggest that lower SES is consistently linked to higher exposure to hazardous materials and limited access to health care services. These findings stress the importance of securing the needed medical care to vulnerable groups (Hasan et al. 2022).

Further Reading

Barber, Megan R. W., Titilola Falasinnu, Rosalind Ramsey-Goldman, and Ann E. Clarke. 2023. "The Global Epidemiology of SLE: Narrowing the Knowledge Gaps." *Rheumatology (Oxford)*, 62(Suppl 1): i4–i9. doi: 10.1093/rheumatology/keac610.

CDC. 2024. "Symptoms of Lupus." https://www.cdc.gov/lupus/signs-symptoms/?CDC_AAref_Val=https://www.cdc.gov/lupus/basics/symptoms.htm.

Fatoye, Francis, Tadesse Gebrye, and Chidozie Mbada. 2022. "Global and Regional Prevalence and Incidence of Systemic Lupus Erythematosus in Low- and Middle-

Income Countries: A Systematic Review and Meta-Analysis." *Rheumatology International, 42*(12): 2097–107. doi: 10.1007/s00296-022-05183-4.

Gergianaki, I., A. Fanouriakis, C. Adamichou, G. Spyrou, N. Mihalopoulos, S. Kazadzis, L. Chatzi, P. Sidiropoulos, D. T. Boumpas, and G. Bertsias. 2019. "Is Systemic Lupus Erythematosus Different in Urban versus Rural Living Environment? Data from the Cretan Lupus Epidemiology and Surveillance Registry." *Lupus*. doi: 10.1177/0961203318816820.

Hasan, Bilal, Alice Fike, and Sarfarz Hasni. 2022. "Health Disparityies in Sysstemic Lupus Erythematosus—A Narrative Review." *Clinical Rheumatology, 41*: 3299–311. https://link.springer.com/article/10.1007/s10067-022-06268-y.

Johns Hopkins Lupus Center. https://www.hopkinslupus.org/lupus-info/lupus/.

Lupus Foundation of America. https://www.lupus.org.

Pan, Qingjun, Yanning Li, Ling Ye, Zhenzhen Deng, Lu Li, Yongmin Feng, Weijing Liu, and Huafeng Liu. 2014. "Geographical Distribution, A Risk Factor for the Incidence of Lupus Nephritis in China." *BMC Nephrology, 15*: 67. doi: 10.1186/1471-2369-15-67.

Tian, Jingru, Dingyao Zhang, Xu Yao, Yaqing Huang, and Qianjin Lu. 2023. "Global Epidemiology of Systemic Lupus Erythematosus: A Comprehensive Systematic Analysis and Modelling Study." *Annals of the Rheumatic Diseases, 82*(3): 351–6. doi: 10.1136/ard-2022-223035.

Impact of Environmental Damages on Health

Alberta Struggles to Contain Health Risks from Oil Sands

Canada is the third-largest exporter of oil in the world, following Saudi Arabia and Russia. In 2022, Canada exported approximately $123 billion worth of oil, which accounted for 8.48 percent of global oil exports. Of this amount, 95 percent was exported to the United States (Twin 2024).

Canada's oil sands deposits yield bitumen, an asphalt-like material, which is a thick form of petroleum formed from marine organisms that once inhabited ancient seas covering Alberta. The extraction process is both energy-intensive and polluting. Despite these challenges, the profitability has been significant. Over the past three decades, the oil sands industry has become not only a lifeline for Canada's GDP but also a major driver of Alberta's economy. However, this economic benefit is overshadowed by health risks, particularly cancer risks, for communities located near oil sands operations.

Historically, the mining of oil sands began in the 1700s with the arrival of European settlers. By the twentieth century, federal and provincial governments took an interest in developing this resource, assisting the establishment of

PFAS Pollution

PFAS (Per- and Polyfluoroalkyl Substances) were first developed in the 1930s, with functional PFAS appearing in the 1940s and rapidly expanding in industrial and consumer applications by the 1950s due to their unique chemical and physical properties. PFAS are highly resistant to heat, pressure, and chemical reactions. Combined with water- and oil-repelling capabilities, PFAS has become widely used across numerous industries.

PFAS molecules are highly stable and can withstand extreme conditions. Known as "forever chemicals," PFAS persist in the environment and in living organisms, resisting natural degradation processes, which has led to widespread contamination and bioaccumulation in humans and wildlife. Since 1999, the CDC's National Health and Nutrition Examination Survey has detected PFAS in human blood, with certain compounds found in over 99 percent of individuals tested.

PFAS are used in a vast array of popular products, including non-stick cookware, water-repellent clothing, stain-resistant fabrics and carpets, food packaging materials, firefighting foams, cleaning products, and cosmetics like sunscreens. Studies link PFAS exposure to health issues, including developmental, immune, cardiovascular, and liver damage, with recent studies showing testicular and kidney cancers having the strongest evidence of association with PFAS exposure.

PFAS in drinking water, along with other serious contamination cases, has become a major focus of federal investigations in the United States. Several major companies have faced lawsuits and significant settlements due to PFAS contamination of drinking water. In 2023, DuPont de Nemours, Inc., Chemours Company, and Corteva, Inc. settled for $1.18 billion over PFAS-related claims in U.S. drinking water. Tyco Fire Products, which manufactured firefighting foam containing PFAS that contaminated water sources near military bases and training sites, agreed to a $750 million settlement in 2023. In 2024, 3M Company agreed to pay up to $12.5 billion over thirteen years to address PFAS contamination in public water systems.

Further Reading

Centers for Disease Control and Prevention. 2024. "PFAS and Worker Health." *CDC*. https://www.cdc.gov/niosh/pfas/about/index.html.

Gaines, Linda G. T. 2022. "Historical and Current Usage of Per-and Polyfluoroalkyl Substances (PFAS): A Literature Review." *American Journal of Industrial Medicine*. doi: 10.1002/ajim.23362.

Miller, Ronald V. 2024. "PFAS Water Contamination Lawsuit." *Lawsuit Information Center.* https://www.lawsuit-information-center.com/pfas-water-contamination-lawsuit.html.

Steenland, Kyle and Andrea Winquist. 2021. "PFAS and Cancer, A Scoping Review of the Epidemiologic Evidence." *Environmental Research.* doi: 10.1016/j.envres.2020.110690.

commercial pilot plants in the 1940s. Over the years, Indigenous communities, known as First Nations, signed impact benefit agreements with developers. These agreements included quotas for hiring Indigenous labor and direct payments to the nations. However, these communities soon witnessed the deterioration of their own way of life, such as hunting and fishing, as the landscape changed and health risks rose.

Today, ExxonMobil and the Canadian company Suncor have expanded the excavation site to a vast area larger than New York City. Aerial view shows a bleak scene of a barren mining zone, crisscrossed with truck routes and dotted with lakes holding make-up water used to wash oil sands. Tens of billions of gallons of water have been drawn from the region's sources and from underground wells. This water, also known as tailings, is laced with hydrocarbons, naphthenic acids, and a number of carcinogenic heavy metals, and they are not easily treatable with current technology. Elevated levels of these pollutants have been detected in the water and the atmosphere near mining sites. The extensive expansion of the operation has been denounced by advocates as "ecocide" (Kusnetz 2021).

Bitumen, which has an asphalt-like quality, is extracted from the ground using two primary methods: "open-pit" mining and "in-situ" extraction. For shallow deposits, large excavators dig out the sands, which are loaded onto heavy-duty trucks and transported to processing plants, where the bitumen is separated from the sandy material. For deeper oil sands, bitumen is extracted through wells by injecting high-pressure steam underground to melt the bitumen, allowing it to pool and be pumped to the surface. Related video clips are available on YouTube.

The operation has been reported to release nitrogen oxides, sulfur oxides, and polycyclic aromatic hydrocarbons (PAHs), traces of which have been detected in soils and snow in the vicinity. Both modes of production yield tailing water that carries carcinogenic compounds detected in drinking aquifers and wildlife. When this wastewater evaporates into the atmosphere, the released volatile organic compounds (VOCs) can form PM2.5 particles, which cause respiratory diseases (Biello 2013).

PAHs, such as anthracene and naphthalene, are particularly concerning because many are known to cause cancer and other health effects in animals and humans. The contaminants being found in waters directly downwind of oil sands mining operations indicates that the pollutants have been carried around by the wind. Researchers from Environment and Climate Change Canada, in collaboration with Yale University conducted real-time measurements and found that oil sands operations are emitting between twenty and sixty-four times more air pollution than reported. The trickier part, however, is that it is difficult to assess how much of the hydrocarbon and other polluting compounds came from the natural oil sands deposits, which favors arguments that downplay risks from mining (Biello 2013).

Establishing direct links between cancer and various types of environmental pollution is a complex process requiring extensive time for data collection and analysis. Additionally, the lack of comprehensive data can undermine the accounts and observations of local residents (Lawrynuik 2019). Meanwhile, residents of the Athabasca Chipewyan First Nation, Mikisew Cree First Nation, and the hamlet of Fort Chipewyan have reported elevated cancer rates among neighbors and family members. Certain cancers, such as bile-duct cancer, which affects only one in 100,000 people, are particularly rare. The proximity of these communities to the mouth of the Athabasca River, which flows through oil sands operations, raises concerns about potential correlations. However, these anecdotal reports have not yet convinced governments and industries of the cancer risks associated with mining operations, which are projected to continue into the 2030s (Kusnetz 2021).

The struggle has been intense. Dr. John O'Connor of Fort McKay, who provided medical care to Chipewyan residents, conducted his own research on cancer rates in the area. In 2014, he traveled to Washington, DC to testify before the U.S. Senate, presenting his findings that the elevated cancer rate in Fort Chipewyan was linked to contamination of the Athabasca River from oil sands operations. In 2015, Dr. O'Connor was dismissed from his position with the local health authority where he worked (Lawrynuik 2019).

For advocates, the experiences of Alberta's Indigenous population expose the complex interplay between economic interests, public health, and the lack of environmental justice. Over 170 doctors signed a letter urging the Canadian government to elevate environmental and public health concerns to issues of environmental justice. The letter states:

Is this a country that treats all peoples with respect? If so, now is the time to bring the best of Canada's health and environmental research capacity to respond to the reasonable concerns of the peoples who live in the area of the oil sands and who have stewarded these lands for millennia. (CAPE 2020)

Meanwhile, oil sands mining continues to expand. However, it is clear that respecting Indigenous rights, developing technology to effectively reverse pollution, and advancing alternative energy sources are urgent steps for sustaining Alberta's energy economy.

Further Reading

Biello, David. 2013. "Oil Sands Raise Levels of Cancer-Causing Compounds in Regional Waters." *Scientific American*. https://www.scientificamerican.com/article/oil-sands-raise-levels-of-carcinogens-in-regional-waters/#:~:text=And%20sediments%20from%20oil%20sands,effects%20in%20animals%20and%20people.

CAPE. 2020. "Letter to Minister Wilkinson and PM on Tech Mine." *CAPE*. https://cape.ca/wp-content/uploads/2020/02/Teck-Letter-Feb-2020.pdf.

Kamnitzer, Ruth. 2024. "Canada Oil Sands Air Pollution 20-64 Times Worse Than Industry Says: Study." *Mongabaay*. https://news.mongabay.com/2024/05/canada-oil-sands-air-pollution-20-64-times-worse-than-industry-says-study/.

Kusnetz, Nicholas. 2021. "Indigenous Groups Say Big Oil's Pollution Threatens Their Existence in Canadian Forest." *NBC News*. https://www.nbcnews.com/news/world/indigenous-groups-say-big-oils-pollution-threatens-existence-canadian-rcna5946.

Lawrynuik, Sahah. 2019. "Downstream of Oilsands, Death by Cancer Comes Too Often." *Canada's National Observer*. https://www.nationalobserver.com/2019/12/17/news/downstream-oilsands-death-cancer-comes-too-often.

Twin, Alexandra. 2024. "The World's 10 Biggest Oil Exporters." *Investopedia*. https://www.investopedia.com/articles/company-insights/082316/worlds-top-10-oil-exporters.asp.

Could Lab Leaks Pose Serious Threats to Public Health?

Research has shown that zoonotic origins are the most common sources of infectious diseases worldwide. The transmission of pathogens between humans and animals, known as spillover, has been increasingly influenced by factors such as deforestation, habitat encroachment, wildlife trade, and climate change, particularly in recent decades.

It is estimated that over 60 percent of known infectious diseases in humans are zoonotic (transmitted from animals to people), and three out of four emerging infectious diseases in humans originate from animals (CDC). According to a 2024 report by the World Health Organization (WHO), more than thirty new human pathogens have been identified over the past three decades, with 75 percent originating in animals.

Furthermore, a 2024 study by Goldberg and colleagues revealed that spillover is not a one-way process; humans can also transmit diseases to animals. The study detected SARS-CoV-2 RNA in various wildlife species across Virginia and Washington, DC, including white-tailed deer, mice, raccoons, groundhogs, and bats, suggesting the possibility of animal-to-animal transmission within these populations. Additionally, the study identified novel mutations in the SARS-CoV-2 virus, including one in the receptor-binding domain of the spike protein which may enhance its ability to bind to the ACE2 receptor or increase resistance to neutralizing antibodies.

The complexity of transmission pathways challenges the simplistic notion that new pathogens emerge solely from forests. One lesser-discussed pathway of spillover but increasingly scrutinized during the Covid-19 pandemic is lab leaks. Reports show that, despite safety measures in laboratories where viruses are studied, accidents can occur, resulting in dangerous infections. Between 2000 and 2021, 309 cases of lab-acquired infections were reported across 94 incidents involving 51 pathogens of varying hazard levels. Some of these infections were fatal, and in certain instances, they spread from lab workers to others in the community. Many incidents were not reported (Ross et al. 2023).

Additionally, certain research methods have raised worries among the general public, one of which is known as "gain of function" (GOF). GOF involves artificially enhancing a pathogen's functions in the laboratory to understand how it might evolve under environmental pressures. While this research can offer valuable insights for vaccine development and the prevention of infectious diseases, it also raises biosafety and biosecurity concerns in the public. These concerns are particularly acute in less developed countries, where regulatory oversight may be limited, but they are also relevant in countries like the United States (American Society for Microbiology).

Furthermore, new lines of research are compounding existing concerns. One such project focuses on creating "mirror" bacteria—organisms whose molecular building blocks are reversed in chirality compared to natural life. By engineering bacterial components that are non-superimposable mirror images, scientists aim to develop innovative medical and industrial applications, such as enzymes that resist degradation or new forms of drug delivery. Thirty-eight scientists from nine countries have warned about the potential dangers of lab-created bacteria in biosecurity and ecological impacts: these bacteria could be impervious to standard antibiotics or containment methods, posing an "unprecedented risk" if accidentally released or misused (Hunt 2024).

Pathogen escapes from laboratory settings are rare events, largely due to advancements in lab technology. However, when lab leaks do occur, the underlying mechanisms can vary, with some scenarios being more common than others. Human error has been identified as the most significant factor in many lab leaks. These errors may include improper handling of pathogens, failure to adhere to safety protocols, or accidental exposure to infectious agents by laboratory personnel.

Failures in equipment, such as ventilation systems, autoclaves, and containment units, can also result in the accidental release of pathogens. Additionally, violations of biosecurity protocols—whether intentional or unintentional—pose another significant risk. These may include inadequacies in decontamination processes, improper use of personal protective equipment (PPE), and lapses in containment procedures.

Nearly 70 percent of known laboratory accidents have been attributed to procedural errors that could be mitigated, while the causes of some incidents remain unidentified (Ross et al. 2023). The following incidents serve as examples of such scenarios.

The 1979 Anthrax Release in Sverdlovsk, Soviet Union (now Russia)

The 1979 anthrax release in Sverdlovsk (now Yekaterinburg), Russia, stands as one of the most infamous examples of a laboratory accident leading to a severe public health crisis. In this incident, *Bacillus anthracis*, the bacterium responsible for anthrax, was accidentally released from a Soviet biological weapons facility. The accident reportedly occurred due to the removal of a critical safety filter in the facility's exhaust system. The filter, which had been taken out for cleaning, was not promptly replaced. When the ventilation system was reactivated, anthrax spores were dispersed into the air and carried downwind, contaminating the surrounding areas.

The contamination resulted in sixty-eight confirmed deaths, with victims suffering from inhalational anthrax, a severe and often fatal form of the disease. Livestock in the surrounding areas also succumbed to anthrax, highlighting the extensive spread of the spores. The spores traveled downwind, primarily impacting individuals living or working in the wind's direct path. It is believed that the consequences could have been far more catastrophic had the wind direction been toward the city center.

The Soviet government initially denied that the outbreak was due to a lab leak, attributing the cases to contaminated meat from local markets. Authorities removed and altered medical records to support the cover story, complicating later investigations. The final breakthrough came only at the end of 1991 when the Soviet Union had ceased to exist, and Boris Yeltsin personally admitted to the existence of the Soviet bioweapons program and the anthrax outbreak (Wampler et al. 2001).

2003 SARS Lab Leaks

In 2003 and 2004, there were several incidents where the Severe Acute Respiratory Syndrome coronavirus (SARS-CoV) leaked from laboratories, leading to the reappearance of the deadly virus. These releases occurred in Singapore, Taiwan, and Beijing (Demaneuf 2020).

In the Singapore case, in September 2003, a student researcher at the National University of Singapore was infected with SARS-CoV due to improper experimental procedures and failure to wear proper PPE. The student subsequently developed a high fever, was hospitalized, and eventually recovered from the SARS infection. Following the SARS leak event, the Minister of the Environment of Singapore apologized. Since 2002, Singapore has introduced legislation and regulations to govern the handling of high-risk infectious agents in lab settings.

The leaking event in Taiwan occurred in Taipei in December 2003. A researcher working on SARS-CoV violated biosafety procedures and decontamination protocols. Furthermore, the researcher, symptomatic at the time, traveled to Singapore for a conference, raising concerns about potential international spread. Initially, the researcher self-quarantined but eventually sought hospital treatment at the urging of relatives. Fortunately, there were no secondary transmissions. The Taiwanese government, along with international experts, conducted a detailed investigation, identifying several breaches in laboratory safety protocols.

The SARS leak in Beijing occurred in April 2004, involving two separate incidents at the Chinese Institute of Virology. These incidents resulted in the infection of two researchers with SARS-CoV, traced to lapses in biosafety protocols and improper virus inactivation. The infections subsequently led to eleven additional cases, including health care workers and family members of the researchers, with one fatality. In response, the institute was temporarily shut down, and a thorough review of biosafety practices in Chinese laboratories was conducted.

2007 Foot-and-Mouth Disease Outbreak in the UK

In August 2007, an outbreak of foot-and-mouth disease (FMDV) occurred in Surrey, England. FMDV primarily affects cloven-hoofed animals such as cattle, sheep, and pigs. Investigations traced the outbreak to the Pirbright Institute, a high-containment laboratory facility shared by the Institute for Animal Health and Merial Animal Health, a commercial vaccine production company. The outbreak was attributed to a breach in biosecurity, specifically faulty drainage systems that allowed the virus to escape from the laboratory, potentially spreading through vehicle transport or surface water.

The outbreak caused significant economic losses due to culling, trade restrictions, and the loss of livestock. A nationwide ban on livestock movement was imposed to curb the spread of the virus, and quarantine zones were established around the affected area. The UK government, in collaboration with veterinary and agricultural authorities, undertook extensive measures, including surveillance, culling of infected and at-risk animals, and thorough disinfection procedures, to contain the outbreak. Multiple investigations were conducted to identify the source and prevent future incidents. Key findings emphasized the need for enhanced infrastructure and stricter biosecurity measures at laboratories handling dangerous pathogens (Anderson 2008).

2019 SARS-CoV-2

The origin of SARS-CoV-2, the virus responsible for Covid-19, remains under investigation, with no direct evidence conclusively supporting either of the two primary hypotheses—the natural zoonotic origin hypothesis or the lab-origin hypothesis.

The natural zoonotic origin hypothesis suggests that the initial outbreak of Covid-19 was linked to the Huanan Seafood Wholesale Market in Wuhan, China, where various live wild animals were sold. According to this hypothesis, SARS-CoV-2 virus may have passed through an intermediate host species before infecting humans, though this host has yet to be definitively identified. One of the studies was conducted by Worobey and 17 of his colleagues (Worobey et al.

2022). Their study indicated that, in December 2019, early SARS-CoV-2 traces were concentrated around Wuhan's Huanan market, especially in the western section where live mammals were sold. Environmental samples from the market tested positive for the virus and matched early human infections. No signs of an earlier outbreak were found elsewhere in Wuhan, including at research labs. Geospatial analysis pointed to the market as the likely origin, supporting a natural spillover from animals to humans. Another study by Pekar and 23 researchers (Pekar et al. 2022) published a few months later in *Science* supported Worobey et al.'s findings. Their study concludes that SARS-CoV-2 likely originated from at least two separate animal-to-human spillover events, not from a single introduction. Early viral lineages A and B, both present in Wuhan in December 2019, appear to have stemmed from distinct transmissions, likely involving animals sold at the Huanan market. Their genetic differences are too great to have arisen quickly in humans, reinforcing the case for multiple zoonotic jumps. The virus's evolutionary patterns show no signs of a lab-related origin, according to the researchers.

The lab-origin hypothesis suggests that SARS-CoV-2 may have accidentally leaked from a laboratory, such as the Wuhan Institute of Virology (WIV), which conducts coronavirus research. Proponents of this hypothesis point to the proximity of WIV to the outbreak's epicenter, reports of safety concerns at certain laboratories, and allegations of gain-of-function (GOF) research being conducted in the lab (Keiser 2021). Gain-of-function research is a type of scientific experiment in which an organism, such as a virus, is genetically altered to enhance its abilities, such as increasing transmissibility, virulence, or host range, in order to better understand potential threats and develop countermeasures. There are reports indicating that GoF was conducted at WIV, and involving international collaboration (BBC 2021; Menachery et al. 2015). To date, however, no direct evidence has been reported that SARS-CoV-2 originated from a lab leak, including from the Wuhan Institute of Virology.

In conclusion, laboratory leaks remain a potential pathway for virus transmission and warrant serious attention. They underscore the inherent risks of working with high-risk pathogens and the critical need for robust biosafety and biosecurity practices. Preventing such incidents requires strict adherence to safety protocols, transparent reporting, and stronger international collaboration.

Further Reading

American Society of Microbiology. "Gain of Function Research." https://asm.org/getmedia/24ebbde0-d618-4a8a-901c-6e297e6f92aa/HD-918-ASM-GoF-FactSheet-final.pdf.

Anderson, Ian. 2008. "Foot and Mouth Disease 2007: A Review and Lessons Learned." London: The Stationery Office. https://assets.publishing.service.gov.uk/media/5a7c7289e5274a5255bceb57/0312.pdf.

BBC. 2021. "Coronavirus: Was US Money Used to Fund Risky Research in China?" *BBC*. https://www.bbc.com/news/57932699.

Centers for Disease Control and Prevention (CDC). 2025. "About Zoonotic Diseases." https://www.cdc.gov/one-health/about/about-zoonotic-diseases.html. Accessed August 5, 2024.

Demaneuf, Gilles. 2020. "The Good, the Bad and the Ugly: A Review of SARS Lab Escapes." *Medium*. https://gillesdemaneuf.medium.com/the-good-the-bad-and-the-ugly-a-review-of-sars-lab-escapes-898d203d175d.

Goldberg, Amanda R., Kate E. Langwig, Katherine L. Brown, et al. 2024. "Widespread Exposure To SARS-Cov-2 In Wildlife Communities." *Nature Communications*, 15: 6210. doi: https://doi.org/10.1038/s41467-024-49891-w.

Hunt, Katie. 2024. "Scientists Warn of 'Unprecedented' Risks of Research into Mirror Life." *CNN*. https://www.cnn.com/2024/12/16/science/mirror-bacteria-research-risks/index.html.

Keiser, Jocelyn. 2021. "NIH Says Grantee Failed to Report Experiment in Wuhan That Created a Bat Virus That Made Mice Sicker." *Science.org*. https://www.science.org/content/article/nih-says-grantee-failed-report-experiment-wuhan-created-bat-virus-made-mice-sicker.

Maxmen, Amy, and Smriti Mallapty. 2021. "The Covid Lab-Leak Hypothesis: What Scientists Do and Don't Know." *Nature*. https://www.nature.com/articles/d41586-021-01529-3.

Menachery, Vineet D., Boyd L. Yount Jr, Kari Debbink, Sudhakar Agnihothram, Lisa E. Gralinski, Jessica A. Plante, Rachel L. Graham, Trevor Scobey, Xing-Yi Ge, Eric F Donaldson, Scott H Randell, Antonio Lanzavecchia, Wayne A. Marasco, Zhengli-Li Shi, and Ralph S. Baric. 2015. "A SARS-Like Cluster of Circulating Bat Coronaviruses Shows Potential for Human Emergence." *Nature Midicine*, 21: 1508–13. https://www.nature.com/articles/nm.3985.

Pekar, Jonathan E., Andrew Magee, Edyth Parker, Niema Moshiri, et al. 2022. "The Molecular Epidemiology of Multiple Zoonotic Origins of SARS-Cov-2." *Science*, 377(6690): 960-966. doi:10.1126/science.abp8337.

Ross, Emma and David R. Harper. 2023. "Laboratory Accidents and Biocontainment Breaches—Policy Options for Improved Safety and Security." *Global Health Programme*. https://www.chathamhouse.org/sites/default/files/2023-12/2023-12-12-laboratory-accidents-biocontainment-breaches-ross-and-harper.pdf.

Wampler, Robert A. and Thomas S. Blanton. 2001. "Volume V: Anthrax at Sverdlovsk, 1979." *The National Security Archive*. https://nsarchive2.gwu.edu/NSAEBB/NSAEBB61/.

World Health Organization. "Zoonotic Disease: Emerging Public Health Threats in the Region." https://www.emro.who.int/about-who/rc61/zoonotic-diseases.html. Accessed August 5, 2024.

Worobey, Michael, Joshua I. Levy, Lorena Maplica Serrano, Alexander Crits-Christoph, and Kristian, et al. 2022. "The Huanan Seafood Wholesale Market in Wuhan Was The Early Epicenter of The Covid-19 Pandemic." *Science, 377*(6609): 951–9. doi: 10.1126/science.abp8715.

Deforestation and Increasing Risks of Lyme Disease

Lyme disease is a common tick-borne illness in the United States, caused by the bacterium *Borrelia burgdorferi*. It is transmitted to humans through the bite of infected black-legged ticks (*Ixodes scapularis*), commonly known as "deer ticks." The bacterium is named after Willy Burgdorfer, the scientist who first identified it in the 1980s.

The disease is most prevalent in the Northeast, mid-Atlantic, and upper Midwest regions of the United States, and it takes its name from Lyme, Connecticut, where it was first diagnosed. According to the Centers for Disease Control and Prevention (CDC), these high-incidence areas account for approximately 90 percent of all reported cases. Infections typically peak during late spring, summer, and fall, when outdoor activities are most common. In 2022, 62,551 new cases were reported, marking a 68.5 percent increase compared to the 2017–19 average.

Lyme disease poses significant health risks in many countries, with cases reported in Canada, Russia, Germany, Austria, Slovenia, Sweden, and China. In northern and central Europe, the two primary strains of the *Borrelia* bacterium are *Borrelia afzelii* and *Borrelia garinii* (Marques et al. 2021). These strains have also been identified as the leading causes of Lyme disease in China (Stark et al. 2022). Variations in *Borrelia* strains may account for differences in the clinical manifestations of Lyme disease, which can range from mild to severe (Marques et al. 2021). Chinese reports enlist a wider range of hosts of the bacterium, including more than thirty species of wild animals including mice, deer, rabbits, foxes, wolves; and over forty species of birds and various domestic animals, including dogs, cattle and horses, have been identified as potential hosts for this disease (NHC 2019).

According to the CDC, a common clinical manifestation of Lyme disease in the United States is a slowly expanding skin lesion called erythema migrans, often referred to as a bull's-eye rash, which develops at the site of the tick bite. This rash is frequently accompanied by flu-like symptoms such as malaise, fatigue, headache, joint pain, muscle aches, fever, and swelling of nearby lymph nodes. Lyme disease is typically treated with antibiotics, however, vaccines are only available for animals, but not yet for humans at this time. Early diagnosis and prompt treatment are critical to preventing severe complications.

If left untreated, Lyme disease can progress to more serious symptoms, including meningitis with episodic headaches and mild neck stiffness, subtle encephalitis leading to cognitive impairments, inflammation of nerve roots causing sharp, shooting pain and other neurological damage, and occasionally facial palsy. Even with treatment, some patients may develop prolonged or recurring symptoms known as Post-Treatment Lyme Disease Syndrome (PTLDS), according to the CDC.

Studies suggest that the spread of Lyme disease, like most vector-borne diseases, is closely linked to environmental factors, which can either promote or inhibit disease transmission. Research indicates that white-tailed deer serve as the primary reproductive hosts for ticks, and higher deer populations are associated with greater tick abundance. In a study conducted in Mumford Cove, Connecticut, controlled hunts reduced deer density by 92 percent, from approximately 100 to 12 deer per square mile. As a result, the number of Lyme disease cases in the area declined significantly, dropping from thirty to fewer than five within three years (Stafford III 2014).

The mechanism of disease transmission suggests that fragmented forests, created for residential or recreational purposes, may play a more significant role in the spread of the bacterium that causes Lyme disease. While white-tailed deer are the primary carriers of deer ticks, however, they are not reservoirs for the bacterium. Instead, the white-footed mouse (*Peromyscus leucopus*) is the principal reservoir. Larval ticks acquire *Borrelia burgdorferi* by feeding on infected white-footed mice. As these ticks mature into nymphs and feed on blood, they can transmit Lyme disease to humans and other animals. Therefore, the density of infected white-footed mice is a stronger indicator of Lyme disease risk than the density of white-tailed deer (Allan 2000).

A study examining the correlation between forest fragmentation and the abundance of white-footed mice found that these mice can reach high densities in small woodlots of one to two hectares, typically created for residential or recreational purposes. In these fragmented areas, the absence of predators and competitors allows mouse populations to grow unchecked. Additionally, smaller wood patches were found to harbor high densities of infected black-legged ticks (deer ticks). These findings suggest that preventing deforestation, particularly in regions with high rates of Lyme disease, could be an effective control measure (Allan 2000).

Studies suggest that climate change has significantly contributed to the spread of Lyme disease. Warming temperatures have been linked to the expanded range of ticks; for instance, ticks are now thriving in parts of Canada where they previously could not survive (Dumic et al. 2018). Deer ticks are most active when temperatures exceed 45°F, and their populations thrive in areas with humidity levels of 85 percent or higher. As a result, a warmer and wetter climate can prolong tick activity and expand their geographic range, increasing human exposure and the risk of contracting Lyme disease (EPA 2021).

These observations suggest that addressing climate change and managing deforestation can help limit tick populations and reduce the risk of human infection. In the broader perspective, maintaining balanced ecosystems is an effective approach to controlling the spread of Lyme disease.

Further Reading

Allan, Brian F. 2000. "The Effect of Forest Fragmentation on Lyme Disease Risk." https://www.caryinstitute.org/sites/default/files/public/reprints/Allan_2000_REU.pdf.

CDC. 2024. "Signs and Symptoms of Lyme Disease." https://www.cdc.gov/lyme/signs-symptoms/index.html.

Dumic, Igor and Edson Severnini. 2018. "Ticking Bomb: The Impact of Climate Change on the Incidence of Lyme Disease." *Canadian Journal of Infectious Diseases and Medical Microbiology, 2018*: 5719081. doi: https://doi.org/10.1155/2018/5719081.

Iowa State University. 2021. "Lyme Disease." https://www.cfsph.iastate.edu/Factsheets/pdfs/lyme_disease.pdf.

Marques, Franc Strle and Gary P. Wormser. 2021. "Comparison of Lyme Disease in the United States and Europe." *Perspective*. https://wwwnc.cdc.gov/eid/article/27/8/20-4763_article.

National Health Commission of the People's Republic of China (NHC). 2019. "Diagnosis of Occupational Lyme Disease." http://www.nhc.gov.cn/wjw/pyl/201902/7bebbb45926347df843fab12490dc607/files/3a92b8f14083499d8347c328c28db944.pdf.

Stafford, Kirby C., III. 2014. "Deer, Ticks, and Lyme Disease." https://www.beaconfalls-ct.org/sites/g/files/vyhlif4141/f/uploads/deer_ticks_fact_sheet.pdf.

Stark, James H., Xiuyan Li, Ji Chun Zhang, Leah Burn, Srinivas R. Valluri, Jiaxin Liang, Kaijie Pan, Mark A Fletcher, Raphael Simon, Luis Jodar, and Bradford D.

Gessner. 2022. "Systematic Review and Meta-Analysis of Lyme Disease Data and Seropositivity for Borrelia burgdorferi, China, 2005–2020." *Emerging Infectious Diseases.* https://doi.org/10.3201/eid2812.212612.

Steere, Allen C. 2021. "Lyme Disease." *New England Journal of Medicine.* doi: 10.1056/NEJM200107123450207.

United States Environmental Protection Agency (EPA). 2021. "Climate Change Indicators: Lyme Disease." *EPA.gov.* https://www.epa.gov/climate-indicators/climate-change-indicators-lyme-disease.

Dengue Fever and Runaway Urbanization in Asian Cities

Dengue fever, also known as "breakbone fever," is a mosquito-borne illness caused by the dengue virus (DENV), part of the *Flavivirus* genus. This group includes other well-known viruses, such as Zika, West Nile, yellow fever, and several that cause encephalitis. Dengue is transmitted to humans through the bite of infected *Aedes* mosquitoes, which are most active during the day, particularly around dawn and dusk. The disease is prevalent in tropical and subtropical regions worldwide, and its incidence has risen sharply over the past few decades. Dengue is now endemic in over 100 countries, affecting an estimated 400 million people and causing around 22,000 deaths annually. Nearly half of the world's population lives in areas at risk of dengue (Roy et al. 2021; CDC).

Dengue fever is especially prevalent in cities across South and Southeast Asia, where similar climates favor the breeding of *Aedes* mosquitoes, the primary vectors of the dengue virus. Urban and semi-urban areas in these regions are particularly vulnerable to outbreaks due to high population density and rapid urbanization. The widespread presence of standing water and inadequate waste management create ideal breeding grounds for mosquitoes. Countries such as Thailand, Vietnam, the Philippines, Malaysia, Singapore, India, and Bangladesh report high numbers of dengue cases each year. Additionally, factors like increased international travel, climate change, and challenges in public health infrastructure contribute to the disease's prevalence and spread. The monsoon season further exacerbates the situation by opening a seasonal window for the mosquitoes to multiply (Kolimenakis et al. 2021).

Historical Chinese medical records suggest that dengue-like illnesses occurred as early as the tenth century AD. However, the first recognized epidemics of dengue fever were documented in the late eighteenth century, with a widespread outbreak resembling dengue fever reported across Asia, Africa, and North America (Gubler 2006). A significant outbreak also occurred in the U.S. in 1780 in Philadelphia (Roy et al. 2021).

The dengue virus was first isolated during the dengue epidemic in Japan in 1943 and later in Hawaii. This marked a significant advancement in understanding the disease, leading to further research on its transmission and effects. It was not until the twentieth century that the *Aedes aegypti* mosquito was confirmed as the primary vector for dengue virus. The global distribution of dengue fever expanded dramatically after the Second World War due to increased urbanization, global travel, and the spread of its mosquito vectors, particularly *Aedes aegypti*. The latter half of the twentieth century saw the emergence of more severe forms of the disease, such as dengue hemorrhagic fever (DHF) and dengue shock syndrome (DSS). The first reported epidemic of DHF occurred in the Philippines in 1953 (Messina et al. 2013).

Symptoms of dengue fever range from mild to severe. Mild cases may cause high fever, severe headache, pain behind the eyes, joint and muscle pain, rash, and mild bleeding, such as nosebleeds or gum bleeding. Severe cases can progress to dengue hemorrhagic fever or dengue shock syndrome, which can be life-threatening. These severe forms of dengue are characterized by bleeding, blood plasma leakage, and a low platelet count. There is no specific treatment for dengue fever; management focuses on relieving symptoms (CDC).

The first dengue vaccine, Dengvaxia (CYD-TDV), was developed and licensed in several countries beginning in 2015. However, its use has been restricted to individuals who have previously been infected with the dengue virus due to concerns about the risk of severe dengue in those without prior exposure (WHO 2018). One of the latest advancements in dengue vaccination is the phase 3 trial of the single-dose tetravalent (four-strain) Butantan-Dengue Vaccine (Butantan D-V), which demonstrated an 80 percent protection rate among participants with no prior dengue exposure and an 89 percent protection rate in those with a history of dengue exposure (Kallás et al. 2024).

In some countries, dengue vaccines are available and recommended for individuals living in areas with high rates of dengue transmission. For others, prevention focuses on measures to avoid mosquito bites, such as using mosquito repellent, wearing long-sleeved clothing and pants, sleeping under mosquito nets, and eliminating standing water where mosquitoes breed (Kolimenakis et al. 2021).

Mosquito-borne diseases highlight the interconnectedness of human, animal, and environmental health, transcending physical borders. This concept, known as "One Health," is essential for managing the emergence and re-emergence of zoonotic diseases in urban settings (Villarroel et al. 2023).

Lessons learned from dengue surveillance in multiple countries provide valuable insights. Vector control is of primary importance, and effective measures include eliminating standing water where mosquitoes breed and using insecticides. Public health strategies must be comprehensive and coordinated, integrating vector control, surveillance, early warning, community engagement, and health care preparedness. Cooperation is essential across various sectors and disciplines, including urban planning, water management, and education. Public health planning must also address the changing patterns of vector-borne diseases due to wetter and warmer seasons. Finally, dengue is a global challenge that requires international cooperation. Sharing knowledge, resources, and best practices among countries and regions is crucial for effectively managing and preventing dengue epidemics (Sharp et al. 2019).

Further Reading

Centers for Disease Control and Prevention (CDC). "Dengue." https://www.cdc.gov/dengue/index.html.

Gubler, Duane J. 2006. "Dengue/Dengue Haemorrahagic Fever: History and Current Status." *Novartis Found Symp*. doi: 10.1002/0470058005.ch2.

Kallás, Esper G., Monica A.T. Cintra, José A. Moreira, et al. 2024. "Live, Attenuated, Tetravalent Butantan-Dengue Vaccine in Children and Adults." *The New England Journal of Medicine, 390*(5): 397–408. doi: 10.1056/NEJMoa2301790.

Kolimenakis, Antonios, Sabine Heinz, Michael Lowery Wilson, Volker Winkler, Laith Yakob, Antonios Michaelakis, Dimitrios Papachristos, Clive Richardson, and Olaf Horstick. 2021. "The Role of Urbanization in the Spread of Aedes Mosquitoes and the Diseases They Transmit—A Systematic Review." *Plos Neglected Tropical Diseases, 15*(9): e0009631. doi: https://doi.org/10.1371/journal.pntd.0009631.

Messina, Jane P., Oliver J. Brady, Thomas W. Scott, et al. 2013. "Global Spread of Dengue Virus Types: Mapping the 70 Year History." *Trends Microbiol, 22*(3), 138–46. doi: 10.1016/j.tim.2013.12.011.

Roy, Sudipta Kumar, and Soumen Bhattacharjee. 2021. "Dengue Virus: Epidemiology, Billogy, and Disease Aetiology." *Canadian Journal of Microbiology, 67*(10):687–702. doi: 10.1139/cjm-2020-0572.

Sharp, Tyler M., Kyle R. Ryff, Gilberto A. Santiago, Harold S. Margolis, and Stephen H. Waterman. 2019. "Lessons Learned from Dengue Surveillance and Research, Puerto Rico, 1899–2013." CDC. https://wwwnc.cdc.gov/eid/article/25/8/19-0089_article.

Shukla, Rahul, Viswanathan Ramasamy, Rajgokul K. Shanmugam, Richa Ahuja, and Navin Khanna. 2020. "Antibody-Dependent Enhancement: A Challenge for Developing a Safe Dengue Vaccine." *Front Cell Infect Microbio*. doi: 10.3389/fcimb.2020.572681.

Villarroel, Paola Mariela Saba, Nuttamonpat Gumpangseth, Thanaphon Songhon, Sakda Yainoy, Arnau Monteil, Pornsawan Leaungwutiwong, and Dorothée Missé. 2023. "Emerging and Re-emerging Zoonotic Viral Diseases in Southeast Asia: One Health Challenge." *Frontiers, 11*. https://doi.org/10.3389/fpubh.2023.1141483.

World Health Organization. 2018. Dengue vaccine: WHO position paper, September 2018—recommendations. *Vaccine*. doi: 10.1016/j.vaccine.2018.09.0632019.

Radioactive Contamination due to Mining—What Can Be Learned?

Radioactive contamination from mining activities poses serious risks to public health and the environment. Extracting uranium and other radioactive materials often releases harmful substances into the air, water, and soil, causing severe long-term damage. This discussion focuses on three prominent cases of radioactive contamination caused by mining: The Church Rock Uranium Mill Spill in the United States, the Wismut Uranium Mining in Germany, and the Ranger Uranium Mine in Australia.

The Church Rock Uranium Mill Spill (1979)

The uranium mining spill that occurred on July 16, 1979, in Church Rock, New Mexico, is one of the largest leaks of radioactive materials in U.S. history. The disaster unfolded when a dam containing uranium mill tailings failed, releasing over 1,000 tons of solid radioactive waste and 93 million gallons of acidic, radioactive tailings solution into the Puerco River (Moore-Nall 2015).

The contamination spread 80 miles downstream, impacting the Navajo Nation, a Native American territory. The Puerco River, a vital water source for livestock and agriculture, was heavily polluted. Elevated levels of radioactive isotopes, including uranium, thorium, and radium, were detected, causing significant environmental damage.

The public health consequences were catastrophic. Residents reported higher rates of cancer, kidney disease, and other illnesses linked to radiation exposure. Livestock, a critical source of livelihood for many Navajo families, suffered from radiation poisoning, causing severe economic hardships for the community. One firsthand account described the devastation caused by the surge of radioactive waste as follows:

> The water, filled with acids from the milling process, twisted a metal culvert in the Puerco and burned the feet of a little boy who went wading. Sheep keeled over and

died, and crops curdled along the banks. The surge of radiation was detected as far away as Sanders, Arizona, fifty miles downstream. (Jennings 2014)

Public opinion holds that the Church Rock incident exposed a lack of oversight and insufficient waste containment strategies in mining operations. It also reflected historical failures by the U.S. government—the sole purchaser of uranium ore since the 1940s—to protect the health and safety of uranium miners and the environment. In 1990, the U.S. Congress enacted the Radiation Exposure Compensation Act, acknowledging the mistreatment of uranium miners. The legislation was amended in 2000 to address lingering inequities from earlier decisions (Brugge et al. 2002).

Wismut Uranium Mining (1946–90)

The Wismut Uranium Mining operations in East Germany were conducted under Soviet control from 1946 until German reunification in 1990. Managed by the Soviet military, the company focused exclusively on exploiting East German uranium deposits for the Soviet nuclear program. During this period, it mined over 23,000 tons of uranium, making it one of the world's largest uranium producers. However, poor safety standards and environmental mismanagement resulted in catastrophic environmental and health consequences.

After the Federal Republic of Germany assumed control of the area, the government initiated a comprehensive and costly remediation program. During this effort, previously unknown levels of contamination were uncovered (Lersow et al. 2006). For example, the mining activities had released vast amounts of radioactive dust and radon gas, contaminating the air, water, and soil. Uncovered tailings and waste rock piles further contributed to widespread environmental pollution. High concentrations of radon gas, a known carcinogen, were pervasive in the mining regions, causing increased rates of lung cancer among miners and local residents.

According to a report by a German environmental organization, radiation exposure in the Wismut region was first measured in 1956, but the results were kept secret under Soviet rule. In 2006, the German Federal Office for Radiation Protection released the largest study ever conducted on uranium workers, involving 59,000 former Wismut miners. The findings revealed a 50–70 percent increase in lung cancer rates, resulting in over 7,000 radiation-induced deaths among the surveyed subjects accounting for nearly 12 percent. The study also noted that the risk of lung cancer was highest fifteen to twenty-four years after uranium exposure, indicating that new cases will likely continue to emerge for years to come. Communities surrounding Wismut also suffered severe health issues, including respiratory diseases, cancers, and other radiation-related conditions (Hibakusha-Worldwide 2024).

Ranger Uranium Mine (1980–Present)

The Ranger Uranium Mine, located in Kakadu National Park, Australia, has been operational since 1980. Despite being regarded as one of the world's most regulated uranium mines, it has experienced numerous contamination incidents, raising serious concerns about the environmental and health impacts of uranium mining. The mine produces 4,000 tons of uranium oxide annually but generates an alarming 1.5 million tons of mine tailings and radioactive waste each year, according to a report by nuclear-risks.org.

The same agency also reported that since 1981, over 120 accidents involving leaks and spills have been reported, highlighting the inherent challenges of managing radioactive materials even under stringent regulations. One of the most significant incidents occurred in 2013 when a leach tank burst, releasing approximately 1 million liters of acidic radioactive slurry. This disaster posed a grave threat to the ecosystems within Kakadu National Park, a UNESCO World Heritage site renowned for its extraordinary biodiversity and cultural significance.

Although the immediate public health impacts were mitigated due to the mine's remote location, the environmental consequences were severe. Contaminants jeopardized the park's pristine water bodies and habitats, potentially endangering its rich biodiversity. The traditional owners of the land, the Mirarr Aboriginal people, have repeatedly expressed concerns about long-term health impacts, including reports of stillbirths and elevated cancer rates in the community (Schultz 2021).

The incidents at Church Rock, Wismut, and the Ranger Uranium Mine illustrate the serious impact radioactive contamination from mining can have on communities and the environment. They demonstrate the need for strong safety measures, careful environmental management, and genuine community involvement. These cases also show that while nuclear power is cleaner than fossil fuels in terms of emissions, managing its associated risks remains a considerable challenge.

Further Reading

Brugge, Doug and Rob Goble. 2002. "The History of Uranium Mining and the Navajo People." *American Journal of Public Health, 92*(9): 1410–19. doi: 10.2105/ajph.92.9.1410.

Hibakusha Worldwide. 2024. "Wismut Region, Germany—Uranium Mining." *Hibakusha-worldwide.org.* https://hibakusha-worldwide.org/en/locations/wismut-region.

International Atomic Energy Agency (IAEA). 2009. "Environmental Consequences of Uranium Mining in Wismut." *IAEA Bulletin, 51*(1): 15–20.

Jennings, Trip. 2014. "Remembering the Largest Radioactive Spill in U.S. History." New Mexico In-Depth. https://nmindepth.com/2014/remembering-the-largest-radioactive-spill-in-u-s-history/.

Lersow, M, and P. Schmidt. 2006. "The Wismut Remediation Project." In AB Fourie, and M Tibbett (eds), *Mine Closure 2006: Proceedings of the First International Seminar on Mine Closure.* Australian Centre for Geomechanics, Perth, pp. 181–90. https://doi.org/10.36487/ACG_repo/605_10.

Moore-Nall, Anita. 2015. "The Legacy of Uranium Development on or Near Indian Reservations and Health Implications Rekindling Public Awareness." *Geosciences, 5*(1): 15–29. doi: https://doi.org/10.3390/geosciences5010015.

Nuclear-risks.org. 2021 (last update). "Ranger, Australia—Uranium Mining Site." Nuclear-risks.org. https://www.nuclear-risks.org/en/hibakusha-worldwide/ranger.html.

Schultz, Rosalie. 2021. "Investigating the Health Impacts of the Ranger Uranium Mine on Aboriginal People." *The Medical Journal of Australia, 215*(4): 157–9. https://doi.org/10.5694/mja2.51198.

2

Population Health and Well-Being

Global aging, lifestyle-related health challenges, health care efficiency, and education are central themes shaping public health and well-being in our time. These interconnected issues influence how societies address health disparities, adapt to demographic shifts, and foster sustainable health care systems. By examining these themes through diverse contexts, we can uncover insights into how cultural, economic, and systemic factors impact health outcomes worldwide.

The rapid aging of populations is one of the most pressing challenges for public health. By 2050, the global population aged sixty years and older is expected to increase dramatically, placing immense pressure on health care systems, economies, and social structures. Countries like Japan, where declining birth rates and rising life expectancies are reshaping demographics, face unique challenges in managing this transition. Societies that value elders, such as those in Japan and Greece, provide stronger social and mental support, contrasting with youth-focused cultures where aging can be seen as a burden. Integrating cultural perspectives into aging policies can promote respect for older adults while enhancing societal cohesion.

Health challenges associated with aging, including dementia and Parkinson's disease, further illustrate the strain on public health systems. Dementia, affecting 55 million people globally, is projected to rise by 10 million cases annually, with significant burdens in countries like Japan and the United States. While Japan emphasizes community-based programs like Dementia Supporters, the United States relies on family and institutional caregiving. Parkinson's disease, which impacts over 8.5 million people worldwide, highlights the role of environmental and genetic factors in age-related conditions. Preventive strategies, such as reducing exposure to environmental toxins, remain essential as societies contend with these neurodegenerative diseases.

Broader factors, including geography, socioeconomic status, and genetics, play crucial roles in shaping aging outcomes. Environmental issues like pollution and extreme weather disproportionately harm older adults in vulnerable regions, while socioeconomic disparities affect access to health care and longevity. Wealthier individuals benefit from better resources and longer lifespans than disadvantaged groups, while genetic predispositions may increase the risk of conditions such as Alzheimer's and cardiovascular diseases across the broader population. Addressing these disparities requires targeted interventions, including socioeconomic support, and advancements in public health research.

Education emerges as a key tool in addressing the broad and complex challenges every individual is faced with, fostering health literacy and promoting healthier behaviors and public health policies backed by science. Comprehensive Sexuality Education (CSE) illustrates the importance of education in improving population health. Despite resistance in regions like East Asia, where cultural and political barriers persist, CSE has demonstrated potential to improve youth health, promote gender equality, and address issues such as sexually transmitted infections and unintended pregnancies. Similarly, education plays a critical role in countering xenophobia, as demonstrated during the Covid-19 pandemic. Anti-Asian sentiment fueled by misinformation emphasized the need for media literacy and cultural understanding to foster inclusivity and resilience.

Programs like Japan's *Shokuiku* initiative highlight how education can integrate cultural values into public health strategies. *Shokuiku* promotes balanced diets, sustainability, and mindfulness, fostering lifelong healthy eating habits through school lunches and community programs. In Africa, where health education faces unique challenges, arts-based interventions such as theater and storytelling deliver culturally resonant health messages that engage communities and reduce stigma. These innovative approaches highlight the adaptability of health education to diverse cultural and social contexts.

Efficient health care systems are another cornerstone of public health. China's health care system, which provides coverage to 95 percent of its population, grapples with challenges such as high costs, corruption, and rural-urban disparities. Reforms focused on primary care, professional training, and financial transparency are critical to advancing the system. Similarly, Africa faces health care challenges rooted in inadequate infrastructure, low health literacy, and external pressures such as brain drain. Investments in education, equitable financing, and systemic improvements are vital for addressing these issues.

Comparative health care systems provide valuable insights into balancing access, equity, and innovation. Japan's universal system emphasizes affordability and preventive care, with remarkable achievements. In contrast, the U.S. multi-payer system prioritizes innovation but struggles with high costs and unequal access, while Canada's single-payer model ensures equity but contends with long wait times. Examining these systems highlights the importance of adapting health care policies to meet the needs of diverse populations. Drug pricing is another area where the United States can learn from countries like Switzerland and Germany, which use centralized agencies, price caps, and value assessments to control costs without sacrificing innovation.

Lifestyle-related health issues further underscore the interconnected nature of public health. In China, dietary shifts and urbanization have driven the rise of metabolic disorders such as fatty liver disease and gout. These conditions, linked to obesity and cardiovascular diseases, stress the importance of prevention through education, regular screenings, and addressing socioeconomic disparities. The surge in e-cigarette use among youth reflects a similar need for regulatory measures and public awareness campaigns to mitigate health risks.

Obesity has become a widespread threat to the health and well-being of populations in our time. Emerging treatments, such as GLP-1 drugs for weight loss and diabetes, showcase the potential of medical innovation in addressing lifestyle-related conditions. These drugs offer significant weight loss and health benefits but face high costs and accessibility barriers. Systemic changes addressing the root causes of obesity, including socioeconomic factors and dietary practices, are essential for achieving long-term impact. Japan's dietary traditions, promoted through initiatives like *Shokuiku*, offer a model for integrating cultural and community-based approaches to health.

Cultural and economic pressures also play a role in public health challenges, as seen in the issue of overwork in Japan and South Korea. Excessive working hours, driven by societal expectations and competitive job markets, contribute to cardiovascular diseases and mental health issues. Reforms such as Japan's Work Style Reform Law illustrate the importance of addressing both policy and cultural attitudes to improve work-life balance and overall well-being.

Traditional Chinese Medicine (TCM) demonstrates the value of integrating holistic practices with modern health care systems. Despite challenges such as limited scientific validation and declining use, TCM's emphasis on prevention and its role in managing chronic diseases underscore its relevance in addressing global health challenges. Its contributions to conditions such as malaria and diabetes highlight the potential for blending traditional practices with Western medicine.

This chapter showcases how global aging, lifestyle-related health challenges, health care efficiency, and education collectively shape public health and well-being. By addressing these interconnected themes through culturally sensitive policies, systemic reforms, and innovative strategies, societies can create healthier, more resilient populations equipped to face the complexities of the modern world.

Aging and Health Challenges

Cultural Perspectives on Aging

The global population is aging at a rapid pace, a trend that is particularly evident in developed countries due to declining birth rates. Japan, where 30 percent of the population is over sixty years, has become the world's oldest nation, according to the World Health Organization (WHO). Meanwhile, developing countries are also witnessing a sharp increase in the proportion of older adults. For instance, China's population has been overtaken by India's, driven by a steep drop in birth rates. The United Nations projects that by 2050, one in six people worldwide will be over sixty-five years, compared to one in eleven in 2019. This demographic shift poses challenges for health care systems, the underlying economies, and social support networks globally. Addressing health issues and ensuring that populations live longer, healthier lives has become a top priority for governments.

From a biological perspective, aging is characterized by the gradual decline of various bodily functions, leading to a progressive loss of mental and physical abilities, and eventually resulting in death. Common age-related conditions include hearing loss, cataracts, back and neck pain, osteoarthritis, chronic obstructive pulmonary disease, diabetes, depression, and dementia (WHO 2022). Some age-related diseases are more prevalent and severe than others. For instance, in the United States, six million people currently live with Alzheimer's disease, a number projected to rise to 13 million by 2050 (Mather 2024). Healthy aging refers to predictable biological changes in physical and cognitive functioning that occur with age. These changes are generally perceived similarly across cultural and ethnic groups (Löckenhoff et al. 2009).

In the United States, the population aged sixty-five years and older is projected to grow from 58 million in 2022 to 82 million by 2050, representing a 47 percent increase. During this period, the share of this age group within the total population is expected to rise from 17 percent to 23 percent. Experts suggest that federal budget cuts and tax increases may become unavoidable as more members of the sizable baby boomer generation reach retirement age and qualify for entitlement programs (Mather et al. 2024).

Understandably, adapting to an aging society is a costly process largely due to health care expenses. Hence, levels of economic development and personal income play a key role in the provisions of necessary resources. Low- and middle-income countries will face more challenges than wealthy countries. According to the WHO, by 2050, two-thirds of the world's population over sixty years will live in these countries, and assuring material sufficiency will be critical.

On the other hand, aging isn't just a biological process; it is also a cultural one (Coughlin 2017). Age-related changes perceived through socioemotional and social economic status lenses are culture-dependent and may vary greatly (Löckenhoff et al. 2009). Different cultures have various attitudes and practices around aging and death, significantly affecting the experience of getting older. Supportive cultural contexts are complementary to medical care and they are indispensable for an aging society, as they influence how societies perceive and handle aging. In cultures that value and respect the elderly, older individuals often experience better mental health and social support. Conversely, in cultures that prioritize youth, older adults may face isolation and ageism. Understanding these cultural nuances is crucial for creating supportive environments and effective policies for aging populations worldwide.

Decades of cross-cultural studies have provided valuable insights into cultural values and psychological traits. Most of these studies focus on comparing Eastern/Asian cultures with Western ones (Giles et al. 2000). For example, Asian societies influenced by Confucian values and traditions such as ancestor worship often foster positive perceptions of aging and show greater respect for older adults.

A study conducted by Karasawa and colleagues (2011) found that Japan's age-supportive cultural environment and practices nurture perceptions of personal growth among its aging adults, whereas in the United States, the older groups tend to show diminished profiles of personal growth relative to midlife adults.

Japanese traditions are deeply rooted in Buddhist, Confucian, and Taoist philosophies, which view aging as a stage of maturity and a time of social value. Old age is even seen as a "spring" or "rebirth" following the demanding years of work and raising children. This perspective encourages individuals to develop a deeper, more transcendent understanding of life, embracing death with equanimity and becoming impartial contributors to social interactions.

The Confucian principle of filial piety, which emphasizes the duty of children to honor and care for their parents, reinforces the importance of respecting and supporting elderly family members. Age-related roles and responsibilities are also prominent in social practices. For example, many women participate in government-supported, age-specific neighborhood groups. Milestone celebrations, such as the 60th, 77th, 88th, and 99th birthdays, are significant events, sometimes marked by monetary gifts from mayors for those over eighty. Additionally, the use of age-specific terms to address older individuals further fosters a cultural acceptance and appreciation of aging.

These findings are supported by other studies indicating that similar reverence for the elderly exists in non-Asian cultures. For example, in Greece, elders, including abbots and abbesses, are respectfully addressed as "Geronda" and "Gerondissa," titles that convey spiritual reverence. In Greek culture, old age is highly honored and associated with wisdom and spiritual closeness. Similarly, Native American elders hold great respect within their communities which encompass over 500 distinct nations. In many tribal societies, elders are valued for their wisdom and life experiences. It is a common tradition in Native American families for elders to pass down their knowledge and teachings to younger generations (Coughlin 2017).

Löckenhoff and colleagues (2009) investigated various cultural and psychological traits related to perceptions of aging across twenty-six cultures. These traits included attitudes toward aging, physical attractiveness, learning and daily task performance capabilities, increases in wisdom and knowledge, respect received, family authority, and life satisfaction. Their findings indicated that cross-cultural differences in perceptions of aging were particularly linked to levels of education, values, and national character stereotypes. The researchers found that these associations were stronger for societal views on aging and perceptions of socioemotional changes than for perceptions of physical and cognitive changes. For example, the study found that societies with a higher proportion of educated population tend to favor the view that wisdom increases with age.

The global demographic shift toward an aging population poses profound challenges for health care, economic, and societal structures worldwide. Addressing this trend requires proactive and strategic efforts from governments and communities to optimize health care resources and improve the quality of life for older adults. Incorporating cultural perspectives on aging can inspire more effective and compassionate approaches, ensuring that older individuals are respected, valued, and supported within their communities. Additionally, integrating an understanding of the complex interplay between biological factors and cultural attitudes toward aging into education systems is essential. Creating a supportive environment for the elderly is not merely a policy priority but a crucial step in promoting societal well-being and preserving cultural heritage, enriching the lives of all generations.

Further Reading

Coughlin, Emma. 2017. "7 Cultures That Celebrate Aging and Respect Their Elders." *HuffPost*. https://www.huffpost.com/entry/what-other-cultures-can-teach_n_4834228.

Giles, Howard, Kim Noels, Hiroshi Ota, et al. 2000. "Age Vitality across Eleven Nations." *Journal of Multilingual and Multicultural Development, 21*(4): 308–23. https://doi.org/10.1080/01434630008666407.

Karasawa, Mayumi, Katherine B. Curhan, Hazel Rose Markus, Shinobu S. Kitayama, Gale Dienberg Love, Barry T. Radler, and Carol D. Ryff. 2011. "Cultural Perspectives on Aging and Well-Being: A Comparison of Japan and the U.S." *International Journal of Aging & Human Development, 73*(1): 73–98. doi: 10.2190/AG.73.1.d.

Löckenhoff, Corinna E., Filip De Fruyt, Antonio Terracciano, et al. 2009. "Perceptions of Aging across 26 Cultures and Their Culture-Level Associates." *Psychology and Aging, 24*(4): 941–54. doi: 10.1037/a0016901.

Mather, Mark and Paola Scommegna. 2024. "Fact Sheet: Aging in the United States." *PRB.org*. https://www.prb.org/resources/fact-sheet-aging-in-the-united-states/.

World Health Organization. 2022. "Ageing and Health." https://www.who.int/news-room/fact-sheets/detail/ageing-and-health.

Combatting Dementia—What Japan and the United States Can Share to Improve Care and Innovation

According to 2023 data from the World Health Organization (WHO) and data published by the Alzheimer's Association in 2024, dementia is a widespread age-related neurological condition, affecting 55 million people globally. Alarmingly, the disease is expected to grow by 10 million new cases annually. Dementia is characterized by cognitive impairments that impact language, problem-solving, general intelligence, orientation, and social skills. As it advances, individuals may lose essential bodily functions, such as mobility and the ability to eat or drink independently. It is now the seventh leading cause of death worldwide and a significant contributor to disability and dependency among older adults. Dementia affects people across all ethnic and socioeconomic groups, particularly those aged sixty-five and older. Unfortunately, there is currently no known cure for the disease.

Can Education Protect the Brain from Dementia?

A 2024 study by Gonzalez-Gomez and colleagues, published in *Alzheimer's & Dementia*, examined how education protects brain function against dementia in Latin America (LA) and the United States. The study analyzed whether years of formal education correlated with differences in brain structure and function among 1,412 participants, including 625 healthy controls, 385 Alzheimer's disease patients, and 402 frontotemporal lobar degeneration patients.

Using neuroimaging techniques such as voxel-based morphometry and resting-state functional connectivity MRI, the researchers assessed gray matter volume and connectivity, controlling for factors like age, sex, and intracranial volume. Results showed higher education levels were linked to greater gray matter volume in key areas associated with memory and cognition, such as the hippocampus, temporal gyri, and orbitofrontal cortices. These regions are critical for cognitive functions and are often the first to degenerate in dementia.

The protective effect of education was more pronounced in U.S. participants, the study found, who generally had higher educational attainment. However, in the LA group, where education levels were lower due to socioeconomic disparities, higher education still correlated with better-preserved brain structure. The findings confirm that education strengthens brain resilience against neurodegeneration and highlight the need to address educational disparities as a strategy for reducing dementia risk globally. The researchers advocate incorporating educational background into dementia care and prevention for more effective outcomes.

Further Reading

Gonzalez-Gomez, Raul, Augustina Legaz, Sebastian Moguilner, et al. 2024. "Educational Disparities in Brain Health and Dementia Across Latin America And the United States." *Alzheimer's & Dementia, 20*(9): 5815–6664. https://doi.org/10.1002/alz.14085.

Dementia is often mistakenly equated with Alzheimer's disease. In reality, dementia is a broader term encompassing a range of cognitive symptoms, with Alzheimer's being the leading cause, accounting for 60 percent to 80 percent of cases, according to the Alzheimer's Association. Other significant contributors to dementia include cerebrovascular disease, frontotemporal degeneration (FTD), hippocampal sclerosis (HS), Lewy body disease, mixed pathologies, and Parkinson's disease (PD). In the United States, 5 percent of individuals aged 65 to 74 years, 13.2 percent of those aged 75 to 84, and 33.4 percent of those aged eighty-five or older have Alzheimer's dementia. Studies show that among people aged sixty-five years and older, the average survival period after an Alzheimer's diagnosis is four to eight years, though some may live up to twenty years, according to the Alzheimer's Association.

Developed countries like the United States and Japan are more severely affected by dementia due to longer life spans and the ongoing demographic changes. Studies have shown that old age is the dominant risk factor for Alzheimer's. According to the U.S. Census Bureau, the number of Americans aged sixty-five years and older is projected to grow from 58 million in 2022 to 82 million by 2050. By 2030, the entire baby-boom generation (born between 1946 and 1964) will have reached the sixty-five years and older age category, which is the most vulnerable to dementia. Currently, it is estimated that over 6.9 million Americans are living with Alzheimer's dementia. Studies show that almost two-thirds of Americans with Alzheimer's are women, primarily because women live longer on average than men.

Dementia is also highly prevalent in Japan. The Japanese population is well-known for its record-breaking longevity. Of the 125 million people, approximately 29 percent are aged sixty-five years and older, making Japan the oldest society in the world. Japan also has one of the highest rates of dementia globally. It is projected that by 2025, one-fifth of the population will be living with dementia, and by 2060, one-third will be affected by dementia (Ishihara et al. 2024).

For both Japan and the United States, the burden of dementia extends far beyond economic losses, which are in the billions and trillions of dollars. More significantly, the disease's impact on people's health is devastating. The extensive period of illness before death greatly affects the quality of life for those living with dementia. Scientists have developed measures for calculating the years of life lost due to progressive disability, such as disability-adjusted life years (DALYs). These measures indicate that dementia is a highly burdensome disease, affecting not only individuals with the condition but also their families, informal caregivers, and communities at large. Alzheimer's and other dementias have risen to the fourth highest cause of years of life lost due to disease or injury, according to Alzheimer's Association.

Caring for dementia patients is a challenging responsibility for families, caregivers, and society as a whole. Approaches to caregiving vary widely across societies, influenced by cultural norms, economic conditions, and differences in health care systems.

In the United States, a significant number of dementia patients are cared for in specialized facilities designed to meet their needs. According to a Harvard study, between 30 percent and 40 percent of adult Americans with dementia reside in nursing homes, and approximately 70 percent of Americans with dementia will die in a nursing home (Jett 2018). However, most caregiving activities, up to 83 percent, are provided by family members and friends and are unpaid, according to Alzheimer's Association. Typical caregiving activities for people with dementia include getting in and out of bed, dressing, bathing or showering, feeding, using the toilet, and managing incontinence. In the United States, more than 11 million Americans provide unpaid care for people with Alzheimer's or other dementias, and approximately one in three dementia caregivers are women, compared to one in five in Japan and other OECD countries. The high levels of emotional, physical, and social stress on caregivers have become an important research topic for scientific studies (Kiecolt-Glaser et al. 1991).

Additionally, families need to rely on paid caregivers to supplement or provide primary care. Temporary relief for primary caregivers is available through respite care services. Institutional care is expensive and primarily relies on coverage from a mixed system of private insurance, Medicare, Medicaid, and out-of-pocket expenses. Long-term care insurance is commonly purchased by families to cover the costs of nursing homes. Many families incur significant out-of-pocket expenses for dementia care, according to Alzheimer's Association.

In most aspects, dementia care in Japan shares similar practices with the United States. For example, in both systems, cultural norms place a strong emphasis on family responsibility for caregiving. While long-term care facilities are widely used, families play an essential role in providing care and maintaining privacy. However, there are differences due to cultural and social traditions. One such difference is the scale of societal engagement. In Japan, in addition to strong government support through universal health care, society is broadly involved not just in caregiving but also in integrating people with dementia as full members of the community with dignity and respect. "To facilitate this process," Ishihara and colleagues write, "as a society we need to see beyond the abilities lost because of dementia and utilize the residual abilities of people with dementia" (Ishihara et al. 2024).

The Japanese government provides resources and support to help family caregivers, including respite care, training programs, and financial assistance. Japan's universal health care system offers long-term care insurance, introduced in 2000 through the Long-term Care Insurance Act (Ishihara et al. 2024). The coverage includes home care, daycare, and institutional care for people of all income levels. This system reduces the financial burden on families and ensures access to necessary services on a larger scale than in the United States.

Japanese society, characterized by an emphasis on community and collectiveness, views dementia care as a responsibility of the entire society. For example, Dementia Supporters is a national training program funded by the government, offering events through schools, police stations, and workplaces, and involving tens of millions of participants. Salespeople, bus drivers, and store employees commonly wear orange bracelets, a symbol of support. Team Orange is a community-based intervention aimed at providing mental and daily life support and monitoring to people diagnosed with dementia. These teams coordinate with businesses, such as banks, hair salons, and grocery stores, to better serve people with dementia. In efforts of prevention, support groups organize events to help elderly people stay active, including physical exercise, hobby groups, and social gatherings.

A notable program in Japan known as "Dementia Barrier-free" was initiated in 2019, involving nearly 100 organizations from various business services, medical facilities, and local governments. The aim is to provide dementia-friendly products and services, and to address issues such as fraud targeting people with dementia, traffic safety, and helping people with dementia make critical decisions in their daily lives.

This contrast in caregiving approaches shows strengths of both countries. The American model leans heavily on institutional and family-based support, while Japan prioritizes social integration and community-based solutions. As aging populations grow in both nations, the shared challenge lies in building high-quality, accessible systems to address the complexities of dementia care. By drawing insights from each other's practices, the United States and Japan can develop more effective strategies to support individuals living with dementia and their caregivers.

Further Reading

Alzheimer's Association. 2024. "Alzheimer's Disease Facts and Figures." https://www.alz.org/alzheimers-dementia/facts-figures.

Ishihara, Miwa, Sanae Matsunaga, Rubana Islam, Ogusa Shibata, and Ung-Il Chung. 2024. "A Policy Overview of Japan's Progress on Dementia Care in a Super-Aged Society and Future Challenges." *Global Health & Medicine,* 6(1): 13–18. doi: 10.35772/ghm.2023.01047.

Jett, Lauren. 2018. "Nursing Homes with Dementia Special Care Units Provide Better Quality of Care." *Harvard Medical School.* https://hcp.hms.harvard.edu/news/nursing-homes-dementia-special-care-units-provide-better-quality-care#:~:text=Around%20750%2C000%20individuals%20in%20nursing,die%20in%20a%20nursing%20home.

Kiecolt-Glaser, J. K., J. R. Dura, C. E. Speicher, O. J. Trask, and R. Glaser 1991. "Spousal Caregivers of Dementia Victims: Longitudinal Changes in Immunity and Health." *Psychosom Med.* doi: 10.1097/00006842-199107000-00001.

U.S. Census Bureau. 2023. "2023 National Population Projections: Downloadable Files." https://www.census.gov/data/tables/2023/demo/popproj/2023-summary-tables.html.

World Health Organization. "Dementia." https://www.who.int/news-room/fact-sheets/detail/dementia#:~:text=Key%20facts,injuries%20that%20affect%20the%20brain.

Global Aging—Exploring the Role of Geography, Genetics, and Socioeconomic Factors

As the global population continues to age, scientists are striving to identify the key factors that influence both life expectancy and quality of life. Research from the Centers for Disease Control and Prevention (CDC) and other institutions highlights three critical areas: geographical and environmental conditions, socioeconomic status, and genetic predispositions. Studies show that these factors often overlap and exacerbate one another, and in unfavorable contexts they may contribute to shorter lifespans and poorer health outcomes. However, targeted public health strategies, policy reforms, and community-based support can help mitigate these negative effects and promote healthier aging worldwide.

Geographical and Environmental Factors

Extreme climate patterns can significantly increase mortality rates, particularly among older adults who are more susceptible to temperature-related health issues. For instance, the UN Environmental Program identifies the historic 2003 European heatwave as one of the deadliest natural disasters in recent history. Spanning from June to August, the heatwave brought temperatures exceeding 40°C (104°F) in some areas, resulting in approximately 70,000 excess deaths across Europe, the majority of whom were elderly. France was among the hardest-hit countries, with about 14,802 excess deaths, primarily affecting older individuals who were especially vulnerable to the extreme heat.

In fact, the frequency and intensity of heat waves have been increasing as climate change worsens. For example, multiple heatwaves hit Europe in the summer of 2019, breaking temperature records in several countries. Paris recorded an all-time high of 42.6°C (108.7°F), according to AccuWeather. In 2021, the Pacific Northwest experienced an unprecedented heatwave in June, with temperatures reaching up to 49.6°C (121.3°F) in Lytton, British Columbia, Canada. Extreme weather conditions disproportionately affect elderly individuals, resulting in higher mortality and morbidity rates compared to younger populations (White et al. 2023).

Furthermore, climate models predict that heatwaves will become even more frequent and intense in the coming decades if global greenhouse gas emissions are not significantly reduced. The IPCC forecasts that, under high emissions scenarios, heatwaves that currently occur once every twenty years could occur as frequently as every 2–3 years by the end of the twenty-first century.

In addition to extreme climate events, high levels of pollution can exacerbate health problems in the elderly, such as respiratory issues and cardiovascular diseases. Research indicates that elderly individuals exposed to high levels of PM2.5 and ozone have a higher risk of mortality. A study on a U.S. population found that for older dialysis patients residing in areas with high PM2.5, a 10 μg/m3 increase in PM2.5 was associated with a 1.16-fold increased risk of mortality (Feng et al. 2021). The elderly population bears a significant portion of this burden due to higher rates of preexisting health conditions. The European Environment Agency (EEA) reports that, in 2021, air pollution caused more than 253,000 premature deaths across Europe. The elderly population is particularly affected, with a significant proportion of these deaths occurring among individuals aged sixty-five years and older.

Research has also found that geographic regions with better health care infrastructure and favorable cultural traditions generally see their elderly populations enjoy better health and longer lives. In contrast, rural or isolated areas often have limited access to medical services, which can affect the prevention and management of age-related diseases. Different cultures have varying attitudes toward the elderly, impacting how they are treated and supported. Societies with strong familial support systems and community engagement for the elderly often see better mental and physical health outcomes among their aging populations.

Socioeconomic Factors

Research indicates that higher income levels generally correlate with better access to health care, healthier lifestyles, and longer life expectancy. Conversely, lower socioeconomic status can be linked to reduced access to health care, nutritious food, and safe living environments. According to a study by the Brookings Institution, there is a significant gap in life expectancy between the richest and poorest Americans. Men in the top 10 percent of the income distribution live approximately twelve years longer than men in the bottom 10 percent, and women in the top 10 percent live about ten years longer than women in the bottom 10 percent (Burtless 2016).

The CDC reports that individuals with lower SES are more likely to suffer from chronic conditions such as heart disease, diabetes, and obesity. For instance, adults with a family income below the federal poverty level are five times more likely to report fair or poor health compared to those with an income at or above 400 percent of the federal poverty level (Woolf et al. 2015).

The AARP Foundation reported that older adults with lower SES are more likely to experience social isolation and loneliness, which are linked to increased risks of depression, anxiety, and even early mortality. Socially isolated older adults face a 29 percent increased risk of heart disease and a 32 percent increased risk of stroke (Anderson et al. 2018).

Genetic Factors

Studies show that genetic factors play a crucial role in the aging process and the health outcomes of an aging society. These factors affect longevity, vulnerability to age-related diseases, and the biological mechanisms underlying aging.

Genetic predisposition is known to be associated multiple common diseases. Certain genetic variations, such as those affecting cholesterol metabolism, familial hypercholesterolemia as an example, can increase the risk of cardiovascular diseases, which are a leading cause of death among older adults. Genome-Wide Association Studies (GWAS) have identified numerous genetic loci associated with heart disease, hypertension, and other cardiovascular conditions.

Certain neurodegenerative diseases have been identified as being associated with genetic conditions. Variants in the *APOE* gene, particularly the *APOE* ε4 allele, are strongly linked to an increased risk of developing Alzheimer's disease. This genetic risk factor influences both the onset and progression of the disease. Additionally, mutations in several genes, including *LRRK2* and *SNCA*, have been linked to an increased risk of Parkinson's disease, affecting the neurological health of the aging population (Giau et al. 2019).

Inherited mutations in genes such as *BRCA1* and *BRCA2* have been associated with increased risk of certain cancers, including breast and ovarian cancer. Genetic factors play a significant role in cancer prevalence among older adults, studies indicate. According to the National Cancer Institute (NCI), women with a *BRCA1* mutation have between a 55 percent and 72 percent lifetime risk of developing breast cancer, and women with a *BRCA2* mutation have between a 45 percent and 69 percent lifetime risk of developing breast cancer (DePolo 2023).

As societies around the world face aging populations, addressing social and environmental factors is essential. This includes reducing pollution, adapting infrastructure to withstand extreme weather, and improving access to health care. Socioeconomic strategies should focus on providing financial support for lower-income populations. Addressing genetic factors requires advancing genetic research, promoting personalized medicine, and implementing public health initiatives that encourage healthy lifestyles. Equally important is ensuring the inclusion of diverse populations in genetic research, studies show. Enhancing the quality of life and health outcomes for aging populations demands a coordinated effort across all levels of society.

Further Reading

Anderson, G. Colette Thayer Oscar. 2018. "Loneliness and Social Connections: A National Survey of Adults 45 and Older." *AARP Research*. https://www.aarp.org/research/topics/life/info-2018/loneliness-social-connections.html.

Burtless, Gary. 2016. "The Growing Life-Expectancy Gap between Rich and Poor." *Brookings.edu*. https://www.brookings.edu/articles/the-growing-life-expectancy-gap-between-rich-and-poor/.

Centers for Disease Control and Prevention. 2016. "Health, United States, 2016." https://www.cdc.gov/nchs/data/hus/hus16.pdf#033.

Congressional Research Service. 2021. "The Growing Gap in Life Expectancy by Income: Recent Evidence and Implications for the Social Security Retirement Age." https://crsreports.congress.gov/product/pdf/R/R44846#:~:text=Recent%20studies%20provide%20evidence%20that,in%20the%20lowest%20income%20quintile.

DePolo, Jaime. 2023. "Breast Cancer Risk Remains High for Women with Braca Mutations after Age 50." *Breastcancer.org*. https://www.breastcancer.org/research-news/brca-risk-older-women.

European Environment Agency. 2024. "Air Pollution." *EEA*. https://www.eea.europa.eu/en/topics/in-depth/air-pollution?activeTab=07e50b68-8bf2-4641-ba6b-eda1afd544be.

Feng, Yijing, Miranda R. Jones, Nadia M. Chu, Dorry L. Segev, and Mara McAdams-DeMarco. 2021. "Ambient Air Pollution and Mortality among Older Patients Initiating Maintenance Dialysis." *Am J Nephrol, 52*(3): 217–27. https://doi.org/10.1159/000514233.

Giau, Vo Van, Vorapun Senanarong, Eva Bagyinszky, Seong Soo A. An, and SangYun Kim. 2019. "Analysis of 50 Neurodegenerative Genes in Clinically Diagnosed Early-Onset Alzheimer's Disease." *International Journal of Molecular Sciences*, *20*(6): 1514. doi: 10.3390/ijms20061514.

IPCC. 2021. "Climate Change Widespread, Rapid, and Intensifying." *IPCC*. https://www.ipcc.ch/2021/08/09/ar6-wg1-20210809-pr/.

SOA Research Institute. 2022. "Mortality by Socioeconomic Category in the United States." https://www.soa.org/globalassets/assets/files/resources/research-report/2020/mort-socioeconomic-cat-report.pdf.

UNEP. 2003. "Impacts of Summer 2003 Heave Wave in Europe." *UNISDR.org*. https://www.unisdr.org/files/1145_ewheatwave.en.pdf.

White, Rachel H., Same Anderson, James F. Booth, et al. 2023. "The Unprecedented Pacific Northwest Heatwave of June 2021." *Nature Communications, 14*: 727. https://doi.org/10.1038/s41467-023-36289-3.

Woolf, Steven, Laudan Aron, Lisa Dubay, et al. 2015. "How Are Income and Wealth Linked to Health and Longevity?" *Urban.org*. https://www.urban.org/sites/default/files/publication/49116/2000178-How-are-Income-and-Wealth-Linked-to-Health-and-Longevity.pdf.

Zeliadt, Nicholette. 2010. "Live Long and Proper: Genetic Factors Associated with Increased Longevity Identified." *Scientific American*. https://www.scientificamerican.com/article/genetic-factors-associated-with-increased-longevity-identified/.

Environmental Triggers of Parkinson's Disease—Insights for Prevention and Management

Parkinson's disease (PD) is a neurodegenerative disorder that primarily affects individuals aged sixty-five years and older, with the incidence of new cases increasing with age. According to Parkinson.org, more than one million Americans are currently living with PD, and 90,000 new cases are diagnosed annually. The combined direct and indirect costs associated with the disease are estimated at nearly $52 billion per year. As the population continues to age, the number of people living with PD in the United States is projected to reach 1.2 million by 2030. On a global scale, PD has also been on the rise. The World

Health Organization (WHO) reports that 8.5 million people were living with PD in 2019, a figure that had doubled over twenty-five years.

PD is symptomatically characterized by the progressive loss of dopaminergic neurons responsible for dopamine transmission. Individuals with PD often exhibit a distinctive shuffling gait and struggle with maintaining balance. Spontaneous facial movements are significantly reduced, giving rise to a mask-like, expressionless appearance. Additional symptoms may include fatigue, hallucinations, delusions, lightheadedness, and cognitive impairments affecting attention, planning, language, or memory. While there is no cure for PD, available medications aim to stimulate dopamine levels in the brain. Unlike Alzheimer's disease, which is marked by relentless neurodegeneration of vital brain functions and often leads to death within four to eight years of diagnosis, PD generally progresses more slowly. The extent of brain damage varies among individuals, and many patients can live for years while maintaining a good quality of life (Parkinson.org).

The direct causes of PD have not been identified; however, scientists believe that both environmental and genetic factors can contribute to its development. Research indicates that genetics account for only up to 15 percent of all cases. The majority are categorized as sporadic, meaning they are not inherited and could be triggered by factors such as age, lifestyle, and the environment. This suggests that in the future PD could be largely prevented by identifying and controlling many of the causal elements (Dorsey et al. 2024).

Among genetic factors, scientists have identified mutations in genes such as *LRRK2, SNCA,* and DJ-1, as mutations commonly associated with PD worldwide. These mutations, whether inherited or developed later in life, result in the production of abnormal proteins. One such protein which is essential to the onset of PD and several other neurodegenerative disorders including Alzheimer's is an abnormal form of the α-synuclein protein encoded by the *SNCA* gene. The mutated forms of alpha-synuclein are prone to aggregation and can form Lewy bodies. The accumulation of these aggregates contributes to neuronal dysfunction and cell death. The depletion of dopaminergic neurons in the substantia nigra region is responsible for the classic motor symptoms of PD, including bradykinesia, resting tremor, muscular rigidity, and postural instability. Additionally, non-motor manifestations such as autonomic dysfunction, olfactory impairment, mood disorders, cognitive deficits, and sleep disturbances are frequently present in PD (Gómez-Benito et al. 2020). Genetic mutations have been associated with different phenotypes of PD, affecting either motor or non-motor symptoms. The prevalence of mutations has also been found to vary among different ethnic groups, making these groups susceptible to different phenotypes of the disease (Ben-Joseph et al. 2020).

Approximately 85 percent of PD cases are sporadic rather than genetically driven, prompting extensive research into potential environmental factors. A promising area of study focuses on the role of epigenetics and epigenetic mechanisms in PD, uncovering numerous potential connections. In this context, epigenetics refers to changes in gene activity without alterations to the genetic code itself. Research suggests that the onset of PD is likely triggered by exposure to pesticides and heavy metals. These toxic substances, commonly used in agriculture, have been widely linked to mitochondrial dysfunction, oxidative stress, and impaired protein degradation.

Research has also shown that occupational exposure to copper and lead can increase PD risks by more than twofold. Drug use, particularly cocaine, amphetamine, and methamphetamine, which affect dopamine transport (a key area of neurodegeneration in PD), has been shown to increase PD risk nearly threefold. Demographic factors, including age, gender, and ethnicity, suggest that age is a major risk factor related to both onset time and severity, with those aged sixty years and older being the most vulnerable. Ethnicity studies have found that Caucasians and Hispanics have an increased risk compared to Asians and Blacks, possibly associated with skin color and melanin levels (Tsalenchuk et al. 2023).

Geographical studies conducted in highly populated urban areas have found significant correlations between industrial airborne heavy metal pollution and ambient air pollution from traffic and an increased risk of PD onset (Ball et al. 2024). One study, for example, argues that there is a "Parkinson disease belt" with high prevalence and incidence of PD in the Midwest and Northeast regions of the United States, due to industrial by-products, highlighting the environmental influence on the pathogenesis of PD (Willis et al. 2010).

It is also noteworthy that exposure to certain environmental factors has been found to have protective benefits against PD. The consumption of tobacco and caffeine has been associated in some studies with a lower risk of both disease onset and progression. The presence of caffeine and eicosanoyl-5-hydroxytryptamide (EHT) in coffee has been found to enhance the activity of protein phosphatase 2A (PP2A), which is responsible for the dephosphorylation of α-synuclein, resulting in reduced aggregation (Tsalenchuk et al. 2023).

A hypothesis presented by Dorsey and colleagues (2024) brings a new perspective on the origins and spread of PD integrating environmental toxicants into existing brain-first and body-first models. The study suggests that inhalation or ingestion of environmental toxins like pesticides, dry cleaning chemicals (trichloroethylene and perchloroethylene), and air pollution can lead to the development of PD. These toxins may enter the brain via the olfactory system or the gastrointestinal tract, causing the misfolding of the alpha-synuclein protein and forming Lewy bodies associated with PD. The study brings new understanding of the etiology of the disease as well as hope for effective prevention (Dorsey et al. 2024).

As with most neurological disorders, pinpointing the direct causes of PD is challenging. While correlations do not equate to direct causation, the studies introduced above offer valuable insights for daily life and provide important guidance for ongoing scientific research.

Further Reading

Ball, Nicole, Wei-Peng Teo, Shaneel Chandra, and James Chapman. 2024. "Parkinson's Disease and the Environment." *Frontier in Neurology, 10*: 218. doi: 10.3389/fneur.2019.00218.

Ben-Joseph, Aaron, Charles R. Marshall, Andrew J. Lees, and Alastair J. Noyce. 2020. "Ethnic Variation in the Manifestation of Parkinson's Disease: A Narrative Review." *Journal of Parkinson's Disease*. doi: 10.3233/JPD-191763.

Dorsey, Ray E., Briana R. De Miranda, Jacob Horsager, and Per Borghammer. 2024. "The Body, the Brain, the Environment, and Parkinson's Disease." *Journal of Parkinson's Disease, 14*(3): 363–81. doi: 10.3233/JPD-240019.

Gómez-Benito, Mónica, Neolia Granado, Patricia Garic-Sanz, Anne Michel, Miereille Dumoulin, and Rosario Moratalla. 2020. "Modeling Parkinson's Disease with the Alpha-Synuclein Protein." *Frontiers, 11*. https://www.frontiersin.org/journals/pharmacology/articles/10.3389/fphar.2020.00356/full.

Parkinson.org. 2018. "10 Interesting Facts about Parkinson's Disease." https://www.parkinson.org/blog/awareness/10-facts.

Prenger, Margaret T. M., Rachael Madray, Kathryne Van Hedger, Mimma Anello, and Penny A. MacDonald. 2020. "Social Symptoms of Parkinson's Disease." *Wiley Online Library, 2020*: 8846544. https://onlinelibrary.wiley.com/doi/10.1155/2020/8846544.

Tsalenchuk, Maria, Steve M. Gentleman, and Sarah J. Marzi. 2023. "Linking Environmental Risk Factors with Epigenetic Mechanisms in Parkinson's Disease." *NPJ Parkinsons Dis, 9*: 123. https://doi.org/10.1038/s41531-023-00568-z.

Willis, Allison Wright, Bradley A. Evanoff, Min Lian, Susan R. Criswell, and Brad A. Racette. 2010. "Geographic and Ethnic Variation in Parkinson Disease: A Population-Based Study of US Medicare Beneficiaries." *Neuroepidemiology, 34*(3): 143–51. doi: https://doi.org/10.1159/000275491.

World Health Organization. 2023. "Key Facts." https://www.who.int/news-room/fact-sheets/detail/parkinson-disease#:~:text=Parkinson%20disease%20.

Why Societies Must Be Prepared for Population Aging

In the twenty-first century, the world is undergoing a major demographic shift known as global aging. By 2050, the proportion of the global population aged sixty years and older is projected to increase from 12 percent to 22 percent, according to the World Health Organization (WHO 2022). This global trend is fueled by various factors, including advances in health care and living standards, declining fertility rates, and longer life expectancies driven by medical innovations.

This shift carries profound implications for economies, health care systems, and social structures. Aging-related diseases will place heavy burdens on society, affecting the quality of life for individuals and their families. Research on the prevalence and impact of cardiovascular disease (CVD), dementia, and osteoarthritis (OA) underscores the need for all societies to prepare for this demographic transformation.

Cardiovascular Disease

Cardiovascular disease (CVD) is the leading cause of death among aging-related illnesses, surpassing cancer and other conditions in mortality rates, according to the Centers for Disease Control and Prevention (CDC). In 2021, heart disease was responsible for approximately 695,000 deaths, accounting for one in every five deaths in the United States. The prevalence of heart disease increases with age, with the highest rates observed among individuals aged seventy-five years and older—24.2 percent of this age group reported having heart disease. The annual economic burden of heart disease was estimated at $239.9 billion between 2018 and 2019, including the costs of health care services, medications, and lost productivity.

Studies have identified the primary causes of CVD to include atherosclerosis (the buildup of plaque in the arteries), hypertension, lifestyle factors such as smoking, poor diet, physical inactivity, excessive alcohol consumption, and genetic inheritance. Numerous studies have established a strong correlation between lower socioeconomic status (SES) and higher rates of CVD. Limited access to health care can lead to inadequate prevention, early detection, and management of cardiovascular risk factors such as hypertension, diabetes, and high cholesterol. Lower SES is also associated with lifestyle factors that increase the risk of heart disease, including poor diet, physical inactivity, smoking, and excessive alcohol consumption. Additionally, people with lower SES often experience higher levels of stress due to financial instability, job insecurity, and challenging living conditions. Chronic stress can contribute to hypertension and other cardiovascular conditions. Geographically, the Southern United States, including Alabama, Mississippi, Louisiana, and Arkansas, have some of the highest rates of cardiovascular health issues and related deaths, according to the CDC and the American Heart Association.

Dementia

Dementia is responsible for a substantial number of deaths in the aging population. Alzheimer's dementia, the most common form of dementia, accounts for more than 60 percent of all dementia cases and is a significant cause of death among older adults. In 2021, Alzheimer's dementia was the fifth leading cause of death among people sixty-five years and older, according to the Alzheimer's Association. Alzheimer's disease leads to severe cognitive decline, loss of independence, and increased reliance on caregiving as the disease progresses.

Data from the Alzheimer's Association indicate that the risk of developing Alzheimer's dementia increases dramatically with age. Nearly 5 percent of people aged 65–74 years live with dementia. This percentage rises to 13.2 percent among those aged 75–84 and reaches 33.4 percent for those aged eighty-five and older. Approximately one in nine aged sixty-five years and older in the United States has Alzheimer's, a staggering number.

As the baby-boomer generation reaches age sixty-five years, Alzheimer's cases are expected to increase significantly. Currently, nearly 7 million Americans are living with Alzheimer's, a number that is projected to rise to nearly 13 million by 2050, according to the Alzheimer's Association.

Research indicates that gender and socioeconomic status are linked to the onset of dementia. According to the Alzheimer's Association, two-thirds of Americans with Alzheimer's are women, largely due to their longer life expectancy. The prevalence of Alzheimer's also varies based on socioeconomic factors, with older Black and Hispanic Americans being one to two times more likely to develop dementia than older White Americans.

Osteoarthritis

Osteoarthritis (OA) is the most common form of arthritis, characterized by the degeneration of cartilage, the smooth tissue that cushions the ends of bones in the joints. Unlike other forms of arthritis, such as rheumatoid arthritis and gout, which are attributable to immunological or chemical causes, OA results from the mechanical wear and tear of the joints over time, affecting the hands, knees, hips, and spine. Obesity and injuries have been identified as major causes; however, OA is primarily an aging disease. Over 32 million adults in the United States live with OA, and nearly half of those with the condition are sixty-five years or older, according to the CDC.

More than half of the people with knee osteoarthritis (OA) will undergo a total knee replacement during their lifetime. Nearly 1 million knee and hip replacements are performed each year, according to estimates. In 2013, OA was the second most costly health condition treated in hospitals in the United States, CDC data indicates.

Socioeconomic data shows that 62 percent of individuals with OA are women, according to the CDC. Latinos are more likely to report greater pain, functional limitations, and work limitations than non-Latino whites. Additionally, studies indicate that osteoarthritis is associated with several mental health comorbidities. People with OA are at a greater risk for depression and anxiety due to the increased disability and fatigue associated with their pain. Social isolation and loneliness are also common among people with osteoarthritis and other chronic musculoskeletal diseases, as reported by Osteoarthritis Action Alliance.

Burdens on Economy and Quality of Life

The cost of managing aging-related diseases can be substantial. Health and long-term care costs for people living with dementia are estimated to be $360 billion in 2024 and are projected to reach $1 trillion by 2050. Additionally, about one-third of the care provided is unpaid, valued at nearly $350 billion, according to Alzheimer's Association.

Cardiovascular disease imposes a substantial economic burden globally. In developed economies such as the United States, the estimated direct and indirect costs of heart disease alone were approximately $252.2 billion annually as of 2019–20, with projections indicating that these costs could surpass $1 trillion by 2035, according to the American Heart Association and the CDC.

The overall economic burden associated with osteoarthritis in the United States is nearly $136.8 billion annually, a figure that has more than doubled over the last decade. Direct medical costs reach $65 billion annually, according to the Osteoarthritis Action Alliance.

The actual burden of CVD, OA, and dementia extends beyond quantitative losses. Rising demand for caregiving leads to labor shortages and decreased productivity, impacting overall economic output. Long-term care is essential for managing these chronic conditions, and health care systems may become overwhelmed if not adequately prepared. There is also a need for more health care professionals, necessitating investment in education and training programs. Without sufficient preparation, health care systems may face severe workforce shortages.

The U.S. Congress has taken significant steps to address the challenges posed by aging population through various policies and programs. Historically, key federal initiatives include Older Americans Act (OAA), Administration on Aging (AoA), both originated in the 1960s, and the National Plan on Aging introduced in 2023 contributed to improving health and living conditions of the elderly population. On May 30, 2024, the U.S. Department of Health and Human Services (HHS) released a comprehensive action plan "Aging in the United States: A Strategic Framework for a National Plan on Aging." The report outlines a coordinated effort among public and private sectors, caregivers, and stakeholders to promote healthy aging and age-friendly communities. It aims to advance best practices in service delivery, strengthen partnerships, and address barriers to health and independence for older adults. Developed by experts from sixteen federal agencies and input from community partners, this framework sets the stage for a comprehensive national aging plan. These government-led initiatives play a crucial role in helping society address one of the greatest challenges of our time.

Further Reading

Alzheimer's Association. 2024. "Alzheimer's Disease Facts and Figures." https://www.alz.org/alzheimers-dementia/facts-figures.

American Heart Association. "What Is Cardiovascular Disease?" https://www.heart.org/en/health-topics/consumer-healthcare/what-is-cardiovascular-disease.

Centers for Disease Control and Prevention. 2024. "Heart Disease Facts." https://www.cdc.gov/heart-disease/data-research/facts-stats/index.html.

Department of Health and Human Services (HHS) released. 2024. "Aging in the United States: A Strategic Framework for a National Plan on Aging." https://acl.gov/sites/default/files/ICC-Aging/StrategicFramework-NationalPlanOnAging-2024.pdf.

Osteoarthritis Action Alliance. 2024. https://oaaction.unc.edu/oa-module/oa-prevalence-and-burden/.

World Health Organization. 2022. "Ageing and Health." https://www.who.int/news-room/fact-sheets/detail/ageing-and-health.

Education and Public Health

The Revival of TCM: Heritage, Health, and the Role of the State

Traditional Chinese Medicine (TCM) has long been an essential part of China's health care system and cultural identity. With origins dating back thousands of years, TCM is grounded in Chinese philosophical concepts such as *yin* and *yang*, the five elements, and the idea of *Qi*, the life force that flows through the body. Historically, TCM played a dominant role in Chinese medical practices and enjoyed widespread trust among the population.

In the 1950s, TCM gained significant ideological importance as part of efforts to establish a nationwide health care system. At the time, China faced the challenge of providing health care to its large population, especially in rural areas with limited infrastructure and medical personnel. TCM, with its affordable herbal and acupuncture-based treatments, became both a practical and ideological solution, representing traditional Chinese health care practices in contrast to the criticized Western influence (Shi et al. 2020).

However, the status of TCM began to shift in the late 1970s when China initiated market reforms and an "open-door" policy under Deng Xiaoping. These reforms marked a transition toward modernization, industrialization, and greater integration with the global economy. As China's health care system evolved, Western medicine, with its emphasis on experimental and evidence-based standards, gained prominence, shaking TCM's dominance (Shi et al. 2020).

As these socioeconomic changes took hold, the utilization of TCM doctors in urban areas dropped significantly—from 25 percent in 1991 to 14 percent in 2004—while the use of Western medicine doctors rose from 69 percent to 80 percent. In cities where modern health care services were more accessible, the decline in TCM was even more pronounced. Meanwhile, rural areas, with limited access to Western medicine, saw a slower, but still noticeable, reduction in the use of TCM in the early 2000s (Lei 2010).

The decline of TCM also led to diminishing job prospects for graduates of TCM programs. Despite efforts to integrate Western medicine into TCM curricula, many graduates found themselves underqualified in the eyes of employers. This hybrid training, intended to provide a balance of traditional and modern medical skills, often left students with unclear or inadequate qualifications. Reports indicated that TCM graduates frequently had their resumes dismissed by recruiters, who expressed concerns about unclear practice scopes and regulatory limitations on what TCM practitioners could legally do, such as performing surgeries or prescribing Western medications. In provinces like Fujian, for example, lower-tier hospitals and health centers openly refused to hire TCM graduates, adding to the frustration and confusion faced by job seekers (Tian 2009).

This decline in TCM's role in modern Chinese health care has sparked extensive debate on platforms like Sohu.com, where commentators offer a wide range of perspectives on the reasons behind the fading of one of China's most iconic traditions. The most common opinions are outlined below.

Lack of Scientific Rigor

Some critics argue that TCM lacks the scientific foundation of Western medicine, which is supported by clinical trials and empirical data. As China's public health care system expanded to address a broader range of diseases, evidence-based medicine became the standard. In contrast, TCM's theoretical framework is often viewed as mystified and difficult to verify scientifically, focusing on abstract elements rather than on practical and universally applicable concepts. Critics suggest that this conservatism, emphasizing tradition over innovation, has hindered TCM's adaptability in modern times.

Low Potential for Market Profitability

Another factor contributing to TCM's decline appears to be its limited financial potential. While the low cost of TCM treatments was once an advantage, in today's market-driven health care system, it has become a drawback. Western medicine, with its specialization in various fields and reliance on expensive medical equipment, creates more opportunities for profit. Hospitals find it more profitable to hire doctors trained in Western medicine who can prescribe both Western and Chinese medicines, perform surgeries, and use advanced equipment—all of which contribute to the hospital's revenue. In contrast, TCM doctors, often restricted by regulations, are unable to generate the same level of income for hospitals.

Insufficient Manufacturing and Quality Control

The availability and quality of natural ingredients essential to TCM have become a growing concern. With the shortage of wild medicinal herbs, TCM products have suffered in both quantity and quality. Many herbs used in today's market are cultivated and may contain pesticide residues, while counterfeit herbs further compromise the industry. The increasing use of genetically modified herbs adds another layer of complexity, as many TCM practitioners are reluctant to use them due to concerns over their safety and efficacy. These challenges in quality control have created a bottleneck for the development of TCM.

Talent Shortage

The decline of skilled professionals is another critical issue facing TCM. As a discipline that requires significant practical expertise, TCM depends on highly qualified doctors, yet such talent is becoming increasingly scarce. Critics point to the inconsistent standards in TCM education across different regions and institutions, with some programs focusing more on rote memorization of classical formulas than on a deeper understanding of TCM principles. This lack of comprehensive education may hinder the effective application of TCM in modern clinical practice.

Lifestyle Changes

In today's fast-paced world, TCM's slower treatment methods are often overshadowed by the quicker results of Western medicine. TCM's philosophy of balancing internal organs and harmonizing with nature is still embraced by many, but an increasing number of people prefer the fast and targeted treatments offered by Western medicine, despite potential side effects. Critics argue that while TCM addresses the root causes of illness, its treatments take longer to show results, which makes Western medicine more appealing to those seeking immediate relief.

TCM's Economic Viability

In times of economic prosperity, non-essential products and services like TCM may thrive. However, during financial downturns, demand for TCM-related products—such as herbal medicines, acupuncture, moxibustion patches, and medicinal diets—tends to decline, further threatening the industry.

Lack of Cultural Confidence

Official media have attributed TCM's decline to the influence of Western culture. An article titled "Cultural Confidence in Traditional Chinese Medicine," published by *The People's Daily*, argued that the rejection of TCM reflects a broader lack of cultural confidence, shaped by China's modern history of defeat and the perceived superiority of Western ideals. The article emphasized that for TCM to thrive, the people must believe in its effectiveness and value, which are deeply rooted in Chinese tradition. True cultural confidence, the article argued, is key to TCM's global acceptance and growth (Wang 2012).

Despite these challenges, critics generally agree that TCM holds irreplaceable value. Its holistic and preventive approach to health care is becoming increasingly relevant as the world faces rising rates of chronic diseases and aging populations. A large segment of the Chinese population remains culturally tied to TCM, and its growing global recognition suggests it will continue to play a vital role in managing chronic conditions. Outcomes like pain relief, improved sleep, or reduced anxiety are simply valuable in themselves, even if the precise biological mechanism is not fully understood or proven in Western terms. With diverse medical treatment options across cultures, TCM's alternative therapies provide a promising complement to modern medicine, supporting long-term wellness and easing the burden of chronic illnesses. Many proponents of traditional Chinese medicine believe that education can better enhance understanding and appreciation of its value—perhaps more effectively than government propaganda, as reflected in various blogs.

Further Reading

Burke, Adam, Yim-yu Wong, and Zoe Clayson. 2002. "Traditional Medicine in China Today: Implications for Indigenous Health Systems in a Modern World." *American Journal of Public Health, 93*(7): 1082–4. doi: 10.2105/ajph.93.7.1082.

Dalianbeimingzi. 2024. "Why Doesn't the State Vigorously Promote Traditional Chinese Medicine (TCM)? Understanding the Considerations behind the Policy." 365doc.com. http://www.360doc.com/content/24/0105/17/57220774_1110062985.shtml. Accessed September 24, 2024.

Lei, Jin. 2010. "From Mainstream to Marginal? Trends in the Use of Chinese Medicine in China from 1991 to 2004." *Social Science and Medicine, 71*(6): 1063–7. doi: https://doi.org/10.1016/j.socscimed.2010.06.019.

Li, Changqing. 2023. "Should You Study Traditional Chinese Medicine (TCM) in the Face of a Challenging Job Market?" (in Chinese language). *Xys.org*. http://www.xys.org/xys/ebooks/others/science/dajia24/zhongyi6.txt. Accessed September 24, 2024.

Shi, Xuefeng, Dawei Zhu, Stephen Nicholas, Baolin Hong, Xiaowei Man, and Ping He. 2020. "Is Traditional Chinese Medicine 'Mainstream' in China? Trends in Traditional Chinese Medicine Health Resources and Their Utilization in Traditional Chinese Medicine Hospitals from 2004 to 2016." *Evidence Based Complementary and Alternative Medicine, 2020*: 9313491. doi: 10.1155/2020/9313491.

Tian Guolei. 2009. "Employment for TCM Graduates Faces Legal Obstacles" (in Chinese language) China Youth. July 15. https://zqb.cyol.com/content/2009-07/15/content_2757981.htm. Accessed September 24, 2024.

Wang, Junping. 2012. "Chinese Medicine Depends on Cultural Confidence" (in Chinese language). *People's Digest*. http://paper.people.com.cn/rmwz/html/2012-10/01/content_1137121.htm?div=-1. Accessed September 23, 2024.

Wang, Xiao. 2023. "The Eight Reasons Why Traditional Chinese Medicine (TCM) Has Been Suppressed and Developed Slowly: Capital Is the Driving Force behind It" (in Chinese language). https://www.sohu.com/a/711302971_121124549. Accessed September 23, 2024.

Yang, Xuetao. 2020. "Traditional Chinese Medicine (TCM) Is Valuable, But Many TCM Graduates Are Struggling to Find Jobs" (in Chinese language). https://www.sohu.com/a/378478174_120597763. Accessed September 23, 2024.

Zihaojun. 2022. "Why Has Traditional Chinese Medicine (TCM), Once a Major Pillar of Healthcare, Fallen into Decline Today?" https://www.163.com/dy/article/HOPFCD2H0553MUOM.html. Accessed September 24, 2024.

Comprehensive Sexuality Education in China, Japan, and Korea—Cultural Challenges and Reforms

Comprehensive Sexuality Education (CSE), as outlined in the 2018 International Technical Guidance on Sexuality Education—An Evidence-based Approach by the United Nations Educational, Scientific and Cultural Organization (UNESCO), is a curriculum based framework designed to educate children and adolescents about the cognitive, emotional, physical, and social aspects of sexuality. CSE empowers young people to understand their rights, respect others, and make informed decisions about their health, relationships, and bodies. Its goal is to provide the knowledge and skills necessary for safe and healthy development.

The Guidance highlights alarming global statistics: over one-third of women experience physical or sexual violence in their lifetime, which increases their risk of HIV infection and unintended pregnancies. Each year, approximately 3 million girls aged 15–19 years undergo unsafe abortions. Moreover, an estimated 120 million girls have been subjected to sexual violence, while child sexual abuse affects 20 percent of women and 5–10 percent of men. Female genital mutilation (FGM) has impacted 200 million women and girls, and early marriage remains widespread, with 40 percent of girls in sub-Saharan Africa married before the age of eighteen.

LGBTI individuals face heightened levels of violence and stigmatization, particularly in school settings. Despite awareness efforts, only 36 percent of young men and 30 percent of young women globally have accurate knowledge of HIV prevention, according to the UNESCO 2018 Guidance.

CSE seeks to reduce the negative factors that jeopardize the well-being of young people. It advocates for gender equality and human rights, fosters respectful relationships, and challenges harmful societal norms. The curriculum covers critical topics such as violence prevention, health-related skills, and the biological aspects of sexuality, providing young people with the knowledge they need to make informed decisions. Furthermore, CSE breaks down taboos surrounding puberty and reproduction, empowering youth to approach these natural processes with confidence and understanding.

The promotion of CSE faces resistance in some Asian countries where traditional ideologies, such as Confucianism, and contemporary conservative politics dominate. In societies like China, Japan, and Korea, discussions about sexuality are often implicit or avoided, as they are considered inappropriate and believed to potentially encourage early sexual activity (Ma et al. 2021). Despite these challenges, educators in these countries are striving to advance CSE through educational reforms, seeking to balance cultural sensitivities with the imperative for comprehensive sexual health education.

Sex education in China has historically faced substantial challenges and cultural resistance. Following the establishment of the People's Republic in 1949, discussions about sexuality were progressively suppressed. During the Cultural Revolution (1966–76), sexuality became a taboo topic, absent from social discourse, arts, and literature. However, the 1980s marked a shift when China, influenced by the Reform and Opening Up policy, began to embrace the idea of sex education. Government officials started to acknowledge its importance, leading to its gradual inclusion in school curricula.

Despite this progress, sex education remained a marginal aspect of pre-college education, primarily taught as part of biology classes. Its focus was often more aligned with enforcing family planning policies than fostering a comprehensive understanding of sexual health or rights (Qin et al. 2023).

The enduring influence of Confucianism, which emphasizes male dominance, female obedience, and filial piety within the family, continues to shape societal attitudes and sexual behaviors (Gao et al. 2012). Within this cultural context, sexuality and reproductive health (SRH) education is often indirect, delivered through subtle methods such as cartoons or family conversations. Most adolescents lack access to formal SRH education or essential services, largely due to cultural norms that prioritize sexual propriety and moral values, making public discussions on these topics uncomfortable.

Although efforts have been made to provide SRH education—such as expert-led lectures or the distribution of informational leaflets—these initiatives frequently lack cohesive frameworks that link educational content to specific outcomes. Moreover, they offer limited standardized materials for widespread implementation.

Sex education in China began making strides in integrating into school curricula during the 1990s. However, research indicates that the term "sex education" was still frequently associated with shame, leading to the more common use of the term "puberty education." While attitudes toward sex education have become more progressive in the twenty-first century, many Chinese teachers remain reluctant to address topics related to sexuality due to enduring cultural taboos.

Systemic challenges, combined with economic disparities, further impede the effective implementation of sex education, particularly in underdeveloped regions where even basic compulsory education is not consistently available. As a result, many adolescents face difficulties in addressing sexual health issues, including managing risky behaviors both offline and online. Meanwhile, the incidence of sexually transmitted infections (STIs) and HIV/AIDS in China has been rising steadily since the 2000s (Ma et al. 2021).

More notable progress was made in the 2000s in adopting UNESCO's CSE guidelines, though full implementation is still far lagging. In 2022, China introduced its own adaptation of UNESCO's International Technical Guidance on Sexuality Education (ITGSE), tailored to align with local laws, policies, and cultural norms. This customized framework aims to deliver scientifically accurate, age-appropriate, and culturally sensitive sexuality education through an integrated approach within subjects such as physical education, biology, and ethics. China's adaptation primarily focuses on urgent issues such as unintended pregnancies, sexually transmitted infections (STIs), and youth violence. However, cultural and governmental resistance, particularly toward topics like sexual rights and gender diversity, continues to pose significant obstacles.

This resistance is exacerbated by the fact that over 64 percent of Chinese parents do not support CSE. Scholars argue that China lacks the necessary social backing to fully implement comprehensive sex education (Shi et al. 2022). In a country where education is tightly controlled by the government, the successful promotion of CSE relies on clear and consistent governmental endorsement. Unfortunately, such strong and sustained support for CSE is still lacking (Liu et al. 2023).

Similar to China, the promotion and implementation of CSE in Japan is strongly shaped by political conservatism and deeply entrenched Confucian values that influence societal norms. The conservative Liberal Democratic Party (LDP), which has dominated Japanese politics for decades, has consistently opposed progressive reforms in sex education. Many conservatives perceive CSE as a challenge to traditional family structures and values, leading to significant political resistance against including topics such as sexual consent, gender diversity, and explicit discussions about sexual intercourse.

A striking example of this resistance is the 2003 controversy at Nanao Special Needs School, where teachers faced criticism for using anatomically correct dolls to teach human reproduction. Conservative groups deemed the methods inappropriate, sparking public backlash and creating a climate of caution among educators. This incident has discouraged many teachers from providing comprehensive sex education, particularly on sensitive topics such as sexual rights and gender diversity, out of concern for potential political or social repercussions (Harel et al. 2024; Ishiwata 2011).

The Confucian value system, which emphasizes social harmony, respect for authority, and the primacy of the family unit, significantly influences Japan's approach to CSE. Its focus on modesty and propriety limits open discussions about sexuality in public and educational settings. This influence is evident in the preference for terms such as "purity education" or "puberty education" over "sex education," mirroring earlier practices in China. As a result, sexual health education in school curricula remains constrained (Harel et al. 2024). Studies suggest that Confucian ideals prioritizing family cohesion and social order often promote a conservative, abstinence-focused approach to sex education rather than one centered on sexual rights or individual autonomy (Noguchi et al. 2024).

Parental attitudes toward CSE in Japan are mixed. While some parents in urban and liberal areas support comprehensive sex education, many remain cautious, viewing CSE as unsuitable for younger children. These parents often prefer a risk-avoidance model focused on preventing sexually transmitted diseases (STDs) and unintended pregnancies (JHPN 2017). Unlike China's selective integration of UNESCO's CSE guidelines with family planning policies, Japan's approach is more fragmented. This inconsistency has resulted in uneven implementation of CSE across regions, with local practices heavily influenced by traditional values and political climates (Noguchi et al. 2024).

The situation of CSE in Korea shares many similarities with that in China and Japan, rooted in traditional ideologies. CSE in Korea faces cultural stigma, inconsistent implementation, and resistance to open discussions about sexuality. Many teenagers report feeling embarrassed about purchasing condoms, reflecting societal disapproval of minors engaging with sexual matters. In some cases, stores even refuse to sell condoms to minors. A 2021 survey revealed that 34.5 percent of sexually active middle and high school students reported inconsistent or no use of birth control, while only 67.8 percent of students received any sex education that year—a decline from 78.6 percent in 2018 (UNESCO 2023; Shin 2023).

Sex education in Korea often consists of vague lessons, with teachers avoiding sensitive topics. One teacher noted that while textbooks explain how eggs meet sperm to result in pregnancy, they omit details on how that process occurs. Although the Ministry of Education recommends fifteen hours of sex education annually, it is not mandatory in the official curriculum, and schools often prioritize other academic subjects, such as math. Teachers who attempt to provide more detailed sex education frequently face backlash from parents (Shin 2023).

In conservative societies like China, Japan, and Korea, cultural resistance to CSE remains strong due to traditional values that remain unquestioned and political conservatism. However, from a broader perspective, there is a growing consent that tailoring content to local norms, and emphasizing health, human rights, and gender equality can help shift attitudes. Most educators agree that reframing CSE as a tool to safeguard youth health could lead to its gradual acceptance.

Further Reading

Gao, Ersheng, Xiayun Zuo, Li Wang, Chaohua Lou, Yan Cheng, and Laurie S. Zabin. 2012. "How Does Traditional Confucian Culture Influence Adolescents' Sexual Behavior in Three Asian Cities?" *Journal of Adolescent Health, 50*(3): S12–S17. doi: 10.1016/j.jadohealth.2011.12.002.

Harel, Sinai, and Beverley Anne Yamamoto. 2024. "Comprehensive Horizons: Examining Japan's National and Regional Sexuality Education Curricula." *Sex Education, 25*(2). doi: 10.1080/14681811.2024.2320399.

Ishiwata, Chieko. 2011. "Sexual Health Education for School Children in Japan: The Timing and Contents." *Journal of the Japan Medical Association, 54*(3): 155–60. https://www.med.or.jp/english/activities/pdf/2011_03/155_160.pdf.

Japan Health Policy Now (JHPN). 2017. "Women's Health: Best Practices in Sex Education Implemented by Local Governments." *JHPN*. https://japanhpn.org/en/wh-1-3-2-2/.

Liu, Wenli, Jiayang Li, Hongyan Li, and Haoran Zheng. 2023. "Adaptation of Global Standards of Comprehensive Sexuality Education in China: Characteristics, Discussions, and Expectations." *Children*, *10*(2): 409. doi: https://doi.org/10.3390/children10020409.

Ma, Xing, Yuanyuan Yang, Ka Ming Chow, and Yuli Zhang. 2021. "Chinese Adolescents' Sexual and Reproductive Health Education: A Quasi-Experimental Study." *Public Health Nursing, 39*(1): 116–25. doi: 10.1111/phn.12914.

Noguchi, Takako, Mieko Tashiro, Yoshimi Marui, Shuhei Horikawa, and Iryna Zablotska-Manos. 2024. "Initiation and Delivery of Comprehensive Sexuality Education in Japanese Schools." *Sex Education*, August: 1–19. doi: 10.1080/14681811.2024.2368022.

Qin, Qian, and Jiali Zhang. 2023. "Sex Education in China: Actors and Dynamics of China's Policies and Practices, Cogent Education." *10*(2): 2270289. doi: 10.1080/2331186X.2023.2270289.

Shi, Wen, Yuxuan Lin, Zihan Zhang, and Jing Su. 2022. "Gender Differences in Sex Education in China: A Structural Topic Modeling Analysis Based on Online Knowledge Community." *Zhihu*. Children 2022, *9*: 615. doi: https://doi.org/10.3390/children9050615.

Shin, Min-Hee. 2023. "Why Is Sex Still a Taboo Subject in Korea." *Korea JoongAng Daily*. June 24. https://koreajoongangdaily.joins.com/2023/06/24/why/why-sex-education-nadaum/20230624070009147.html.

UNESCO. 2018. "International Technical Guidance on Sexuality Education—An Evidence-based Approach." https://www.unfpa.org/publications/international-technical-guidance-sexuality-education.

UNESCO. 2023. "Republic of Korea—Comprehensive Sexuality Education." https://education-profiles.org/eastern-and-south-eastern-asia/republic-of-korea/~comprehensive-sexuality-education.

The Power of Words and the Stigma of Contagion

Throughout history, pandemics have often been accompanied by fear, misinformation, and the targeting of vulnerable communities. From the Black Plague in the fourteenth century—when Jewish communities were falsely accused of spreading disease—to more recent health crises, these patterns have resurfaced in various forms. During the Covid-19 pandemic, terms such as "China Virus" and "Wuhan Virus" circulated widely in public discourse and coincided with a noticeable rise in anti-Asian sentiment. These labels, though seemingly geographic in nature, often reinforced damaging stereotypes and contributed to social division. In response, members of Asian communities were seen protesting while holding signs that read "I am not a virus" (Mssari 2021; Brown 2020). Yet such expressions of solidarity were not always enough to halt the spread of stigma and fear.

For many Asian Americans, the discrimination experienced during the pandemic echoed a longer history of racial exclusion, including policies like the Chinese Exclusion Act of 1882 and racialized narratives such as the "yellow peril." These legacies resurfaced in modern contexts through renewed suspicion and scapegoating during a time of global uncertainty.

Pandemics tend to amplify existing societal tensions. In moments of crisis, the language used to describe disease can unintentionally link illnesses to specific geographic or ethnic groups, fostering misunderstanding and fear. Historical patterns suggest that during public health emergencies, communities already facing social or economic vulnerabilities may experience heightened scrutiny or marginalization. During the Covid-19 pandemic, this dynamic became visible in increased reports of verbal abuse, discrimination, and even physical violence against individuals of Asian descent.

Education plays a critical role in countering misinformation and prejudice during such times. By teaching historical context and promoting media literacy, societies can better resist fear-based narratives. According to a Pew Research Center study (Ruiz et al. 2023), the use of culturally or ethnically linked language during the pandemic correlated with a measurable rise in anti-Asian bias. These findings were reflected in government and nonprofit data: FBI statistics recorded a sharp increase in anti-Asian hate crimes—from 158 incidents in 2019 to 746 in 2021—while Stop AAPI Hate documented over 11,000 instances of harassment, bullying, and violence.

The scapegoating of minority or immigrant populations during health crises is not new. In 1849, Irish Catholic immigrants in New York's Five Points neighborhood were blamed for a cholera outbreak and suffered a disproportionate number of deaths due to overcrowded and unsanitary living conditions. During the 1892 typhus outbreak, Russian Jewish immigrants arriving at New York's port were quarantined in inadequate facilities, leading to dozens of deaths. In 1916, Italian immigrants were stigmatized during a polio outbreak and subjected to increased surveillance. African American communities bore a heavy burden during the tuberculosis epidemics of the late nineteenth and early twentieth centuries, yet public health efforts to address these disparities were often delayed.

Similar patterns emerged during the 1980s AIDS crisis, when LGBTQ+ individuals, Haitian immigrants, and intravenous drug users were often blamed and ostracized. These examples show how outbreaks can reveal—and sometimes intensify—existing social divisions.

Scientifically, viruses and pandemics do not discriminate; they transcend borders and affect people regardless of background. Framing a disease as the responsibility of a particular community distracts from the complex realities of disease transmission and prevention. It can also hinder public health efforts by undermining trust, dividing communities, and fostering resistance to cooperation.

In moments of fear, some rhetoric may reflect broader anxieties. When terms with geographic or ethnic references are repeatedly used, they can contribute to polarization rather than unity which is evidenced by data from Pew Research Center survey and many other sources (Ruiz et al. 2023; Kurilla 2021). Understanding the consequences can help foster resilience, informed decision-making, and compassion during times of crisis.

Rather than assigning blame, responses to pandemics benefit most from shared responsibility and collective resilience. Encouraging empathy, informed dialogue, and community cohesion helps societies meet public health challenges more effectively.

Ultimately, education remains a cornerstone of this resilience. When students learn the historical roots of stigma and the importance of inclusive, evidence-based discourse, they are better equipped to identify and reject harmful stereotypes. Teaching global citizenship and cultural understanding fosters solidarity and helps prepare future generations to navigate crises with compassion and integrity.

Further Reading

Bhanot, Dvya, Tushar Singh, Sunil K Verma, and Shivantika Sharad. 2021. "Stigma and Discrimination during COVID-19 Pandemic." https://pmc.ncbi.nlm.nih.gov/articles/PMC7874150/.

Brown, Robin Terry. 2020. "Educators Take a Stand against Coronavirus Racism." https://www.nea.org/nea-today/all-news-articles/educators-take-stand-against-coronavirus-racism.

Cohn, Samuel K. 2012. "Pandemics: Waves of Disease, Waves of Hate from the Plague of Athens to AIDS." *Historical Journal*, 85(230): 535–55. doi: 10.1111/j.1468-2281.2012.00603.x.

HealthMatch. 2022. "Pandemics: A History of Discrimination." *HealthMatch*. https://healthmatch.io/blog/pandemics-a-history-of-discrimination.

Kurilla, robin. 2021. "'Kung Flu'—The Dynamics of Fear, Popular culture, and Authenticity in the Anatomy of Populist Communication." *Frontiers*, 6: 2021. doi: https://doi.org/10.3389/fcomm.2021.624643.

Massari, Paul. 2021. "New Hate Old History – Harassment of Asians Is on the Rise in the U.S. It Has Deep Roots in the Country's Past." *Harvard Griffin GSAS News*. https://gsas.harvard.edu/news/new-hate-old-history.

Ozturk, Ayfer. 2021. "'Stigmatization Spreads Faster Than the Virus. Viruses Do Not Discriminate, and Neither Should We.' Combatting the Stigmatization Surrounding Coronavirus Disease (COVID-19) Pandemic." *Perspect Psychiatr Care*, 57(4): 2030–4. doi: 10.1111/ppc.12815.

Ruiz, Neil G., Carolyne Im, and Ziyao Tian. 2023. "Asian Americans and Discrimination during the COVID-19 Pandemic." https://www.pewresearch.org/race-and-ethnicity/2023/11/30/asian-americans-and-discrimination-during-the-covid-19-pandemic/.

Saeed, Fahimeh, Ronak Mihan, S. Zeinab Mousavi, Renate L. E. P. Reniers, Fatemeh Sadat Bateni, Rosa Alikhani, and S. Bentolhoda Mousavi. 2020. "A Narrative Review of Stigma Related to Infectious Disease Outbreaks: What Can Be Learned in the Face of the Covid-19 Pandemic?" *Frontiers in Psychiatry*, 11: 565919. doi: 10.3389/fpsyt.2020.565919. https://pmc.ncbi.nlm.nih.gov/articles/PMC7738431/.

Nutrition Education in Japan

A description of Japanese school lunch menus starts as follows:

> Don't expect to find pizza and pasta for lunch in Japanese schools. Instead, you'll find well-balanced meals with items from each major food group. You can typically expect to see a serving of rice, soup, salad, meat, or fish on a plate. Nearly every day, lunch is served alongside a bottle of milk. (Quintana 2022)

This description reflects the influence of Japan's nutrition education that has been developed for over forty years. In the 1980s, the influence of Westernization led to the popularization of Western foods in Japan, which brought about a rise in lifestyle-related diseases such as obesity and diabetes. The health problems prompted the Japanese government to take intervening actions. In early 2005, Ministry of Agriculture, Forestry and Fisheries (MAFF), established a comprehensive nutrition guideline, known as *Japanese Food Guide Spinning Top*, and in collaboration with other government branches made nutrition education (*Shokuiku*) a national priority. The Basic Law on *Shokuiku*, enacted in 2005, mandated nutrition education at every level of society, particularly in schools. The law emphasizes balanced nutrition, appreciation for traditional Japanese cuisine, and fostering lifelong healthy habits to combat the rise of health issues linked to poor dietary choices.

Can Education Help People Lose Weight?

Obesity is a complex condition often misunderstood as simply a result of lacking willpower or personal discipline in diet and exercise. Many researchers are exploring other factors, such as knowledge and education, as significant predictors in tackling obesity. Statistics indicate that obesity in the United States rose from 30.5 percent to 42.4 percent over the twenty-year period between 1999 and 2018. Associated health risks, such as cardiovascular disease, type 2 diabetes, and premature death, disproportionately affect racial minorities and individuals with lower socioeconomic status (SES). For instance, obesity prevalence is notably higher among non-Hispanic Black adults and Hispanics up to nearly 50 percent and 45 percent, respectively, according to the CDC.

A 2021 study by Lando and colleagues surveyed 2,171 U.S. adults from varied age, race, and SES backgrounds. Results indicated that one in three participants could not accurately estimate their daily calorie needs, and nearly half lacked confidence in their ability to do so. Moreover, the lack of calorie confidence and BMI was inversely related. Those who were overweight or obese reported lower confidence in their calorie knowledge.

These findings suggest that by improving knowledge of caloric intake, public health programs could better support high-risk populations in achieving and maintaining healthier weights.

Further Reading

Centers for Disease Control and Prevention (CDC). 2024. "New CDC Data Show Adult Obesity Prevalence Remains High." https://www.cdc.gov/media/releases/2024/p0912-adult-obesity.html.

Lando, Amy M., Martine S. Ferguson, Linda Verrill, Fanfan Wu, Olivia E. Jones-Dominic, Cecile Punzalan, and Beverly J. Wolpert. 2021. "Health Disparities in Calorie Knowledge and Confidence among the U.S. Adult Population." *Journal of Primary Care & Community Health*, 12: 21501327211002416. doi: 10.1177/21501327211002416.

The *Japanese Food Guide Spinning Top* (Food Guide) is modeled after a traditional Japanese toy and serves as a visual representation of dietary recommendations. It is designed as a rotating inverted cone, divided into layers that depict food groups in cooked form or as dishes. These layers are arranged according to the recommended daily servings. At the top are grain-based dishes like rice, bread, noodles, followed by vegetable-based dishes, including salads, cooked vegetables, and soups. Next come dishes with fish, eggs, and meat, while milk and fruit are placed at the bottom. A running figure at the top of the spinning top symbolizes the importance of physical activity for maintaining good health. The Food Guide also advises consuming plenty of water and tea, and recommends moderating the intake of highly processed snacks, confectionery, and sugar-sweetened beverages.

In addition to promoting a balanced diet, *Shokuiku* emphasizes the integration of traditional and locally sourced foods, which is admittedly a key factor in Japan's remarkable longevity which stands as the highest in the world. This longevity is often attributed to the traditional Japanese diet (*washoku*), which is rich in vegetables, fish, and fermented foods like miso and pickles (Wilcox et al. 2007).

Shokuiku encourages not only healthy eating but also a deep appreciation for the natural world that supports food production. It teaches people to value the efforts of those who grow, harvest, deliver, and prepare the food on the table, fostering gratitude and mindfulness. Additionally, *Shokuiku* promotes responsible consumption by advising against food waste.

Shokuiku is not just about diet, it also carries recommendations for eating behavior that enhance social and mental well-being. It advocates, for instance, for the practice of eating together, emphasizing that communal meals foster togetherness, strengthen relationships, and improve mental health. *Shokuiku* teaches that shared meals are not only a time to nourish the body but also an opportunity to build social bonds and reinforce a sense of community (MAFF 2012).

In promoting *Shokuiku*, every member of Japanese society contributes their efforts. At the government level, the Japanese government actively promotes the Food Guide through national media, including television, magazine ads, web pages, public service announcements, and through distribution of pamphlets, posters, diet self-check sheets, and hand straps for cell phones in public places. Supermarkets, convenience stores, restaurants, and similar vendors are seen as ideal venues for providing information about the Food Guide.

In schools, school lunch programs diligently follow the Food Guide and *Shokuiku*-promoted principles. Japanese school lunch menus feature items from all major food groups. Common foods include grilled fish, fried rice with vegetables, and various soups like miso wakame and tofu seaweed soup. Teachers encourage students to finish everything on their plates. Students participate in the lunch process by serving meals on a rotating duty schedule.

They wear aprons, caps, and masks, and are responsible for setting up and serving lunch in the classroom, as schools typically lack cafeterias. This system is intended to foster responsibility and appreciation. For students not on lunch duty, the routine involves preparing the eating area by pushing tables together and setting out placemats. After receiving their meals, everyone says *itadakimasu* ("I humbly receive"), and students, as a group, plan and distribute leftovers, reinforcing the importance of portion control and avoiding food waste (Quintana 2022).

Reports comparing Japanese and American school lunches highlight several interesting differences (Korteman 2022; Quitana 2022; Tokyo Restaurant Guide 2024; Mortazavi 2014):

In menu composition, Japanese lunches focus on traditional foods like rice, noodles, fish, and vegetables, with seasonal ingredients and desserts reserved for special occasions. In contrast, American lunches often feature processed options like pizza, burgers, or pasta, alongside raw vegetables and fruit, with snacks like chips or cookies being common. Healthier options are sometimes rejected by students.

Regarding the nutritional approach, Japanese lunches are part of a broader educational initiative (*Shokuiku*), emphasizing balanced nutrition and the inclusion of vegetables in almost every dish. American lunches, though regulated, still contain processed, high-calorie foods, and efforts to promote healthier choices face resistance.

In terms of attitude toward food, the Japanese concept of *mottainai* which stresses that everything has intrinsic value and wastefulness is shameful encourages students to finish their meals. In the United States, students are more likely to throw away uneaten food, with less concern on waste reduction.

In student involvement, Japanese students take turns serving lunch, fostering responsibility. Some U.S. schools engage students through gardening or cooking initiatives, though this is less common.

When making comparisons, it's important to recognize the cultural context that shapes the acquired insights from global experiences, some analysts suggest. Food traditions, such as how food is prepared, served, and consumed, are deeply tied to cultural identity and shared history. The American school lunch system, as many perceive it, emphasizes cultural diversity and inclusion regarding food and eating habits. The key point is that this focus on diversity keeps the American school lunch system open, rather than closed, to global influences (Mortazavi 2014).

The *Shokuiku* initiative demonstrates Japan's commitment to nutrition education by integrating healthy eating habits with cultural values, sustainability, and social responsibility. This comprehensive approach enjoys broad participation from both the national government and local communities in Japan, and offers much for the global community to learn.

Further Reading

Japan Ministry of Agriculture Forestry and Fisheries. "What Is Shokuiku (Food Education)?" https://www.maff.go.jp/e/pdf/shokuiku.pdf.

Kisaki, Yukiko. 2023. "Japanese Eating Habits and Dietary Guide." https://wawaza.com/blogs/japanese-eating-habits-and-dietary-guide/?srsltid=AfmBOoq0AQxiTOr_oIWC5Mqn1wj_yqwk6cwWTbPO7kL6QnK15INUi8iA. Accessed September 2, 2024.

Korteman, Jessica. 2022. "Japanese School Lunch: Why It's Awesome and One Reason It's Not." *Japanese Food Guide*. https://www.japanesefoodguide.com/japanese-school-lunch/. Accessed September 2, 2024.

Ministry of Agriculture, Forestry and Fisheries (MAFF). 2016. https://www.maff.go.jp/e/policies/tech_res/shokuiku.html.

Ministry of Agriculture, Forestry and Fisheries (MAFF). 2005. "Japanese Food Guide Spinning Top." https://www.maff.go.jp/e/policies/tech_res/shokuiku.html.

Ministry of Agriculture, Forestry and Fisheries (MAFF). 2012. "A Guide to Shokuiku." https://www.maff.go.jp/j/syokuiku/guide/pdf/00_en_guide.pdf.

Ministry of Agriculture, Forestry and Fisheries (MAFF). 2015. "Basic Act on Shokuiku." https://www.maff.go.jp/e/policies/tech_res/attach/pdf/shokuiku-19.pdf.

Mortazavi, Melissa. 2014. "Consuming Identities Law, School Lunches, and What It Means to Be American." *Cornell Journal of Law and Public Policy*, 24(1), Article 1. https://papers.ssrn.com/sol3/papers.cfm?abstract_id=2836289.

Nakamura, Teiji. 2011. "Nutritional Policies and Dietary Guidelines in Japan." *Asia Pacific Journal of Clinical Nutrition*, 20(3): 452–4. https://pubmed.ncbi.nlm.nih.gov/21859666/.

Quintana, Krystina. 2022. "What's for Lunch in Japanese Schools?" *Bokksu*. https://www.bokksu.com/blogs/news/lunch-in-japanese-schools.

Tokyo Restaurants Guide. Undated. "Japanese and American School Lunch: Contents and Culture." https://restaurants-guide.tokyo/column/japanese-and-american-school-lunch-contents-and-culture/. September Accessed 20, 2024.

Willcox, Bradley J., D. Craig Willcox, Hidemi Todoriki, Akira Fujiyoshi, Katsuhiko Yano, Qimei He, J. David Curb, and Makoto Suzuki. 2007. "Caloric Restriction, The Traditional Okinawan Diet, and Healthy Aging: The Diet of the World's Longest-Lived People and Its Potential Impact on Morbidity and Life Span." *Annals of the New York Academy of Sciences*, 1114(1): 434–55. doi: https://doi.org/10.1196/annals.1396.037.

Promoting Health Education in Africa through Artistic Forms

Africa bears a disproportionate share of the global disease impact, encompassing both infectious and non-communicable diseases (NCDs). Despite accounting for less than 20 percent of the world's population, Africa is responsible for 25 percent of the global disease burden. For example, in 2020, 94 percent of the world's malaria cases occurred in Africa, resulting in over 200 million cases. The continent also faces rampant diseases such as tuberculosis, HIV/AIDS, and zoonotic illnesses including Ebola, Lassa fever, and mpox. In addition to these infectious diseases, NCDs such as diabetes, hypertension, cardiovascular diseases, and cancers are on the rise. The World Health Organization (WHO) anticipates that, by 2030, NCDs are expected to account for 46 percent of all deaths in Africa (Niohuru et al. 2023).

Africa's public health struggle is further exacerbated by socioeconomic conditions, lifestyle changes, and low health literacy. With increasing urbanization, many Africans have adopted more sedentary lifestyles and unhealthy dietary habits. The consumption of processed, high-fat, and sugary foods has contributed to the growing prevalence of NCDs. Poverty remains a major driver of disease across the continent. Limited access to health care, clean water, and sanitation makes people more vulnerable to infectious diseases. Additionally, individuals in lower socioeconomic brackets often lack the resources and knowledge needed to prevent or manage these diseases. A significant portion of the population is unaware of preventive measures and available treatment options. Misinformation, cultural misconceptions, and linguistic barriers further complicate disease control efforts, making health interventions even more challenging (Niohuru et al. 2023).

While solutions from various perspectives are needed to address these challenges, experts believe health education plays a vital role in improving medical knowledge and fostering healthier lifestyles. Health literacy, the ability to access, understand, and use health information, is simply crucial for better health outcomes. A study by McClintock et al. (2020) conducted across fourteen sub-Saharan African countries revealed widespread health literacy deficiencies. The study found that 64.23 percent of participants had low health literacy, with many unable to engage with or comprehend essential health information. The study also revealed significant disparities in health literacy where less than 10 percent of individuals with less than a primary education exhibiting high health literacy, compared to more than 80 percent of those with a secondary education.

Their study also shows that health literacy levels varied greatly between countries, ranging from 8.51 percent in Niger to 63.89 percent in Namibia, indicating a broad discrepancy across Africa. The study identified key predictors of low health literacy, including limited education, rural residency, poverty, and restricted access to health care resources. People in rural areas are less likely to receive health information or services, simply because poverty bars access to education and health programs (McClintock et al. 2020).

To promote health education, many experts advocate for greater involvement of African youth in health programs, events, and research. Training and empowering young people to participate in public health initiatives can lead to innovative solutions and create a skilled workforce dedicated to improving health care outcomes. It is expected that peer-led health education can ensure that local challenges are addressed (Adebisi et al. 2024).

Political factors also play a crucial role in the effectiveness of health interventions. Researchers emphasize the importance of global health diplomacy to secure funding and strengthen health care systems across Africa. Governments must prioritize health education and health literacy within national health strategies. By raising public awareness and investing in health literacy programs, governments can promote disease prevention and healthier lifestyles. Incorporating health education into political planning can empower citizens to advocate for better health care policies and hold their governments accountable for health outcomes (Chattu et al. 2021).

A study by Bunn et al. (2020) shows that a promising approach for improving health literacy is the use of arts-based methods. These culturally relevant strategies have proven effective in reaching diverse populations across Africa, especially in communities with low literacy levels. Art forms such as storytelling, music, theater, and visual arts resonate deeply with African cultural traditions and are accessible to people of all ages and social backgrounds. In many communities, oral traditions are central to daily life, making these art forms ideal for delivering important health messages.

Arts-based approaches have demonstrated a potential to foster collective engagement, encouraging open discussions about health issues without stigma. For instance, public theater performances addressing HIV/AIDS and malaria can help dispel myths and encourage preventive actions. The following examples serve to demonstrate the effectiveness of arts-based interventions in Africa.:

Theater in South Africa: The "Soul City" series used drama to educate communities about HIV/AIDS prevention, testing, and safe sexual practices, resulting in a 172 percent increase in voluntary HIV testing in some areas.

Music in West Africa: During the Ebola outbreak, local musicians in Sierra Leone and Liberia composed songs that educated the public on preventing the virus' spread. These songs, broadcast on the radio, reached remote regions where traditional health campaigns had limited impact.

Storytelling in Nigeria: Traditional storytelling was employed to educate communities about malaria prevention, incorporating health messages into familiar tales that emphasized the importance of using bed nets and eliminating mosquito breeding grounds.

Visual Arts in Kenya: Murals and posters promoting family planning and reproductive health were displayed in public spaces, helping to raise awareness and encourage community discussions.

However, it has been observed that arts-based interventions may not always achieve the desired outcomes. Cultural sensitivity is essential, and if the health messages are too complex or the chosen art form does not resonate with the community, the impact may be limited. Additionally, logistical challenges such as insufficient funding or lack of access to platforms can hinder the reach of these initiatives. Without community involvement in the design and execution of the projects, the interventions may fail to address local needs and values effectively (Bunn et al. 2020).

Developing health education in Africa requires an integrated approach to addressing the continent's unique challenges. Health literacy is a critical tool for empowering individuals to make informed decisions about their well-being. Arts-based approaches have offered innovative and culturally relevant methods for promoting health literacy. By combining these methods with formal education strategies, engaging youth, and addressing political challenges, experts believe, African countries can make significant strides in reducing their disease burden and improving public health outcomes.

Further Reading

Adamu, Amanu A., Sewdie Birhanu, and Ameyu Godesso. 2023. "Health Literacy among Young People in Africa: Evidence Synthesis." *Risk Management and Healthcare Policy,* 16: 425–37. doi: 10.2147/RMHP.S399196.

Adebisi, Yusuff Adebayo, Nafisat Dasola Jimoh, Archibong Edem Bassey, et al. 2024. "Harnessing the Potential of African Youth for Transforming Health Research in Africa." *Global Health,* 20: 35. doi: 10.1186/s12992-024-01039-7.

Bunn, Christopher, Chisomo Kalinga, Otiyela Mtema, et al. 2020. "Arts-Based Approaches to Promoting Health in Sub-Saharan Africa: A Scoping Review." *BMJ Global Health,* 5(5): e001987. doi: https://doi.org/10.1136/bmjgh-2019-001987.

Chattu, Vijay Kumar, W. Andy Knight, Anil Adisesh, et al. 2021. "Politics of Disease Control in Africa and the Critical Role of Global Health Diplomacy: A Systematic Review." *Health Promot Perspect*. February 7, 2021, *11*(1): 20–31. doi: 10.34172/hpp.2021.04. PMID: 33758752; PMCID: PMC7967135.

McClintock, Heather F., Julia M. Alber, Sarah J. Schrauben, Carmella M. Mazzola, and Douglas J. Wiebe. 2020. "Constructing A Measure of Health Literacy in Sub-Saharan African Countries." *Health Promotion International*, *35*(5): 907–15. doi: https://doi.org/10.1093/heapro/daz078

Niohuru, Ilha. 2023. "Disease Burden and Mortality. In: Healthcare and Disease Burden in Africa." SpringerBriefs in Economics. Springer, Cham. https://doi.org/10.1007/978-3-031-19719-2_3.

Health Care Systems and Public Health

China's Health Care System—Challenges and Opportunities

Since the launch of economic reforms in the late 1970s, China has achieved significant success in economic growth. It is encouraging that China's health care provision has also made strides alongside the improvement of living standard. However, it is also apparent that China's health care system has much room for improvement, particularly in providing quality and affordable care, and in providing standardized professional and ethical training.

In the 1950s, China's public health care system was entirely managed by the government, with a primary focus on controlling the prevalence of infectious diseases such as tuberculosis, schistosomiasis, and leprosy. During the 1960s and 1970s, Patriotic Health Campaigns effectively targeted rodents, insect vectors, and contaminated drinking water. These initiatives were particularly impactful in rural areas, leading to a significant reduction in diseases such as encephalomyelitis, malaria, measles, and typhoid, while also improving life expectancy.

The health care workforce at the time mainly comprised "barefoot doctors," who received only basic medical training. However, with the onset of economic reforms in 1978, government funding for hospitals was drastically reduced to about 10 percent of previous levels, where it remains today. One of the key effects of marketization was its impact on the health care delivery system.

As of 2017, China had relied on a three-tiered delivery system, spanning rural villages, municipal health care networks, and urban community health care systems. This health care structure, which required patients to first seek care at the local level, became unsustainable due to funding cutbacks. Hospitals were forced to shift the financial burden onto patients, and without effective insurance coverage, rising medical costs rendered health care increasingly unaffordable for a growing portion of the population (Wang et al. 2019).

The current two-part Basic Medical Insurance (BMI) system aims to reduce the financial burden of health care costs. Within this framework, the Employee Basic Medical Insurance (EBMI) program covers 337 million urban employees and is funded through payroll taxes shared by employees and employers, with mandatory enrollment. Meanwhile, the Residents Basic Medical Insurance (RBMI) program, which is voluntary, provides coverage for 1.014 billion individuals, including rural residents and non-working urban residents.

Together, the BMI system covers over 1.35 billion people, accounting for approximately 95 percent of the population. However, this still leaves 5 percent of the population without any health coverage. Despite health care expenditures amounting to 6.6 percent of GDP in 2018—a commendable level considering the size of the population and disparities between provinces—the BMI system remains inadequate. A drawback is that the coverage is thin and out-of-pocket payments are high. High expense thresholds for qualification and the exclusion of long-term care are key limitations. As high as 38 percent of health care expenses are paid out-of-pocket, covering costs such as long-term care, medications, and procedures not included in the approved formulary (Fang 2020).

Experts point to several challenges underlying China's public health care system, including a lack of trust, corruption, and insufficient training for medical providers. Many stem from the unaffordable costs.

The growing mistrust patients feel toward doctors reflects a deteriorating relationship between the two groups and contributes to a broader sense of dissatisfaction in China. Doctors are often perceived as professionals who prioritize financial gain over patient care, frequently being labeled as unethical. This perception has, in some cases, escalated to acts of violence against medical practitioners. A researcher describes this situation as an "ethical dilemma." As Hu (2021) explains, "Patients and their families often respond with suspicion to recommendations for relatively new therapies or drugs, questioning whether the doctors' motivations are financially driven rather than aimed at the patients' best interests."

Medical providers are facing criticism for prioritizing interests other than patient care during treatment. An article points out that doctors do not receive appropriate incentives to ensure the provision of high-quality care, as evidenced by instances of irrelevant drug prescriptions. The article reveals that hospitals are known to inflate drug prices for profit, which leads to patients being overcharged through improper treatment or overmedication, a practice that is "widely observed," according to Zhang (2021).

Some scholars attribute the root of corruption in China's health care system to the country's economic transition and poorly managed regulatory framework. During the era of government-subsidized health care, strict regulatory controls and rigorous accounting procedures left little room for hospitals and doctors to seek personal profit. However, when China's health care system was exposed to market competition, hospitals began prioritizing profit over patient care.

Doctor performance evaluations shifted to focus on metrics such as revenue generated from prescription drugs, bed turnover rates, and the profitability of prescribed medical procedures. Financial incentives, such as awards for revenue generation, often doubled or tripled a doctor's base salary. Meanwhile, the quality of medical care provided by doctors became undervalued.

It has become widely recognized that hospitals often act as sales outlets for drug manufacturers, who incentivize doctors with kickbacks or "grey pay." In this scenario, the real losers are the patients, who often lack the expertise to discern whether the care they receive is appropriate or in their best interest (Hu 2021).

Studies indicate a rise in medical disputes as corruption worsens within the health care system. An analysis of 156 medical dispute cases filed by patients revealed that the overwhelming majority stemmed from deficient medical services. These deficiencies included insufficient examinations, technical errors such as intestinal injuries caused by accidental endoscopy operations, and inadequate diagnoses. Approximately less than half of the disputes were attributed to patient-related factors, such as unmet medical expectations and disruptive behavior. Poor communication between doctors and patients, along with instances of medical disturbance, accounted for approximately one-tenth of the disputes. Additionally, a significant number of conflicts arose from high medical bills (Luo et al. 2022).

Another study found that medical disputes in China increased by 3 percent nationwide from 2019 to 2020. During the same period, Shanghai saw an 11 percent rise in medical disputes, signaling that such conflicts had become a major challenge for the health care system. The study reported that in a tertiary public hospital in Suzhou, approximately 60 percent of disputes were attributed to factors related to health care providers, including communication failures, medical errors, and issues with provider attitudes. Meanwhile, 35 percent of disputes stemmed from patient-related factors, such as unmet expectations and a lack of understanding of doctors and treatment procedures (Wang 2021).

Various initiatives have been proposed to address corruption and create effective solutions. Among these, recommendations include enhancing the training of medical personnel by adopting practices from the American system in areas such as accreditation, management, evaluation, and financial remuneration for doctors (Cui and Wang 2016).

The Chinese government's portal, Xinhua.net, attributes the shortcomings in the health care safety net to resistance toward insurance participation, uneven regional development leading to demographic disparities between wealthier and poorer provinces, and the country's slowing economy. The government advocates for strengthening systematic, top-level planning to reduce discrepancies in practices caused by market dynamics (Xinhua.net 2016).

In 2023, multiple provinces responded to the government's call by initiating crackdowns on medical corruption, employing Mao-era mass campaign tactics. However, experts argue that relying solely on government-led anti-corruption campaigns is unlikely to effectively control corruption or build a robust health care system. Critics also highlight government decisions during the Covid-19 pandemic, such as mandating routine antigen testing and facilitating the mass production of nucleic acid reagents, which allegedly became breeding grounds for corruption (Huang 2023).

Studies suggest that reforms in at least three key areas could bring about noticeable improvements in China's health care system. First, the system must prioritize protecting the poor and rural populations by developing an effective primary care structure. Achieving this requires the government to increase support for training competent medical professionals who can deliver high-quality primary care. Second, a robust monitoring and evaluation system must be implemented to uphold moral and professional standards. Finally, transparency in medical financing is essential. The detrimental influence of drug companies, particularly their practice of inflating drug prices for profit, must be curtailed to safeguard public health (Meng 2019).

Further Reading

Bradsher, Keith. 2023. "How Health Insurance Works in China, and How It's Changing." *New York Times*. https://www.nytimes.com/2023/02/23/business/china-health-insurance-explained.html.

Cui, Yong, and Tianyou Wang. 2016. "From the Residency Training in the United States to See the Challenges and Directions of China Residency Standardized Training." *Chinese Journal of Lung Cancer*, June 2016, *19*(6): 321–7. doi: 10.3779/j.issn.1009-3419.2016.06.03.

Fang, Hai. 2020. "China." *The Commonwealth Fund*. https://www.commonwealthfund.org/international-health-policy-center/countries/china.

Hu, Qimin. 2021. "How Doctors Are Entangled with 'Immorality.'" *Sciencenet.cn*. https://news.sciencenet.cn/htmlnews/2021/5/457126.shtm. Accessed October 7, 2023.

Huang, Yangzhong. 2023. "Anti-corruption Campaign in China's Medical Sector: Unmasking the Hidden Agenda." *Council on Foreign Relations*. https://www.cfr.org/blog/anti-corruption-campaign-chinas-medical-sector-unmasking-hidden-agenda.

Jourdan, Adam. 2016. "Scapled: At China's Creaking Hospitals, Illegal Ticket Touts Defy Crackdown." *Reuters*. https://www.reuters.com/article/us-china-healthcare-scalpers-idUSKCN0X82O1.

Luo, Yong, Pu Chuan, Liu Yiting, Peng Yongsong, and Pi Xing. 2022. "Analysis of Medical Disputes and Solutions." *Healthcare Economy Research*, *39*(12). doi: 10.14055/j.cnki.33-1056/f.2022.12.018.

Meng, Qingyue, Anne Mills, Longde Wang, and Qide Han. 2019. "What Can We Learn from China's Health System Reform?" *BMJ*. doi: https://doi.org/10.1136/bmj.l2349.

Wang, Li, Zhihao Wang, Qinglian Ma, Guixia Fang, and Jinxia Yang. 2019. "The Development and Reform of Public Health in China from 1949 to 2019." *Globalization and Health, 15*: 45. https://doi.org/10.1186/s12992-019-0486-6.

Wang, Ying. 2021. "A Study on Medical Disputes Related to Service Quality and Strategies of Solution." *Jiangsu Medical Management*, *32*(12): 1595–8.

Xinhuanet. 2016. "China's Social Safety Net Faces Four Problems and Five Challenges." *Xinhuanet.com*. http://www.xinhuanet.com/politics/2016-02/17/c_128726709.htm. Accessed October 7, 2023.

Zhang, Yu. 2021. "Identifying the Greatest Shortfall of China's Healthcare System and My Personal Suggestion for Healthcare Reform." *Zhihu*. https://zhuanlan.zhihu.com/p/374935597. Accessed October 14, 2023.

Health Care in Africa—Challenges and Opportunities

The health care situation in African countries, particularly in sub-Saharan Africa, remains a critical global concern. According to the World Health Organization (WHO), the region accounts for 11–13 percent of the world's population, bears 24 percent of the global disease burden, yet has only 3 percent of the global health workforce and less than 1 percent of worldwide health expenditure. Communicable diseases, such as malaria, diarrheal diseases, and lower respiratory infections, remain widespread among both children and adults (WHO 2018).

While the global prevalence of HIV/AIDS has decreased to as low as 1 percent, Africa continues to experience an overall prevalence rate of 7 percent. Furthermore, non-communicable diseases, including diabetes, cardiovascular diseases, and stroke, have been on the rise across the continent (Azevedo 2017). In its 2018 report on the state of health in the African region, WHO highlights that health care accessibility across the region scored just 0.48, indicating that countries can provide only 48 percent of the health and related services their populations require.

The WHO report further indicates:

> The country scores in the Region range from a low of 0.31 to a high of 0.70. Only five countries in the Region have a score above 0.6: Namibia (0.62), Kenya (0.64), South Africa (0.66), Seychelles (0.68) and Algeria (0.70). Algeria, the country with the best score in the Region, is only able to provide 70% of the possible health and heal-related services needed by its population—a worrying situation. (WHO 2018:38)

Efforts in improving Africa's health care have been decades in the making. In 2007, the WHO proposed a framework for action, titled "Everybody's Business," aimed at revamping Africa's dysfunctional public health care. The framework carries six core components—service delivery, health workforce, information system, medical products, vaccines and technologies, sustainable financing and social protection, and leadership and governance (WHO 2007). Studies and surveys indicate that after more than a decade the goals of the component programs were unmet. The leading problems clustered in areas such as leadership and governance, health care financing, training and retaining health care workforce, and health care service delivery (Olerbie et al. 2019). In 2015, the United Nations (UN) adopted another, but more comprehensive framework this time, known as the Sustainable Development Goals (SDGs) with 169 targets encompassing poverty, health, education, and climate actions to be achieved by 2030. A recent study by the Institute for Security Studies indicates that, partly due to Covid-19 breakout in 2020, more Africans fell into extreme poverty, and the SDGs are unlikely to be met as expected (Aikins et al. 2022).

Factors that persistently hamper Africa from developing health care services in a systematic and reliable fashion have been studied in detail. The consensus appears to be that establishing effective public health care hinges on a wider range of economic and social conditions most of which are unfavorable in the African region. A top barrier is poverty. Low-income countries have the poorest access to health services; indebted governments tend to allocate the low priority to health care expenditure. Likewise, low-income individuals can't afford to take care of their health. As one article indicates, poverty and ill health go hand-in-hand: when 75 percent of Africans live on less than $2.00 a day and 46 percent on less than $1.08 a day, health care simply can't be a priority (Azevedo 2017).

However, a greater impediment is corruption and social unrest in African countries. While donations from international charities are a major bloodline of Africa's health cause, financial embezzlement is also endemic. Corrupt officials exploit weaknesses in governments and seek opportunities to benefit themselves. Lack of transparency in health funds' management has resulted in endless cases where funds for disease prevention and treatment are looted by corrupted officials for private use. An illustrative case is the 2019 case of embezzlement of FIFA's funding for Ebola prevention by a high-ranking executive committee member at the Confederation of African Football (Negley 2019). Corruption and social inequality are also a root cause of frequent wars that destroy health care infrastructure and threaten the lives of health care workers who carry out tasks such as vaccinations in conflict zones.

Low level of education is another factor that adversely affects health care efficacy in Africa. Basic hygienic behaviors, such as hand washing and utilization of sanitation services are key to disease prevention. However, lack of education on hygiene in economically distressed communities in Africa, often due to failure of local authorities, has been an important reason why diarrheal diseases remain a leading cause of mortality and morbidity among children. A study describes the lack of access to public toilets serves to reflect the crisis in public hygiene:

> Public toilets in the city are few and the municipalities either do not have the regulations on hygiene and sanitation or simply do not enforce them when they exist. Abidjan (capital of Ivory Coast) is said to be one of the most sanitary major cities, but the figures show that only 10–30% of its population is connected to standard sanitation facilities and with only 20–30% of the urban population having access to improved sanitary structures. Despite its many big rivers such as the Congo and myriad smaller ones, Kinshasa (capital of Democratic Republic of Congo) is also one of the filthiest cities in Africa. Accra, in Ghana, where one finds public signs saying "DO NOT URINATE AGAINST THE WALL," is not as bad in this respect, but it is an exception in West and Central Africa, which is seen as the worse region in sanitation on the continent. About 37% of the population of Ghana has no indoor toilet facilities, and in many areas, where there are latrines, no flush toilets exist or faucet water for people to wash their

hands. Where there are flush toilets, wastes are discharged into the household septic tank. (Azevedo 2017: 62–3)

Several barriers to health care development in Africa can be traced to external influences. The maladaptation of Western aid and globalization has been criticized for its adverse effects, as highlighted by the 2021 Africa Health Agenda International Conference Commission. For instance, the International Monetary Fund's (IMF) Structural Adjustment Programs (SAPs) have been widely condemned for their disruptive impact on the economies of borrowing countries.

Introduced in the 1980s, SAPs aimed to address high inflation, balance of payments deficits, and public debt in developing nations. These programs required countries to implement measures such as shifting from food crops to cash crops for export, abolishing government subsidies, reducing social sector funding, implementing large-scale layoffs, devaluing currency, liberalizing trade, and privatizing public enterprises. However, these policies often resulted in unemployment, heightened poverty, social unrest, riots, rampant inflation, and diminished national sovereignty.

In Kenya, the IMF's influence reportedly led to a hiring freeze in the public sector, including the health sector, along with the introduction of user fees. These measures contributed to the loss of a significant number of nurses and hindered the country's ability to implement effective health interventions. Similarly, in Ghana, efforts to establish community-based primary care were undermined by SAP-related policies, leaving primary care out of reach for many who needed it most (Singh 2022).

Globalization has been criticized as a double-edged sword. On one hand, globalization is recognized as enhancing interconnectivity between countries with respect to integration of health care services, exchange of medical information and products, transfer of skills, and jointly responding to challenges of health care sectors. On the other hand, globalization has facilitated health care professionals to move from poor countries to rich countries. When brain drain happens at a large scale, delivery of health services is negatively impacted (Nolen 2022).

Recognizing the challenges to developing modern health care systems in Africa paves the way for targeted efforts and opportunities. However, given the continent's encompassing challenges, the global community must be ready for sustained and long-term commitment to support Africa in achieving its health care goals, as meaningful change is unlikely to occur in the short term.

Further Reading

Africa Health Agenda International Conference Commission. 2021. "The State of Universal Health Coverage in Africa—Executive Summary Report of the Africa Health Agenda International Conference Commission." https://ahaic.org/download/executive-summary-the-state-of-universal-health-coverage-in-africa/.

Aikins, Enoch Randy, and Jacobus Du Toit McLachlan. 2022. "The Content Will Probably Miss the SDG Poverty Target, But the Right Policies Could Deliver Significant Reductions." *Institute for Security Studies*. https://issafrica.org/iss-today/africa-is-losing-the-battle-against-extreme-poverty.

Azevedo, Mario J. 2017. "The State of Health System(s) in Africa: Challenges and Opportunities." *Historical Perspectives on the State of Health and Health Systems in Africa*, II. 3 February, 2017: 1–73. doi: 10.1007/978-3-319-32564-4_1.

Negley, Cassandra. 2019. "FIFA Bans African Soccer Official 10 Years for Stealing Funds from Ebola Campaign." *Yahoo Sports*. https://sports.yahoo.com/fifa-bans-african-soccer-official-10-years-for-stealing-funds-from-ebola-campaign-182912725.html.

Nolen, Stephanie. 2022. "Rich Countries Lure Health Workers from Low-Income Nations to Fight Shortages." *The New York Times*. https://www.nytimes.com/2022/01/24/health/covid-health-worker-immigration.html.

Oleribe, Obinna O., Jenny Momoh, Benjamin S. C. Uzochukwu, Francisco Mbofana, Akin Adebiyi, Thomas Barbera, Roger Williams, and Simmon D. Taylor-Robinson. 2019. "Identifying Key Challenges Facing Healthcare Systems In Africa And Potential Solutions." *International Journal of General Medicine, 12*: 395–403. https://www.ncbi.nlm.nih.gov/pmc/articles/PMC6844097/.

Singh, Tanupriya. 2022. "Structural Adjustment by Any Other Name: International Financial Institutions and Health in Ghana and Kenya." *Peoples Dispatch*. https://peoplesdispatch.org/2022/11/05/structural-adjustment-by-any-other-name-international-financial-institutions-and-health-in-ghana-and-kenya/.

WHO. 2007. "Everybody's Business: Strengthening Health Systems to Improve Health Outcomes. WHO's Framework for Action." https://iris.who.int/bitstream/handle/10665/43918/9789241596077_eng.pdf?sequence=1.

WHO. 2018. "The State of Health in the WHO African Region." https://www.afro.who.int/sites/default/files/2018-08/State%20of%20health%20in%20the%20African%20Region.pdf.

WHO. 2017. "What Needs to Be Done to Solve the Shortage of Health Workers in the African Region." https://www.afro.who.int/news/what-needs-be-done-solve-shortage-health-workers-african-region.

Japan's Health Care System

Japan's health care system provides universal coverage for its citizens, with non-citizens also eligible if they meet specific criteria. The system is widely praised for its efficient management, where the government determines the costs of medical services. Japan has approximately 3,000 insurance funds divided into three main schemes: employer-based insurance, the residence-based National Health Insurance (NHI), and insurance for individuals aged seventy-five and older.

By law, Japanese hospitals and clinics operate as public and nonprofit entities. Privately owned clinics typically focus on elective and cosmetic procedures. Nursing care budgets are established by the forty-seven regional and municipal governments, with citizens over forty contributing 2 percent of their salary toward long-term care costs.

Over 90 percent of citizens and residents participate in the public health care system, enabling the government to cover 70 percent of medical expenses. Many also have secondary private insurance to cover supplementary services, such as orthodontics and the 30 percent co-pay not covered by the government. The NHI provides extensive coverage, particularly catering to the growing number of retirees and low-income individuals, according to Japan Health Policy Network (JHPN).

All residents of Japan are required to have health insurance, either through an employer-based plan or through a community-based scheme for the self-employed, unemployed, or retired. This universal coverage ensures access to a broad range of health care services with minimal out-of-pocket expenses. The cap on out-of-pocket costs is adjusted based on age and income levels, resulting in health care expenses that are relatively low compared to those in other developed countries.

Japan's health care system has several distinctive features, with a strong emphasis on preventive care and regular health checkups. This approach facilitates the early detection and treatment of diseases. The system is supported by an extensive network of hospitals and clinics, providing patients with high levels of access to health care providers.

One notable difference from other OECD countries is that Japanese patients typically bypass primary care triage and go directly to the specialist or doctor of their choice. While this can lead to longer wait times, most patients in Japan seem unbothered by the delays.

Another key distinction is the uniformity of benefit packages across insurance plans. Unlike in the United States, where benefits vary by plan, Japan's health care coverage includes hospital care, outpatient services, mental health care, prescription drugs, home health care, and dental services. Co-payments are standardized across all plans, with discounts available for children and seniors aged above seventy. Additionally, out-of-pocket expenses are capped based on age and income, offering robust financial protection (JHPN).

Controlling high drug prices is a significant challenge for health care systems in the United States and EU. In contrast, Japan's system benefits from the government's direct role in price determination, ensuring swift and universal market access for new medicines. Newly approved drugs in Japan typically receive a price within three months of regulatory approval, making it one of the fastest processes globally. In the United States, similar negotiations often take considerably longer. This rapid introduction of new medicines allows Japanese patients to access innovative treatments more quickly than in most other countries.

Once approved, drugs in Japan are reimbursed by the NHI, with patients paying minimal out-of-pocket costs. In the United States, however, out-of-pocket expenses vary significantly depending on individual insurance plans.

To maintain the sustainability of the NHI, Japan employs an aggressive repricing strategy to control drug costs. This includes measures such as mid-year repricing and market expansion repricing, allowing the government to regularly evaluate and adjust drug prices as new treatments become available. While effective in keeping costs manageable, these repricing strategies have drawn criticism from pharmaceutical companies for placing continuous pressure on their ability to innovate (Chen and Cheng 2023).

Japan's universal health coverage was established in the 1960s during a period of rapid industrialization and urbanization, which propelled the country to become the world's second-largest economy by 1968. Since then, successive governments have consistently expanded health care benefits, focusing on reducing out-of-pocket costs for low-income individuals and citizens aged sixty-five and older. This robust health care system has arguably contributed to Japan's aging population, making it the oldest country in Asia. However, this success has brought the significant challenge of managing the increasing economic burden required to sustain universal coverage.

The Long-Term Care Insurance (LTCI) system, introduced in 2000, for example, provides coverage for both home-based and institutional care for individuals over sixty-five, based on their assessed level of disability. Between 2000 and 2018, the number of LTCI users tripled from 1.49 million to

4.74 million, representing nearly 35 percent of Japan's population. Sustaining LTCI adds to Japan's economic burden.

At the same time, Japan's prolonged economic stagnation following the bubble economy collapse in the early 1990s has adversely affected employment. By 2018, health care spending had grown to be several times larger than expenditures on education, science, and technology. To address these financial pressures, the government increased the consumption tax to 10 percent in 2019, though this remains significantly lower than rates in OECD countries like Germany (19 percent) and France (19.6 percent) (Nakatani 2019; Matsuda 2019).

Whether Japan can successfully resolve population aging crisis will be critical to the country's future. Statistics shows a worrisome trend: between 1981 and 2016, the population of sixty-five years and older in Japan rose from 9.1 percent to 27.3 percent. The total fertility rate, however, decreased from 1.75 percent to 1.44 percent. An aging society means the number of households with elderly members is increasing. From 1971 to 2015, households with elderly couples increased from 13.1 to 31.1 percent. This means long-term care has become a major medical service that is broadly needed. Disease pattern has changed from predominately acute to chronic diseases. Today, the three major causes of death in Japan are cancer, heart diseases, and cerebrovascular diseases, account for 60 percent of all deaths (Matsuda 2019).

The Japanese government perceives population aging and decrease of working population as a persistent threat to future development of the country. To resolve these challenges, the Japanese government has initiated a number of changes which included expanding medical and nursing care support at the community level, training more medical providers specializing in chronic diseases, transforming service provisions to reduce acute care and increase care for chronic diseases, and preparing all prefectures to plan and transform services provisions ahead of 2025 when baby boomers become over seventy-five. Additionally, during Shinzo Abe's prime ministership (2012–20), Japan amended immigration policy to accept more care workers from foreign countries (Nakatani 2019).

Further Reading

Chen, Andrew, and Gary Cheng. 2023. "Drug Pricing in Japan: The Changing Landscape and Futures Prospects." *Health Advances*. https://healthadvances.com/insights/blog/drug-pricing-in-japan-the-changing-landscape-and-future-prospects.

JHPN. Undated. "Health Insurance System." https://japanhpn.org/en/hs1/.

Matsuda, S. 2009. "Health Insurance Scheme for the Aged in Japan—its outline and challenges." *Asian Pacific Journal of Disease Management*, 3(1): 1–9. https://www.jstage.jst.go.jp/article/apjdm/3/1/3_1_1/_pdf/-char/en.

Matsuda, Shinya. 2019. "Health Policy in Japan – Current Situation and Future Challenges." *JMA Journal*, 2(1): 1–10. doi: 10.31662/jmaj.2018-0016.

Ministry of Finance: Japanese Public Finance Fact Sheet—FY2016 Budget. https://www.mof.go.jp/english/budget/budget/fy2016/03.pdf.

Ministry of Health, Labour and Welfare: Comprehensive Survey on living conditions of the People on Health and Welfare 2015. https://www.mhlw.go.jp/toukei/saikin/hw/k-tyosa/k-tyosa15/index.html.

Ministry of Health, Labour and Welfare: Handbook of Health and Welfare Statistics. https://www.mhlw.go.jp/english/database/compendia.html.

Ministry of Internal Affairs and Communications, Statistics Bureau: Current Population Estimates as of October 1, 2017. http://www.stat.go.jp/english/data/jinsui/2017np/index.htm.

Nakatani, Hiroki. 2019. "Population Aging in Japan: Policy Transformation, Sustainable Development Goals, Universal Health Coverage, and Social Determinates of Health." *Global Health & Medicine*, 1(1): 3–10. doi: 10.35772/ghm.2019.01011.

National Institute of Population and Social Security Research: Population Statistics of Japan 2008. http://www.ipss.go.jp/p-info/e/psj2008/PSJ2008.pdf.

How Health Care Systems in the United States and Canada Address Their Challenges Differently

Health care systems in the United States and Canada both strive to provide quality care to their citizens and face the shared challenge of ensuring health care is accessible and affordable for everyone, including those who are underinsured or uninsured. Central to the issue are concerns about costs and wait times. However, due to historical and political differences, the approaches taken by the United States and Canada often vary significantly and are frequently the subject of heated debate.

Health care systems are path-dependent, meaning a country's approach to health care provision is heavily shaped by its historical context. In the United States, there is a strong tradition of private enterprise and market-driven solutions. Attempts to establish a more centralized, publicly funded system have often encountered substantial political resistance, as such measures are seen as opposing the principles of individual choice and free markets. Consequently, the U.S. health care system operates as a multi-payer system, relying primarily on employer-based insurance alongside federal programs

An Overview of Key Health Care Models

Health care systems worldwide can be categorized into four primary models, according to some analysts, each tailored to address specific medical needs and local conditions:

Beveridge Model:

Used in the UK, Spain, and New Zealand, health care is funded through taxes and provided as a public service. The government acts as the sole payer and employs many providers, keeping costs low and access universal. However, resource shortages and long wait times are common challenges.

Bismarck Model:

Adopted in Germany, Japan, and the Netherlands, this system is funded by payroll contributions from employers and employees. Services are delivered by private providers under government-regulated pricing. It promotes competition and reduces wait times but faces rising costs due to aging populations, limiting access for those unable to contribute.

National Health Insurance Model:

Implemented in Canada and South Korea, this model combines public insurance with private health care providers, reducing administrative costs. However, limited resources often result in long wait times for procedures like hip replacements, which can take months.

Out-of-Pocket Model:

Common in low-income countries, individuals pay directly for health care services. While immediate care is available for those who can afford it, many cannot, leading to significant health inequities. Even in countries with universal coverage, such as China, high out-of-pocket costs can impose severe financial burdens.

U.S. Hybrid Model:

The U.S. system blends private insurance, public programs (e.g., Medicare and Medicaid), and out-of-pocket payments. While it offers high-quality care for the insured, it is plagued by high costs, bureaucratic complexity, and millions of uninsured individuals, resulting in unequal access and stark health disparities.

Further Reading

Fang, Hai. 2020. "China." *The Commonwealth Fund*. https://www.commonwealthfund.org/international-health-policy-center/countries/china.

PPHR. 2017. "Health Care Reform: Learning from Other Major Health Care Systems." *Princeton Public Health Review*. https://pphr.princeton.edu/2017/12/02/unhealthy-health-care-a-cursory-overview-of-major-health-care-systems/.

Wallace, Lorraine. 2013. "A View of Health Care around the World." *Annals of Family Medicine, 11*(1): 84. doi: 10.1370/afm.1483.

like Medicare (for individuals aged sixty-five and older), Medicaid (for low-income individuals), and direct out-of-pocket payments (Emanuel 2020).

The U.S. health care system is considerably more complex than those of other countries. Private health insurance companies negotiate prices with hospitals and pharmaceutical companies, sell insurance policies directly to individuals or groups, and compete for customers. Government insurance programs, such as Medicare, Medicaid, and the Children's Health Insurance Program (CHIP), also negotiate their own deals. Unlike many other countries, the United States does not regulate drug prices; instead, the government grants monopolies to pharmaceutical companies through patents and exclusive marketing rights. This contributes to the United States accounting for nearly 50 percent of global pharmaceutical spending, not because Americans use more drugs, but because prices are significantly higher (Emanuel 2020).

Patients bear a substantial financial burden, including co-payments at the point of service, premiums, and deductibles that must be met before insurance coverage applies. Benefit packages vary widely depending on the employer. Despite this, approximately 15 percent of adults aged 18–64 lack any form of insurance coverage (Chiu 2020). Reports have highlighted instances of patients working multiple jobs to cover medical bills and health care providers aggressively suing thousands of patients for overdue payments (Tolan et al. 2023).

According to the Congressional Research Service, 91.4 percent of the U.S. population had health insurance as of 2021, with private health insurance being the primary source, covering approximately three-fourths of the insured population. Government programs also play a significant role: Medicare provides coverage for the elderly, Medicaid and the Children's Health Insurance Program (CHIP) support low-income individuals and children, and Military TRICARE and VA Care serve service members and veterans.

Since the Affordable Care Act (ACA) took full effect in 2016, the percentage of uninsured American adults has decreased from 22.3 percent to 13.3 percent over a decade (Goodnough 2020). However, 8.6 percent of the U.S. population remains uninsured, as reported by the Congressional Research Service.

To assure emergency services to uninsured individuals, the Emergency Medical Treatment and Labor Act (EMTALA), enacted by the U.S. Congress in 1986, reinforced by ACA, requires that emergency room (ER) cannot refuse to treat a patient based on their lack of insurance or inability to pay. EMTALA ensures that any individual with an emergent medical condition, regardless of the patient's citizenship, legal status, insurance status, or financial ability, is provided medical screening, stabilization, and transfer to appropriate hospitals if necessary or provide treatment. If the patient cannot pay, they may be eligible for charity care or financial assistance programs. Hospitals often have financial counselors or social workers who can help navigate these options. However, a hospital that violates EMTALA can face civil monetary penalties and can be sued by patients or other hospitals. Furthermore, violations can also result in a hospital's Medicare provider agreement being terminated, which can be financially devastating for most hospitals.

In contrast, Canada operates a single-payer health care system based on the principle that public health care is a social welfare provision for all citizens. Health care is regarded as a societal responsibility and is managed collaboratively by federal and provincial governments (Government of Canada). Under this publicly funded system, the federal government provides funding to provincial governments in accordance with the Canada Health Act of 1984. This ensures all citizens have access to health insurance through the national health care system.

Patients typically do not pay at the point of service and are not required to meet deductibles. Health care providers are reimbursed directly by the federal government for the services they provide. Consequently, low-income individuals generally do not face financial barriers to accessing essential medical care, such as visits to general practitioners, specialist consultations (with a referral), and hospital stays for medically necessary procedures. Similarly, hospitals treating low-income patients are compensated through the publicly funded health care system.

In Canada, medications administered to patients during a hospital stay are typically covered by the publicly funded health care system. This means that if patients are admitted to a hospital and receive medication as part of their treatment, they generally do not receive a bill for those drugs. However, once discharged, medications required for use at home are not universally covered under the national health care system (SGU 2019).

Coverage for outpatient prescriptions varies by province and territory, as well as by individual factors such as age, income, and specific medical conditions. To address these costs, many Canadians rely on private insurance, often obtained through employers. Provincial programs often reduce, waive, or cover drug costs for low-income individuals, ensuring they have access to necessary medications.

The structural differences between the U.S. and Canadian health care systems are a major source of the distinct advantages and disadvantages experienced by patients. According to Saint George's University Medical School, these differences have shaped unique characteristics in how each country delivers health care services.

Health Care Costs

The U.S. health care system is funded through a combination of private health insurance premiums, out-of-pocket payments, and government funding. This multi-payer system necessitates a large workforce to handle complex billing and reimbursement processes. In 2021, administrative costs reached $1,055 per person, contributing significantly to overall health care expenses (Investopedia 2023). Additionally, Americans spend twice as much on pharmaceutical drugs compared to other developed countries, where governments often regulate drug pricing.

The Canadian health care system, by contrast, is primarily funded through general taxation at both the provincial and federal levels. Canadians have access to medically necessary hospital and physician services without any direct charges at the point of care. While outpatient prescription drugs, dental care, and vision care are not included in the public health care system, their costs are substantially reduced through various government programs.

Service Delivery

In the United States, the quality and availability of health care can vary based on factors such as insurance coverage, geographic location, and the ability to pay. Rural areas often face health care provider shortages, and access to services frequently depends on whether health care providers are within an individual's insurance network. However, studies indicate that wait times for specialist consultations are generally shorter in the United States compared to Canada.

In Canada, while patients are relieved from the financial burden of medically necessary procedures due to the publicly funded health care system, they may experience longer wait times for elective procedures and specialist consultations. The Fraser Institute's 2024 report indicates that the median wait time between a general practitioner's referral and receipt of treatment was 30 weeks, the longest ever recorded and a significant increase from 9.3 weeks in 1993 (Moir et al. 2024).

These extended wait times can limit patients' choices regarding the timing of elective procedures and the selection of specialists. Despite the absence of direct charges at the point of care, the longer wait times in Canada contrast with the generally quicker access to specialist services in the United States.

Innovation and Research

The United States, home to many leading pharmaceutical and biotech companies, serves as a global hub for medical research and innovation. The private-sector-driven nature of its health care system often fuels these advancements. While Canada has made notable contributions to medical research, its scale is smaller compared to the United States. However, the Canadian health care system actively collaborates internationally and supports institutions dedicated to health care research.

Some experts argue that the U.S. health care system could learn from Canada and other industrialized nations, particularly in addressing escalating costs. One proposed solution is increasing government involvement in pharmaceutical price negotiations, ensuring uniform pricing for drugs rather than the wide variability seen today (Emanuel 2022).

On the other hand, some other experts contend that health care systems are deeply rooted in cultural values. They argue that the US approach, which emphasizes creativity and innovation, reflects broader societal norms. "In one sense, what Americans can learn from Canadians is nothing," states Mark Pauly, a professor of Health care Management at the University of Pennsylvania, "because we don't share the same views of society as they do" (Pauly 2017).

Further Reading

Centers for Disease Control and Prevention. "Vital Statistics Rapid Release." https://www.cdc.gov/nchs/data/vsrr/vsrr023.pdf.

Chiu, Jeff. 2020. "How the US Health-Care System Works—And How Its Failures Are worsening the Pandemic." https://theconversation.com/how-the-us-health-care-system-works-and-how-its-failures-are-worsening-the-pandemic-150271.

Congressional Research Service. "U.S. Health Care Coverage and Spending." https://sgp.fas.org/crs/misc/IF10830.pdf.

Emanuel, Ezekiel J. 2022. *Which Country Has the World's Best Health Care?* New York: Public Affairs.

Goodnough, Abby, Reed Abelson, Margot Sanger-Katz, and Sarah Kliff. 2020. "Obamacare Turns 10. Here's a Look at What Works and Doesn't." *The New York Times.* https://www.nytimes.com/2020/03/23/health/obamacare-aca-coverage-cost-history.html.

Government of Canada. "Canada's Health Care System." https://www.canada.ca/en/health-canada/services/canada-health-care-system.html.

Investopedia Team. 2023. "6 Reasons Healthcare Is So Expensive in the U.S." *Investopedia.com*. https://www.investopedia.com/articles/personal-finance/080615/6-reasons-healthcare-so-expensive-us.asp.

Moir, Mackensie and Bacchus Barua. 2024. "Canada's Median Health-Care Wait Time Hits 30 Weeks—Longest Ever Recorded." *Fraser Institute*. https://www.fraserinstitute.org/studies/waiting-your-turn-wait-times-for-health-care-in-canada.

Panchal, Rahul. 2019. "23+ Pros and Cons of Canadian Healthcare System (Explained." *NextFind*. https://thenextfind.com/canadian-healthcare-system-pros-cons/.

Pauly, Mark. 2017. "Is Canada the Right Model for a Better U.S. Health Care System?" *Knowledge at Wharton*. https://knowledge.wharton.upenn.edu/article/lessons-can-u-s-learn-canadian-health-care-system/.

Peter G. Peterson Foundation. 2024. "How Does the U.S. Healthcare System Compare to Other Countries?" http://www.pgpf.org/blog/2023/07/how-does-the-us-healthcare-system-compare-to-other-countries.

Saint George University School of Medicine (SGU). 2019. "Comparing the US and Canadian Health Care Systems: 4 Differences You Need to Know." https://www.sgu.edu/blog/medical/comparing-us-and-canadian-health-care-systems/.

Tolan, Casey, and Ed Lavandera. September 8 2023. "Arkansas Hospital Sued Thousands of Patients over Medical Bills during the Pandemic, Including Hundreds of Its Own Employees." *CNN*. https://www.cnn.com/2023/09/08/us/arkansas-hospital-debt-collections-lawsuits-pandemic/index.html.

What Can the United States Learn from Other Industrialized Countries in Controlling Drug Prices?

According to the Global Prescription Index, as of 2018, the average American spent $1,228.66 on prescription drugs—the highest expenditure among industrialized countries. This marked a 127.19 percent increase since 2000. Following the United States were Switzerland ($893.88), Germany ($883.64), Canada ($865.19), France ($671.40), and the United Kingdom ($526.21) (NiceRx 2023). Notably, the high costs faced by Americans were not due to higher rates of illness or medication use compared to other countries but stemmed from the pricing system in place (Emanuel 2020). A 2021 study found that Medicare could have saved at least $5.1 billion on just six high-cost drugs in 2018 if it had paid the same prices as France (Raimond et al. 2021).

To understand the disparity in drug prices, it's essential to examine how the U.S. prescription drug market operates. A unique aspect of the American health care system is the absence of a centralized authority responsible for evaluating the benefits and cost-effectiveness of pharmaceutical products, whose recommendations could potentially influence drug pricing. While the Food and Drug Administration (FDA) certifies the safety and efficacy of medications, it does not determine their prices. In the United States, pharmaceutical companies benefit from patent protections and marketing exclusivity (Emanuel 2022).

Although the Institute for Clinical and Economic Review (ICER) does evaluate the clinical and economic value of prescription drugs in the United States, it lacks the explicit authority over public or private payers that its counterparts have in other industrialized countries (Baumgartner et al. 2020). Consequently, in the American market-oriented health care system, drug manufacturers set their own prices, and both private insurance companies and Medicare negotiate separate deals with the manufacturers. This occurs without the constraints of government-imposed drug pricing and coverage policies, leading to a situation where drug prices are essentially free-range (Nagar 2022).

Moreover, the broader sociopolitical context plays a crucial role in shaping this issue. One study highlights that the prevailing market-oriented approach in U.S. politics, combined with a decentralized insurance system where each private and public payer negotiates its own coverage and pricing, contributes to the current state of drug costs (Mulligan et al. 2020).

It is worth examining how drug prices are set in other countries such as Switzerland, Germany, Canada, and France, where people enjoy lower per capita spending on prescription drugs compared to the United States.

Switzerland

Since 2001, Switzerland has implemented various strategies to control drug spending. On the patient side, insurance plans require individuals to first meet their deductible by paying the full price of the drug; only after this threshold is reached does their payment decrease to a 10 percent co-pay. This policy aims to discourage unnecessary spending by patients. On the regulatory side, the Federal Office of Public Health (FOPH) acts as a powerful authority with the ability to determine whether a drug qualifies for inclusion on a specialty drug list reimbursed by insurance plans. This decision is based on scientific evidence and cost-effectiveness comparisons with similar drugs. Additionally, the FOPH can mandate price reductions for drugs upon re-evaluation every three years. When making pricing decisions, the FOPH considers drug prices from Austria, Belgium, Denmark, Finland, France, Germany, the Netherlands, Sweden, and the UK. Both international price references and therapeutic cross-comparisons are given equal weight in these evaluations (GLI 2023).

Germany

In Germany, manufacturers can set the prices for new brand-name drugs during their first year on the market. After this initial year, prices are negotiated with the Association of Sickness Funds, a coalition of health insurers. During these negotiations, international pricing is used as a benchmark. The process is guided by the Federal Joint Committee and the Institute for Quality and Efficiency in Health Care, which evaluate whether a new drug provides additional benefits compared to existing treatments. Their assessments influence decisions on coverage by the Association of Sickness Funds. If a drug is deemed to offer additional benefits, the Association negotiates the price directly with the pharmaceutical company (Nagar 2022).

Additionally, German law requires pharmacies to offer discounted drug prices to the Sickness Funds, ensuring consistent medication costs for patients nationwide. Individual Sickness Funds also have the flexibility to negotiate prices directly with manufacturers for generic drugs, such as statins. Moreover, legal regulations cap the markup pharmacies can apply to drug prices, helping to reduce the final cost for consumers (Emanuel 2020).

Canada

In Canada, the Patented Medicine Prices Review Board (PMPRB) oversees drug pricing by setting maximum price ceilings. The PMPRB bases its pricing decisions on objective evidence provided by the Canadian Agency for Drugs and Technologies in Health (CADTH), an independent, not-for-profit organization. The PMPRB also considers international drug prices in selected countries, including France, Germany, Italy, Sweden, Switzerland, the UK, and the United States. Value-for-money assessments are carried out at the provincial level through negotiations between pharmaceutical companies and individual provinces. These negotiations are facilitated by the pan-Canadian Pharmaceutical Alliance (pCPA), a government organization that includes representatives from each province, territory, and the federal government (Nagar 2022; Sokic 2020).

France

In France, the Health Care Products Pricing Committee (CEPS) is responsible for negotiating the maximum price of a drug for a five-year term. CEPS consults with the Transparency Commission, which assesses the therapeutic value of drugs through cost-effectiveness comparisons that take into account factors like mortality, morbidity, and risks associated with similar drugs. French law stipulates that if sales exceed a predetermined cap, manufacturers must pay rebates ranging between 50 percent and 80 percent. After the initial five-year term, CEPS renegotiates prices, often seeking reductions in line with those of generic equivalents. Additionally, CEPS conducts an annual review of high-cost medications within each therapeutic class or group, aiming to align their prices with those of other drugs in the same category (Raimond et al. 2021).

While drug prices in the United States far surpass those in other nations, some argue that this has driven significant investment in innovation. In 2018, U.S. pharmaceutical companies invested $80 billion in drug research, resulting in the development of forty-four new drugs between 2015 and 2019. Notably, 47 percent of these are classified as orphan drugs, targeting only a small patient population. The FDA designated half of these new medications as "first-in-class," and over a quarter as "breakthroughs" (Lieberman et al. 2020).

However, most experts believe that policymakers and regulators need to take steps to rein in soaring drug prices, given successful experience from other countries, and suggest that spending can be reduced without sacrificing innovation. Supporting this perspective is the fact that the majority of new drugs today, such as the mRNA vaccines for COVID-19, have originated from small companies. These are often spin-offs from university labs and are developed on more modest budgets, free from many of the unproductive activities undertaken by larger pharmaceutical companies (Blumenthal et al. 2021).

Further Reading

Baumgartner, Jesse C. and Lovisa Gustafsson. 2020. "Comparative Effectiveness Research, 10 Years after the ACA: Where Do We Go from Here?" *The Commonwealth Fund*. https://www.commonwealthfund.org/blog/2020/comparative-effectiveness-research-10-years-after-aca-where-do-we-go-here.

Blumenthal, David, Mark E. Miller, and Lovisa Gustafsson. 2021. "The U.S. Can Lower Drug Prices without Sacrificing Innovation." *Harvard Business Review*. https://hbr.org/2021/10/the-u-s-can-lower-drug-prices-without-sacrificing-innovation.

Emanuel, Ezekiel J. 2022. *Which Country Has the World's Best Health Care?* New York: PublicAffairs.

Global Legal Insights (GLI). 2023. "Pricing & Reminbursement Laws and Regulations 2023—Switzerland." https://www.globallegalinsights.com/practice-areas/pricing-and-reimbursement-laws-and-regulations/switzerland.

Lieberman, Steven M., Paul B. Ginsburg, and Kavita Patel. 2020. "Balancing Lower U.S. Prescription Prices and Innovation—Part 1." *Brookings*. https://www.brookings.edu/articles/balancing-lower-u-s-prescription-drug-prices-and-innovation-part-1/.

Mulligan, Karen, Darius Kadawalla, Dana Goldman, Jakum Hlavka, Desi Peneva, Martha Rya, Schaffer Center Staff, Peter J. Neumann, Gail R. Wilensky, and Ruth J. Katz. 2020. "Health Technology Assessment for the U.S. Healthcare System." *USC Schaeffer*. https://healthpolicy.usc.edu/research/health-technology-assessment-for-the-u-s-healthcare-system/.

Nagar, Sarosh, Leah Z. Rand, and Aaron S. Kesselheim. 2022. "What Should US Policymakers Learn from International Drug Pricing Transparency Strategies?" *AMA Journal of Ethics*. https://journalofethics.ama-assn.org/sites/journalofethics.ama-assn.org/files/2022-10/msoc2-2211.pdf.

NiceRx. 2023. "The Global Prescription Index—Where in the World Pays the Most for Their Medication?" https://www.nicerx.com/blog/the-global-prescription-index/.

Raimond, Véronique C., William B. Feldman, Benjamin N. Rome, and Aaron S. Kesselheim. 2021. "Why France Spends Less Than the United States on Drugs: A Comparative Study of Drug Pricing and Pricing Regulation." *Milbank Quarterly*. doi: 10.1111/1468-0009.12507.

Rodwin, Marc A. 2019. "What Can the United States Learn from Pharmaceutical Spending Controls in France?" *The Commonwealth Fund*. https://www.commonwealthfund.org/publications/issue-briefs/2019/nov/what-can-united-states-learn-drug-spending-controls-france.

Sokic, Nicholas. 2020. "Drug Pricing in Canada: How It Works and Where It Doesn't." *Healthing*. https://www.healthing.ca/pharma/drug-pricing-in-canada-how-it-works-and-where-it-doesnt/.

Vokinger, Kerstin N. and Hueseyin Naci. 2022. "Negotiating Drug Prices in the US—Lessons from Europe." *JAMA Health Forum*. doi: 10.1001/jamahealthforum.2022.4801.

Lifestyle and Health Issues

China's Struggle with Mental Health Challenges

Major depression is defined by distinct episodes lasting at least two weeks (though most episodes persist much longer), characterized by feelings of sadness, emptiness, irritability, and impaired cognitive abilities that can significantly affect an individual's ability to function (APA 2013). Depression arises from a complex interplay of social, psychological, and biological factors. In the United States, it is a leading cause of mortality, morbidity, and disability. Consequently, mental health care is a heavily invested sector, with over one million professionals, including psychologists, psychiatrists, therapists, counselors, and social workers, according to a recent report (PsychCentral 2023). In contrast, mental health issues in China, historically misunderstood and given low priority for decades, are only now beginning to receive top attention.

The widely recognized mental health crisis in China is closely linked to the nation's rapid socioeconomic transformation. Since the economic liberalization policies initiated in the late 1970s, China has shifted from an agriculture-based economy to a fast-paced, manufacturing-centered one. In 1980, approximately 19 percent of China's population resided in urban areas; by 2023, this figure had risen to about 66 percent, a level comparable to that of developed Western countries (Statista 2023).

China's transition from a planned economy to a market-based economy since the late 1970s has brought profound social and economic changes. These changes have contributed to a reduction in social protections, increased competition, and feelings of instability, which are linked to heightened psychological distress. Intense competition and long working hours have adversely affected people's mental health. While regions with higher levels of marketization tend to have residents with lower psychological distress due to improved economic prospects and optimism, those living in less marketized areas feel more deprived and face worse mental health outcomes. Middle-aged individuals, in particular, report higher distress levels compared to younger or older adults, likely due to challenges adapting to societal changes (Yu 2008).

Moreover, it has taken decades for both society and policymakers to fully grasp the severity of mental health disorders. Experts have warned that depression has become a leading cause of medical consultations and poses a significant burden on China's health care system. According to a study published in *The Lancet*, 16.6 percent of Chinese are at risk of experiencing anxiety and depressive symptoms (excluding dementia) in their lifetime (Huang 2019). Comparatively, the prevalence of mental disorders in China is quickly approaching the level in the United States which stands at 18.5 percent (Lee et al. 2023). Prominent business leaders and celebrities have openly shared their struggles with depression, enhancing public awareness. Additionally, the Covid-19 pandemic has further exacerbated mental health issues, elevating treatment and prevention to a top priority for the first time in history.

The slow recognition of mental health crisis is due to multiple factors. On one hand, mental illnesses carry stigma in Chinese society. The term "mental illness" is often derogatorily conflated with "madness" due to the similar wording in the language (Wang 2023). On the other hand, depressive symptoms have traditionally been sidelined as weakness of the personal character and lack of trust in the system. The stigma raises fear for individuals to seek medical help or share their pain with someone they know. Moreover, medical help is barely available. An article in *China Youth Online* reveals that by 2021, there were only 64,000 mental health doctors nationwide, or 1.49 percent of the total China's medical professionals for a population of 1.4 billion (Ye et al. 2022). This is all but unfamiliar, as China has always allocated priority to what matters the most—national defense and the GDP. Medical schools have prioritized the training of physicians rather than psychiatrists. Moreover, stigma and lower incomes for psychiatric profession are among discouraging factors for medical students to specialize in mental health field (Wang 2012).

The assessment of the prevalence of anxiety and depression in China is still at an early stage. However, research findings have contributed important insights to the pathogenesis and epidemiology of depressive disorders in general, as well as characteristics endemic to China's sociocultural context. Thanks to a broad adoption of standard survey instruments, such as Center for Epidemiological Studies Depression Scale (CES-D) and Patient Health Questionnaire (PHQ-9), China's survey data can be compared on a uniform platform.

Socioeconomic Status (SES) and Mental Health

Many studies have confirmed that SES is intrinsically associated with anxiety and depression. Research has found, for example, that depression is more prevalent in the Appalachian region and the Southern Mississippi Valley region in the United States where poverty, lack of educational attainment, and chronic diseases such as diabetes and cardiovascular diseases are more concentrated compared to other regions (CDC 2023). A 2021 study conducted by Luo et al. on 14,960 households from twenty-five provinces in China during 2010 and 2018 brought new understanding on the relationship between SES and mental disorders. Their study showed that while depression significantly increased during the eight-year period in all groups, the increase of prevalence was notably more rapid among people with higher levels of education and higher family income. The researchers attribute the phenomenon to the drastic slowdown of China's economy from double-digit to single-digit growth and a fast urbanization from 49.5 percent to 60 percent during this period. In such situation, according to the researchers, the better-educated, higher income-earning, and urban-dwelling populations were more exposed to economic and mental stress than the less privileged groups, and were thereby at higher risk of depression. In other words, socioeconomic shifts are more influential to people's mental health than the socioeconomic status *per se*.

Prevalence in Elderly Population

Multiple studies have shown that the prevalence of depression is the highest in Chinese population aged sixty and older which is in contrast with the situation in the United States where age-specific prevalence is the lowest (14.5 percent) among individuals sixty-five and older (Lee et al. 2023). A study investigating the prevalence of depression and associated factors among 7,963 women aged forty-five and older showed that the prevalence rate was 41.52 percent in the age group 45–59, and 45.88 percent among women aged sixty and higher. Higher educational level, living with a spouse, residing in urban area, and having access to the internet are associated with lower rate of depression; while having more dependent children, being indebted, and having difficulties in dealing with daily living activities and instrumental activities are associated with higher rate of depression (Ye et al. 2021).

A broad-scoped meta-analysis examining the data of 439 studies conducted between 2010 and 2019, covering 52,437 Chinese individuals aged sixty and older showed that the overall prevalence of depression was 25.55 percent, with prevalence of females higher than that of males by nearly 6 percent, and residents in urban areas have a lower prevalence of depression than rural residents. The main factor contributing to high prevalence of depression is identified as the rapid sociocultural transition the Chinese elderly population has lived through, which includes rapid industrialization and urbanization, faster pace of life, and the shrinking family size as a result of young people leaving for cities. These changes have resulted in weakened mental, spiritual, and material support to the elderly population (Rong et al. 2020).

Prevalence among High School and College Students

A number of surveys on Chinese adolescent population showed that the prevalence among high school students was as high as 30–40 percent. Academic pressure, failures in exams, emotional setbacks, insomnia, and problems with interpersonal relations are believed to be top contributing factors, with academic pressure being the most impacting factor. Studies further showed that depressive symptoms are more widespread among high school seniors as they face college entrance exams (Li and Zhang 2017; Ma et al. 2020). The prevalence of depression in Chinese adolescent population seems to parallel the rates in the United States where one in five adolescents aged 12–17 have experienced major depressive episodes, and one in three high schools students have experienced depression (CDC 2023).

A meta-analysis of thirty-seven studies conducted between 2009 and 2019 on Chinese college students' mental health showed an overall prevalence of 31.38 percent, with prevalence among female students higher than male students. Pressure from academic work, worries about jobs, and inexperience in coping with emotional setbacks were major influencing factors (Wang et al. 2020). These statistics echoed the general trends in the United States showing that college students are at a very high risk of mental disease. A comprehensive survey conducted by Healthy Minds Network in 2021–22 showed that 44 percent of students in the United States reported suffering from major or moderate depression, 37 percent had anxiety disorder, and 15 percent reported having suicidal thoughts in the past twelve months (Eisenberg et al. 2022).

Impact of Covid-19 on Students' Mental Health

The Covid-19 pandemic and the government-led Zero-Covid policy had a significant negative impact on college students' mental health. An online survey conducted in February 2020 in China, participated by 4,560 students from multiple universities in the Autonomous Region of Inner-Mongolia, showed a prevalence of depression as high as 77 percent; nearly 50 percent of the respondents reporting depressive symptoms had severe depression. Comparatively, in the United States, a study conducted in the same year reported 71 percent of students suffering depression and anxiety due to the Covid-19 pandemic (Eisenbach et al. 2020). China's abrupt relaxation of Zero-Covid policy in November 2022 reduced the prevalence of depression to 25.8 percent, according to a survey conducted from December 2022 to January 2023 with 22,624 responding students. However, the study also showed a high prevalence of PTSD (29.7 percent). Worries about shortage of medication and potential quarantine were believed to be a significant causing factor (Chen et al. 2023).

Treatment and Prevention

During the past ten years, China has been struggling to make up for the severe shortage of mental health professionals, as well as the lack of experience in providing effective psychotherapy.

The government and the medical community are calling on the entire society to fight against stigma, and show love and care for people who suffer from anxiety and depression (Hwang 2022). On the other hand, however, the area of psychotherapy primarily implements ideological indoctrination—hospitals and educational institutions are dependent on the country's experience in conducting ideological campaigns for guidance and counseling. An article describes the ideological approach as follows:

"'To educate people, first instill morality; to instill morality, first straighten their hearts.' Mental health education must foster compassion, enjoyment of life, coping with emotional setbacks, mood management, and valuing life. These elements are commensurate with the socialist value system that includes patriotism, professionalism, honesty, trustworthiness, and friendliness" (Jin et al. 2021).

When addressing mental disorders, culturally and socially tailored approaches are widely recognized as essential. China's efforts in treatment and prevention are anticipated to contribute valuable insights to global practices.

Further Reading

American Psychiatric Association (APA). 2013. *Diagnostic and Statistical Manual of Mental Disorders.* https://doi.org/10.1176/appi.books.9780890425596.

Bitsko, Rebecca H., Angelika H. Claussen, Jesse Lichstein, et al. 2022. "Mental Health Surveillance Among Children—United States, 2013-2019." *MMWR Suppl* 2022, 71(2)(Suppl-2): 1–42. doi: http://dx.doi.org/10.15585/mmwr.su7102a1.

CDC. 2023. "Children's Metal Health: Understanding an Ongoing Public Health Concern." https://www.cdc.gov/childrensmentalhealth/features/understanding-public-health-concern.html#:~:text=Among%20adolescents%20aged%2012%E2%80%9317,%25)%20seriously%20considered%20attempting%20suicide.

Chen, Hongguan, Haoou Feng, Yiyang Liu, Shaoshuai Wu, Hui Li, Guowei Zhang, Peiyue Yang, and Konglai Zhang. 2023. "Anxiety, Depression, Insomnia, and PTSD among College Students after Optimizing the Covid-19 Response in China." *Journal of Affective Disorders, 337*: 50–6. doi: 10.1016/j.jad.2023.05.076.

Eisenbach, Gunter, Guy Fagherazzi, and John Torous. 2020. "Effects of Covid-19 on College Students' Mental Health in the United States: Interview Survey Study."

Journal of Medical Internet Research, 22(9): e21279. https://www.ncbi.nlm.nih.gov/pmc/articles/PMC7473764/.

Eisenberg, Daniel, Sarah K. Lipson, Justin Heinze, and Sasha Zhou. 2022. "Healthy Minds Study—2021–2022 Data Report." *The Healthy Minds Network*. https://healthymindsnetwork.org/wp-content/uploads/2023/03/HMS_national_print-6-1.pdf.

Huang, Jieyun. 2023. "The Pathogenesis and Treatment Progress of Depression." Chinese. *Chinese Journal of Convalescent Medicine, 22*(3). https://www.zglyyx.com/CN/abstract/abstract1267.shtml.

Huang, Wei, Rile Wu, Peng Guan, Jie Yan, and Quan Hui. 2016. "Prevalence and Influencing Factors of Depression among Empty-nest Elderly in China." *China Journal Public Health*, September 2016, *32*(9): 1137–40.

Huang, Yeqin, Yu Wang, Hong Wang, et al. 2019. "Prevalence of Mental Disorders in China: A Cross-Sectional Epidemiological Study." *The Lancet Psychiatry*. https://www.thelancet.com/journals/lanpsy/article/PIIS2215-0366(18)30511-X/fulltext.

Hwang, Christine. 2020. "How China Plans to Achieve Depression Awareness among 85% of Students by 2022." *Bridge*. https://bridgebeijing.com/blogposts/china-plans-to-achieve-depression-awareness-among-85-of-students-by-2022-but-how/.

Jin, Zhuyun, Shi Yingfang, and Peng Wenbing. 2021. "An Exploration on the Causes and Prevention of Depression in College Students." *Journal of Southwest Forestry University (Social Sciences), 5*(2): 101–6.

Lee, Benjamin, Yan Wang, Susan A. Carlson, et al. 2023. "National, State-Level, and County-Level Prevalence Estimates of Adults Aged ≥18 Years Self-Reporting a Lifetime Diagnosis of Depression—United States, 2020." *MMWR*. June 16. doi: 10.15585/mmwr.mm7224a1.

Li, Fang, Mei Li, and Ying Wang. 2022. "Prevalence and Influencing Factors of Depression Symptom among Elderly People in China." *Journal of International Psychiatry, 49*(4): 612–15.

Li, Lingfeng, and Zhicheng Zhang. 2017. "Analysis of Prevalence of Depression of High School Students and Influence Factors." *China Health Industry*. doi: 16659/j.cnki.1672-5654.2017.19.006.

Ma, Xiaofeng, Guoquan Hou, and Wenxiu Luo. 2020. "A Survey on Depression and Influencing Factors among Junior High School Students in Jinshan District of Shanghai." *Occupation and Health, 36*(13): 1831–6.

PsychCentral. 2023. "How Many Mental Health Professionals Are There in the U.S.?" *PsychCentral*. https://psychcentral.com/health/mental-health-professionals-us-statistics.

Ren, Shuai, Fan Wang, Guangxia Li, Wenjie Hou, Jiali Liu, Baocui Hu, and Weili Qin. 2020. "Investigation on the Status of Influencing Factors for Depression and Negative Emotions of College Students in Inner-Mongolia during the Prevalence of Novel Coronavirus Pneumonia." *Journal of Baotou Medical College, 36*(8): 70–4.

Rong, Jian, Yanhong Ge, Nana Meng, Tingting Xie, and Hong Ding. 2020. "2010–2019 Meta-analysis of Prevalence of Depression of China's Elderly Population." *Chinese Journal of Evidence-based Medicine*, 20(1): 26–31.

Statista. 2023. "Degree of Urbanization in China in Selected Years from 1980 to 2023." https://www.statista.com/statistics/270162/urbanization-in-china/.

Wang, Fan. 2023. "Coco Lee: Death of Pop Icon Sparks Mental Health Discussion in China." *BBC*. July 7. https://www.bbc.com/news/world-asia-china-66125051.

Wang, Hongyi. 2012. "Country's Mental Health Services Lacking." *China Daily*. May 16. http://usa.chinadaily.com.cn/epaper/2012-05/16/content_15307682.htm.

Wang, Miyuan, Jia Liu, Fu Wu, Lei Li, Xiaodi Hao, Qing Shen, Minting Huang, and Ruihua Sun. 2020. "The Prevalence of Depression among Students in Chinese Universities over the Past Decade: A Meta-Analysis." *Journal of Hainan Medical University*, 26(9). doi: 10.13210/j.cnki.jhmu.20200218.001.

Ye, Haichun, Yajie Yan, and Quan Wang. 2021. "Prevalence and Associated Factors of Depression among Middle-aged and Elderly Women." *Chinese General Practice*, 24(36): 45749.

Ye, Yuting, Zhou Ruisheng, and Liu Ruochen. 2022. "Shortage of Mental Health Professionals Raised Concerns." *China Youth*. December 12. http://m.cyol.com/gb/articles/2022-12/05/content_PbPQJ7hx0j.html#:~:text=%E6%A0%B9%E6%8D%AE%E5%9B%BD%E5%AE%B6%E5%8D%AB%E5%81%A5%E5%A7%94,%E4%B8%87%E4%BA%BA.

Yu, Wei-hsin. 2008. "The Psychological Cost of Market Transition: Mental Health Disparities in Reform-Era China." *Social Problems*, 3: 347–69. https://www.jstor.org/stable/10.1525/sp.2008.55.3.347.

E-Cigarettes and Their Associated Health Risks

E-cigarettes have seen a rapidly growing user base since their introduction. Promoted as an alternative to traditional tobacco products, "vaping" has quickly integrated into modern culture, especially among younger generations. Although initially touted as a safer option, the rising popularity of e-cigarettes has raised significant health concerns and drawn increasing scrutiny from public health authorities.

Although the concept of e-cigarettes dates back to 1963—when Herbert A. Gilbert patented a "smokeless non-tobacco cigarette" that produced vapor rather than smoke—it was not until 2003 that Hon Lik, a Chinese pharmacist, developed the first commercially successful version. Motivated by his father's death from lung cancer, Lik sought to create a safer alternative to traditional cigarettes. His device used a battery-powered heating element to vaporize a liquid containing nicotine, flavors, and other chemicals, providing a smoke-free way to consume nicotine (HHS 2016).

E-cigarettes entered the U.S. and European markets in the mid-2000s, initially promoted as smoking cessation aids. By the 2010s, their use had skyrocketed, especially among young people. In the United States, sales rose from $2.5 billion in 2014 to $3.5 billion in 2015, driven by social media promotions on platforms like Twitter, Facebook, YouTube, and Instagram (HHS 2016). A 2023 CDC report on middle and high school students found that one in ten reported current tobacco product use, and e-cigarettes remained the most commonly used tobacco product among youth. Among these students, 25.2 percent reported vaping daily, and 89.4 percent used flavored e-cigarettes (Birdsey et al. 2023). This rapid rise in popularity has placed e-cigarettes under increasing public health scrutiny.

E-cigarette users, often referred to as vapers, are predominantly young adults and teenagers. Generation Z, in particular, has embraced vaping, drawn to the variety of flavors, sleek device designs, and the perception that it is less harmful than traditional smoking. Social factors also play a major role, as many young people vape in social settings, influenced by peers and a desire to fit in. According to Johns Hopkins Medicine, curiosity, peer pressure, and the appeal of flavored e-liquids are among the primary reasons young people start vaping (Johns Hopkins Medicine 2023).

Vaping has also become part of the social fabric of modern Western life. For many young people, it is not just a habit but a social activity. It is common to see groups of friends sharing devices or trying out new flavors together. This communal aspect, reinforced by portrayals on social media, has cemented vaping's place in youth culture. Influencers and celebrities often promote vaping products, further weaving them into the lifestyles of their followers (Holtermann 2023).

The influence of vaping has expanded beyond social settings and into the realms of art and fashion. The aesthetic appeal of vapor clouds and sleek e-cigarette designs has made vaping a popular subject in contemporary art, where it is used to explore themes of modernity, consumerism, and the intersection of health and lifestyle. In fashion, vaping is often presented as a symbol of the modern, tech-savvy individual, portrayed as a chic and sophisticated alternative to smoking (Vapovor 2024).

Despite their widespread popularity, e-cigarettes are not without risks. Studies have shown several major hazards associated with vaping, with nicotine addiction being the primary concern. Because nicotine is highly addictive, e-cigarettes—especially those containing flavored e-liquids—make it easy for young people to begin using nicotine. In addition, the aerosol produced by e-cigarettes contains harmful chemicals such as heavy metals, volatile organic compounds, and carcinogens. Research indicates that these chemicals can lead to lung damage, cardiovascular problems, and other health issues, according to the U.S. Food and Drug Administration (FDA).

Another major concern is that e-cigarettes may act as a gateway to traditional cigarette smoking. Several studies have shown that young people who begin vaping are more likely to transition to smoking traditional cigarettes than those who do not vape. This is particularly worrying given the high rates of e-cigarette use among teenagers and young adults. This gateway effect has spurred regulations on e-cigarettes, especially those targeting youth (HHS 2016; Johns Hopkins Medicine 2023).

While e-cigarettes are often marketed as a safer alternative to traditional cigarettes, the reality is more nuanced. E-cigarettes generally contain fewer toxic chemicals than combustible tobacco products, and some studies suggest they may be less harmful. For smokers who switch entirely to e-cigarettes, there can be some reduction in harm. However, research shows that nicotine exposure during adolescence can impair brain development, potentially leading to cognitive deficits and mood disorders. Moreover, the chemicals in e-cigarette aerosol can damage the lungs, with some young people developing conditions such as E-cigarette or Vaping Product Use-Associated Lung Injury (EVALI) (CDC 2023).

EVALI, first identified in 2019, represents a significant public health crisis linked to vaping. The outbreak primarily affected young adults and adolescents, many of whom were otherwise healthy. Patients with EVALI experienced symptoms such as coughing, shortness of breath, chest pain, and, in severe cases, respiratory failure. By the end of 2019, the CDC reported over 2,800 cases of EVALI, including sixty-eight deaths. Most cases were associated with e-cigarettes containing THC, particularly those adulterated with vitamin E acetate—a substance used to thicken the oil in some vaping products (CDC 2020).

In response to growing concerns about youth vaping and the related health risks, the FDA extended its regulatory authority to include e-cigarettes.

Manufacturers are now required to submit their products for review and approval before they can be marketed. The agency has also imposed restrictions on the sale of flavored e-cigarettes, particularly those appealing to youth. Additionally, many states and localities have enacted their own regulations, such as raising the minimum purchasing age to twenty-one and banning the sale of flavored e-liquids, according to data compiled by FDA—Vaping: Facts about E-Cigarettes.

The CDC emphasizes that no tobacco products, including e-cigarettes, are risk-free. While e-cigarettes may offer potential benefits for smokers seeking a complete alternative to traditional smoking, none has been approved by the FDA for smoking cessation. The CDC further notes that additional research is needed to fully understand the health impacts of e-cigarettes and their effectiveness in helping adults quit smoking (CDC 2024).

E-cigarettes remain widely popular, especially among youth, yet they pose health risks—such as addiction and a gateway to smoking—deeply tied to social and cultural acceptance. Moving forward, balancing stricter regulations, robust research, and targeted education will be crucial for mitigating harm and reshaping the societal norms that have propelled vaping into mainstream culture.

Further Reading

Birdsey, Jan, Monica Cornelius, Ahmed Jamal, et al. 2023. "Tobacco Product Use among U.S. Middle and High School Students—National Youth Tobacco Survey, 2023." *MMWR Morb Mortal Wkly* Rep 2023; *72*(44): 1173–82. DOI: http://dx.doi.org/10.15585/mmwr.mm7244a1.

Centers for Disease Control and Prevention (CDC). 2024. "E-Cigarettes (Vape)." https://www.cdc.gov/tobacco/e-cigarettes/.

Centers for Disease Control and Prevention (CDC). "E-Cigarettes and Vaping: What's the Bottom Line?" CDC. Last reviewed February 25, 2023. https://www.cdc.gov/tobacco/basic_information/e-cigarettes/severe-lung-disease.html.

Centers for Disease Control and Prevention (CDC). 2022. "E-Cigarette Use among Youth and Young Adults." CDC. October 7. Last reviewed 2024. https://www.cdc.gov/tobacco/e-cigarettes/youth.html.

Centers for Disease Control and Prevention (CDC). 2020. "Outbreak of Lung Injury Associated with the Use of E-Cigarette, or Vaping, Products." CDC. Last reviewed February 25, 2020. https://archive.cdc.gov/#/details?url=https://www.cdc.gov/tobacco/basic_information/e-cigarettes/severe-lung-disease.html. Accessed August 25, 2024.

FDA.GOV. Undated. "Facts about E-Cigarettes." https://www.fda.gov/media/159410/download.
Holtermann, Callie. 2023. "Vapes Get a Gen Z Makeover." *The New York Times*. https://www.nytimes.com/2023/11/06/style/vape-elf-bar-juul.html?searchResultPosition=1.
Johns Hopkins Medicine. 2023. "5 Vaping Facts You Need to Know." *Johns Hopkins Medicine*. Last reviewed August 24, 2023. https://www.hopkinsmedicine.org/health/wellness-and-prevention/5-truths-you-need-to-know-about-vaping.
Mucci, Dan. 2019. "The Culture of Vaping." *Child & Adolescent Behavioral Health*. https://www.childandadolescent.org/the-culture-of-vaping.
U.S. Department of Health and Human Services (HHS). 2016. "E-Cigarette Use among Youth and Young Adults: A Report of the Surgeon General." https://www.cdc.gov/tobacco/sgr/e-cigarettes/pdfs/2016_sgr_entire_report_508.pdf.
U.S. Food and Drug Administration. 2023. "Facts about E-Cigarettes." FDA. Last reviewed June 30, 2023. https://www.fda.gov/news-events/rumor-control/facts-about-e-cigarettes.
Vapovor. 2024. "The Vape: A Cultural Trend in Full Expansion." *Vapovor*. https://www.vapovor.com/en/the-vape-a-cultural-trend-in-full-expansion.htm. Accessed August 24, 2024.

China's Struggle with Fatty Liver Disease and Gout

Since China began its market liberalization in the late 1970s, the country has experienced rapid economic growth and a substantial improvement in living standards. This transformation contrasts sharply with the pre-reform era, when many people lived at subsistence levels. Among the notable changes is a shift in dietary habits, moving away from traditional diets rich in carbohydrates and vegetables to an increased consumption of protein-rich foods, sugary beverages, and alcohol. These dietary changes contribute to higher purine intake and elevated uric acid levels, both of which are associated with the rise of metabolic disorders such as fatty liver disease and gout, particularly in urban areas (Wang et al. 2020). Currently, China reports one of the highest prevalence rates of these conditions globally, placing significant strain on the nation's health care system (Zhou et al. 2020). Combating these metabolic diseases has become a key focus in daily life and public health efforts.

Understanding the Diseases

Fatty liver disease is defined by the excessive accumulation of fat in liver cells. While alcohol consumption is a well-known cause, other factors such as type II diabetes, obesity, and aging can lead to the development of non-alcoholic fatty liver disease (NAFLD). Regardless of its origin, the condition can progress to steatohepatitis, which involves inflammation of liver cells. If left untreated, this can further escalate to fibrosis, cirrhosis, or even liver cancer, according to the Centers for Disease Control and Prevention (CDC).

Recognizing the strong link between fatty liver disease and various metabolic dysfunctions, the Chinese Society of Hepatology (CSH) has adopted the term "metabolic associated fatty liver disease" (MAFLD) to replace NAFLD. This updated terminology, proposed by a group of scientists in 2020, is a broader term emphasizing the metabolic underpinnings of the disease. CSH scientists believe that "MAFLD" can better characterize the specific challenges and realities faced in China (Nan et al. 2021).

Studies indicate a dramatic rise in the prevalence of MAFLD in China since the early 2000s. The prevalence increased from 23.8 percent in 2001 to 32.9 percent in 2018, reflecting a significant public health concern. Globally, China's MAFLD rates are higher than those reported in the Middle East (31.79 percent), South America (30.45 percent), Asia (27.37 percent), North America (24.13 percent), and Europe (23.71 percent) (Yuan et al. 2022).

Gout has followed a trajectory similar to MAFLD, with its prevalence rising alongside lifestyle changes in China. Gout, a metabolic disease, is caused by hyperuricemia—an excess of uric acid in the blood—which crystallizes in joints and leads to inflammatory arthritis. The condition is marked by intense pain, particularly in the big toe, along with redness and swelling, significantly impairing daily activities and work capacity. The onset of gout is strongly linked to the consumption of high-purine foods such as red meat and seafood. Additionally, sugar-sweetened beverages, beer, and alcohol in general are known to increase blood urate levels and trigger gout flares, according to the CDC.

Similar to MAFLD, gout is associated with other metabolic and chronic conditions, including hypertension, obesity, cardiovascular disease, diabetes, chronic kidney disease, and kidney stones, all of which contribute to premature mortality (Dalbeth et al. 2021).

Research shows that between 1990 and 2019, the prevalence of gout in China was reportedly 12.3 percent among men and 3.9 percent among women, with an annual increase of 0.9 percent. These rates exceed global averages of 10.31 percent for men and 3.03 percent for women. In addition to dietary imbalances, factors such as a sedentary lifestyle, aging, and genetic predispositions have also been identified as contributors to gout's rising prevalence (Zhu et al. 2022).

Certain East Asian populations, particularly the Chinese, may have a genetic predisposition that increases their susceptibility to gout. A specific variant of the *ABCG2* gene, which affects uric acid excretion, has been identified in these populations, heightening their risk of developing the condition (Dalbeth et al. 2021). Additionally, the growing trend of sedentary lifestyles, coupled with rising obesity rates, has further elevated the risk of metabolic syndromes.

Obesity, a major risk factor for MAFLD, affects a substantial portion of the Chinese population. Urbanization and Westernization have contributed to the adoption of sedentary habits and increased obesity rates, as studies show, particularly among younger individuals. When obesity is combined with excessive alcohol consumption, it can amplify the prevalence of both MAFLD and gout (Zhu et al. 2021; Yip et al. 2022; Yuan et al. 2022).

The coexistence of MAFLD and gout with cardiovascular diseases (CVD) and diabetes requires careful attention. Shared risk factors, such as obesity and insulin resistance, significantly increase the likelihood of CVD in individuals with MAFLD. Additionally, elevated uric acid levels, if left unmanaged, can further amplify the risks of developing both CVD and diabetes.

Moreover, both gout and MAFLD have been associated with a range of other health conditions, including chronic kidney disease (CKD), hypothyroidism, osteoporosis, and psychiatric disorders such as depression. These associations may be partly explained by metabolic dysfunctions and hormonal imbalances (CDC; Yip et al. 2022; Dalbeth et al. 2021).

Unhealthy Pressures and Lifestyle Shifts Fueling MAFLD and Gout

Urbanization and the rise of middle class have significantly transformed lifestyles in China (Luo 2005; Luo 2019). As the country emerged as the world's manufacturing hub, extended work hours became the norm for many people, often pushing health considerations to the background. This shift has encouraged a fast-paced, grab-and-go approach to meals, favoring calorie-dense foods and increasing the risk of metabolic disorders.

Adding to these challenges is the cultural emphasis on banquet culture in Chinese business and social settings. These gatherings, known for their lavish consumption of rich foods and alcohol, often serve as the backdrop for negotiations and relationship-building. As the saying goes, "No deal is sealed without alcohol." This tradition not only normalizes but also promotes excessive alcohol consumption, further exacerbating the risks of fatty liver disease and gout. Together, these lifestyle changes have created a perfect storm for the rise of metabolic disorders in modern China.

The escalating competition in today's fast-paced environment intensifies anxiety, a known contributor to metabolic disorders, as noted by the CDC. Across academic and professional sectors, the relentless pressure to excel and succeed fosters sleepless nights, irregular meal schedules, and elevated stress levels, all of which contribute to the rise of metabolic diseases. From a young age, students face intense academic competition, leading to reduced physical activity, inconsistent eating habits, and significant stress. Similarly, in the corporate world, the drive to stand out—or simply to keep up—often results in prolonged work hours and minimal rest, creating conditions ripe for health issues like MAFLD.

Compounding these challenges, China's economic changes have widened disparities. Socioeconomic status often influences access to quality food, health care, and information. Individuals in lower income brackets may gravitate toward less nutritious dietary and lifestyle choices due to financial constraints, increasing their risk for conditions like gout and MAFLD. Supporting this, a survey on metabolic disorders related to liver conditions among Beijing residents reported an MAFLD prevalence of 32.40 percent. The study highlights that urban residents with lower economic status and below-college-level education face a significantly higher risk of developing MAFLD (Yuan et al. 2022).

Prevention and Treatment

China is tackling the prevention and treatment of metabolic disorders through a multifaceted approach. Recommendations from the Chinese National Consensus Workshop emphasize the importance of liver screening for patients with obesity and type II diabetes to standardize diagnosis. Additionally, there is a strong focus on educating individuals about adopting healthier lifestyles, including understanding caloric intake, making better dietary choices, and prioritizing regular physical activity. Experts recognize, however, that these initiatives will require time to produce meaningful results (Fan et al. 2018).

Further Reading

Centers for Disease Control and Prevention (CDC). 2024. "Gout." https://www.cdc.gov/arthritis/gout/.

Centers for Disease Control and Prevention (CDC). 2025. "Liver Cancer Basics." https://www.cdc.gov/liver-cancer/about/.

Dalbeth, Nicola, Anna L. Gosling, Angelo Gaffo, and Abhishek Abhischek. 2021. "Gout." *The Lancet*. https://doi.org/10.1016/S0140-6736(21)00569-9.

Estes, Chris, Quentin M. Anstee, Maria Teresa Arias-Loste, et al. 2018. "Modeling NAFLD Disease Burden in China France, Germany, Italy, Japan, Spain, United Kingdom, and United States for the Period 2016–2030." *Journal of Hepatology* 69(4): 896–904. doi: 10.1016/j.jhep.2018.05.036.

Fan, Jian Gao, Lai Wei, and Hui Zhuang. 2018. "Guidelines of Prevention and Treatment of Nonalcoholic Fatty Liver Disease (2018, China)." *Journal of Digestive Diseases,* 20(4): 163–73. doi: 10.1111/1751-2980.12685.

Le, Michael H., Yee Hui Yeo, Xiaohe Li, et al. 2022. "2019 Global NAFLD Prevalence: A Systematic Review and Meta-Analysis." *Clinical Gastroenterol Hepatology,* 20(12): 2809–17. doi: 10.1016/j.cgh.2021.12.002.

Luo, Jing. 2005. *China Today—An Encyclopedia of the People's Republic.* Wesport, CT: Greenwood Press.

Luo, Jing. 2019. *Cities around the World—Struggles and Solutions to Urban Life.* LLC: ABC-CLIO.

Nan, Yuemin, Jihong An, Jianfeng Bao, et al. 2021. "The Chinese Society of Hepatology Position Statement on the Redefinition of Fatty Liver Disease." *Journal of Hepatology,* 75(2): 454–61. doi: https://doi.org/10.1016/j.jhep.2021.05.003.

Wang, Yuying, Pan Weng, Heng Wan, Wen Zhang, Chi Chen, Yi Chen, Yan Cai, Minghao Guo, Fangzhen Xia, Ningjian Wang, and Yingli Lu. 2020. "Economic Status Moderates the Association between Early-Life Famine Exposure and Hyperuricemia in Adulthood." *The Journal of Clinical Endocrinology and Metabolism,* 105(11): dgaa523. doi: 10.1210/clinem/dgaa523.

Yip, Terry Cheuk-Fung, Eudardo Vilar-Gomez, Salvatore Petta, Yusuf Yilmaz, Grace Lai-Hung Wong, Leon A. Adams, Victor de Lédinghen, Silvia Sookoian, and Vincent Wai-Sun Wong. 2022. "Geographical Similarity and Differences in the Burden and Genetic Predisposition of NAFLD." *AASLD.* doi: 10.1002/hep.32774.

Yuan, Qianli, Peigao HuaiWang, Weixin Chen, Min Lv, Shuang Bai, and Jiang Wu. 2022. "Prevalence and Risk Factors of Metabolit-Associated Fatty Liver Disease among 73,566 Individuals in Beijing, China." *International Journal of Environmental Research and Public Health,* 19(4): 2096. doi: 10.3390/ijerph19042096.

Zhang, Han, et al. 2022. "Trend Dynamics of Gout Prevalence among the Chinese Population, 1990–2019: A Joinpoint and Age-Period-Cohort Analysis." *Frontiers.* https://www.frontiersin.org/articles/10.3389/fpubh.2022.1008598/full.

Zhou, Feng, Jianhua Zhou, Wenxin Wang, et al. 2019. "Unexpected Rapid Increase in the Burden of NAFLD in China from 2008 to 2018: A Systematic Review and Meta-Analysis." *Hepatology,* 70(4): 1119–33. doi: https://doi.org/10.1002/hep.30702.

Zhou, Jianghua, Feng Zhou, Wenxin Wang, Xiao-jing Zhang, Yan-Xiao Ji, Peng Zhang, Zhi-Gang She, Lihua Zhu, Jingjing Cai, and Hongliang Li. 2020. "Epidemiological Features of NAFLD from 1999 to 2018 in China." *Hepatology* 71(5): 2020. https://aasldpubs.onlinelibrary.wiley.com/doi/pdf/10.1002/hep.31150.

Zhu, Bowen, Yimei Wang, Weirn Zhou, Shi Jin, Ziyan Shen, Han Zhang, Xiaoyan Zhang, Xiaoqiang Ding, and Yang Li. 2022. "Trend Dynamics of Gout Prevalence among the Chinese Population, 1990–20219: A Joinpoint and Age-Period-Cohort Analysis." *Frontiers in Public Health*. doi 10.3389/fpubh.2022.1008598.

Could GLP-1 Drugs End Obesity?

The emergence of GLP-1 (glucagon-like peptide-1) receptor agonist drugs for treating obesity and diabetes marks a pivotal moment in modern medical science. Prominent examples include Ozempic and Wegovy (both semaglutide products made by Novo Nordisk), as well as Mounjaro (tirzepatide), produced by Eli Lilly. These drugs represent a significant advancement in combating the global obesity epidemic and its associated chronic conditions, such as type 2 diabetes and cardiovascular disease (Gupta 2024).

GLP-1 drugs have demonstrated remarkable efficacy in inducing substantial weight loss, improving glucose control, and reducing cardiovascular risks, providing crucial pharmacological support for millions struggling with obesity and related health challenges. For many, tackling obesity through lifestyle changes alone has been likened to "trying to clear a major snowstorm with a shovel instead of a snowplow" (Powell 2023). Now, GLP-1 drugs—hailed by some as "miracle drugs"—offer a transformative solution (Gupta 2024).

GLP-1 receptor agonists mimic the effects of the naturally occurring hormone GLP-1, which is released in response to food intake and plays a vital role in regulating metabolism. This hormone stimulates insulin secretion from the pancreas when blood glucose levels are elevated, slows gastric emptying, and promotes feelings of fullness by acting on the brain's appetite centers. GLP-1 drugs reduce appetite, leading to decreased caloric intake and weight loss. Additionally, slower gastric emptying helps improve glycemic (blood sugar) control, making these drugs particularly effective in managing type 2 diabetes. The combination of weight loss and better glycemic control also lowers the risk of cardiovascular disease, positioning GLP-1 drugs as a powerful tool for simultaneously addressing several major health conditions (Lenharo 2024; Flynn 2024).

The prevalence of overweight and obesity in the United States has reached alarming levels. According to the Centers for Disease Control and Prevention (CDC), approximately 42.4 percent of U.S. adults are classified as obese, while an additional 31.9 percent are overweight (Fryar et al. 2020). The CDC defines overweight as a body mass index (BMI) between 25 and 29.9, while obesity is classified as a BMI of 30 or higher. Obesity is further categorized, with severe obesity defined as a BMI of 40 or higher. The risk of developing comorbidities increases progressively with higher weight categories.

Results from the 2017–18 National Health and Nutrition Examination Survey (NHANES) estimated that 42.5 percent of U.S. adults aged twenty and older have obesity, including 9.0 percent with severe obesity, while another 31.1 percent are classified as overweight. Obesity prevalence is highest in the South (36.6 percent), followed by the Midwest (35.4 percent), the Northeast (29.9 percent), and the West (28.7 percent) (CDC 2024; Lin and Li 2021).

Globally, adult obesity has more than doubled since 1990, while adolescent obesity has quadrupled, according to the World Health Organization (WHO). Currently, one in eight people worldwide are living with obesity. An estimated 2.5 billion adults aged eighteen and older are classified as overweight or obese, accounting for 43 percent of the global adult population (WHO 2024).

According to the CDC, the primary comorbidities associated with obesity include type 2 diabetes, cardiovascular diseases (such as coronary artery disease and stroke), hypertension, and certain types of cancer. Obesity is also linked to sleep apnea, osteoarthritis, and fatty liver disease. These conditions can be debilitating, significantly reducing quality of life and increasing mortality.

The interrelationship between obesity, diabetes, and heart disease is well-established. Obesity is a major risk factor for type 2 diabetes, as excess body fat contributes to insulin resistance, which elevates blood glucose levels. In turn, high blood glucose and insulin resistance are key factors in the development of cardiovascular diseases, including coronary artery disease and stroke. Therefore, effective management of obesity is critical for preventing diabetes and reducing the risk of heart disease (CDC 2024).

The ability of GLP-1 drugs to simultaneously address weight, glycemic control, and cardiovascular risk makes them a powerful tool for managing interconnected health challenges. However, while these drugs are a promising treatment option, they have limitations in addressing some of the root causes of these conditions, particularly those related to lifestyle factors shaped by socioeconomic conditions.

Individuals with lower socioeconomic status (SES) often face significant barriers to maintaining a healthy lifestyle, including limited access to nutritious foods, safe environments for physical activity, and adequate health care services. These challenges contribute to higher rates of obesity and diabetes among low-income populations. According to the CDC, obesity and diabetes are more prevalent in low-income groups, who are more likely to consume high-calorie, low-nutrient foods due to their affordability and availability. This dietary pattern often leads to weight gain and the development of obesity.

Ethnically, approximately 48 percent of non-Hispanic Black and Hispanic populations are classified as obese (Hales et al. 2017). The U.S. Department of Health and Social Services highlights that factors such as economic stability, social support, access to health care, education, safe housing, and transportation all contribute to health disparities. For example, a study by Oh and colleagues examined the relationships between food deserts, fast-food restaurant density, park access, and the prevalence of obesity and diabetes across 3,108 U.S. counties. They found that exposure to food deserts is positively associated with higher rates of obesity and diabetes, particularly in counties near Alabama, Georgia, and Tennessee. The study emphasizes the importance of considering both food and recreational environments in public health strategies aimed at reducing obesity and diabetes (Oh et al. 2024). Addressing these underlying socioeconomic barriers is essential for achieving long-term health improvements in populations most affected by obesity and its related conditions.

The physical environment presents another significant challenge for low-income populations. Many low-income neighborhoods lack safe spaces for physical activity, such as parks and recreational facilities. For individuals without access to regular physical exercise, maintaining weight loss can be difficult even with the assistance of GLP-1 drugs (Bose 2024).

The high cost of GLP-1 drugs presents a significant barrier. As of this writing, the annual cost of a prescription could exceed $10,000. While this expense may not be a concern for affluent individuals, it is unaffordable for the majority of low-income individuals who may not carry adequate health insurance but urgently need these treatments. Ongoing debates center on when and how these drugs might become more affordable and accessible to a broader population. Efforts to reduce costs, whether through expanded insurance coverage, government subsidies, or other mechanisms, are crucial to making these medications a viable treatment option for those who need them most (Lenharo 2024).

Moreover, GLP-1 drugs are not without shortfalls. Dr. Sanjay Gupta, CNN medical correspondent, emphasizes that "they are not for everyone" (Gupta 2025), pointing to the importance of medical supervision. Additionally, research indicates that weight loss achieved through these drugs is often not sustainable without accompanying lifestyle changes, such as improved diet and increased physical activity (Bose 2024; Powell 2023). Addressing these challenges will be key to maximizing the benefits of GLP-1 drugs for a wider population.

In addition to socioeconomic conditions, GLP-1 drugs cannot address the broader issue of the nation's food environment for children. As one pediatrician insightfully noted, "It's no big surprise or mystery why we have such a problem with obesity. We continue to allow children to be exploited by the beverage and food industry for profit during their formative years, even though we know it's contributing to mortality and suffering" (Powell 2023).

The bottom line is that combating obesity requires not only effective medical treatments but, more importantly, systemic changes that tackle the root causes of overweight and obesity, particularly among vulnerable populations. By combining these efforts, there is greater hope for reversing the obesity epidemic and improving the health of millions worldwide.

Further Reading

Bose, Priyom. 2024. "Exercise, GLP-1 Receptor Agonist, or Combined Approach Explored in Year-long Study." *News Medical Life Science*. https://www.news-medical.net/news/20240229/Exercise-GLP-1-receptor-agonist-or-combined-approach-explored-in-year-long-study.

Centers for Disease Control and Prevention (CDC). 2024. "About Obesity." https://www.cdc.gov/obesity/php/about/index.html#:~:text=These%20include%20high%20blood%20pressure,and%20some%20types%20of%20cancer.

Centers for Disease Control and Prevention (CDC). 2024. "Adult Obesity Prevalence Maps." https://www.cdc.gov/obesity/php/data-research/adult-obesity-prevalence-maps.html.

Department of Health and Social Services (DHSS). "Social Determinants of Health." *Healthy People 2030*. https://health.gov/healthypeople/priority-areas/social-determinants-health.

Flynn, Hanna. 2024. "How Semaglutide and Similar Drugs Act on the Brain and Body to Reduce Appetite." *MedicalNewsToday*. https://www.medicalnewstoday.com/articles/how-semaglutide-and-similar-drugs-act-on-the-brain-and-body-to-reduce-appetite.

Fryar, Cheryl D., Margaret D. Carrol, and Joseph Afful. 2020. "Prevalence of Overweight, Obesity, and Severe Obesity among Adults Aged 20 and Over: United States, 1960–1962 through 2017–2018." *Centers for Disease Control and Prevention (CDC)*. https://www.cdc.gov/nchs/data/hestat/obesity-adult-17-18/overweight-obesity-adults-H.pdf.

Gupta, Sanjay. 2025. Podcast: "Can Weight Loss Drugs Impact Your Joy of Food?" *CNN*. https://www.cnn.com/audio/podcasts/chasing-life/episodes/ad90b9c4-37bb-11ef-8219-bbbc540c1632.

Gupta, Sanjay. 2024. Podcast: "How Ozempic Transformed the Way We Look at Obesity." *CNN*. https://www.cnn.com/audio/podcasts/chasing-life/episodes/ad3d5eb4-37bb-11ef-8219-3bc7a5be33a2.

Hales, Craig M., Margaret D. Carroll, Cheryl D. Fryar, and Cythia L. Ogden. 2017. "Prevalence of Obesity among Adults and Youth United States, 2015–2016." *Centers for Disease Control and Prevention (CDC)*. https://stacks.cdc.gov/view/cdc/49223.

Holland, Kimberly, Rachael Ajmera, and Alina Sharon. 2023. "Obesity Facts." *Healthline*. Updated March 2023. https://www.healthline.com/health/obesity-facts.

Lenharo, Mariana. 2024. "How Blockbuster Obesity Drugs Create a Full Feeling—Even before One Bite of Food." *Nature*. https://www.nature.com/articles/d41586-024-02106-0.

Lin, Xihua and Long Li. 2021. "Obesity: Epidemiology, Pathophysiology, and Therapeutics." *Frontiers, 12*: 2021. https://www.frontiersin.org/journals/endocrinology/articles/10.3389/fendo.2021.706978/full.

Medaris, Anna, and Gabby Landsverk. 2023. "Elon Must Says He Used a Popular Weight-loss Drug to Get 'Fit, Ripped, and Healthy.'" Business Insider. https://www.businessinsider.com/elon-musk-weight-loss-drug-wegovy-semaglutide-fit-ripped-healthy-2022-10.

Oh, Jae in, KangJae Jerry Lee, and Aaron Hipp. 2024. "Food Deserts Exposure, Density of Fast-Food Restaurants, and Park Access: Exploring The Association of Food And Recreation Environments with Obesity and Diabetes Using Global and Local Regression Models." *Plos.org, 19*(4): e0301121. https://doi.org/10.1371/journal.pone.0301121.

Powell, Alvin. 2023. "Are New Weight-Loss Drugs the Answer to America's Obesity Problem?" *The Harvard Gazette*. https://content.news.harvard.edu/gazette/story/2023/07/are-new-weight-loss-drugs-the-answer-to-americas-obesity-problem/.

The World Health Organization (WHO). 2024. "Obesity and Overweight." https://www.who.int/news-room/fact-sheets/detail/obesity-and-overweight.

Japanese Tips for a Healthy Diet   Insights and Practices

Japan is renowned for the exceptional longevity of its population, a characteristic often linked to its healthy diet. Recent demographic data confirms Japan's status as one of the countries with the highest life expectancies globally. As of 2021, Japanese men have an average life expectancy of eighty-one years, while women live an average of eighty-seven years (Japan Cabinet Office 2021). By contrast, life expectancy in the United States is notably lower, with men averaging seventy-five years and women eighty years (CDC 2022).

Studies consistently highlight the health benefits of the traditional Japanese diet, which is rich in vegetables, fish, and rice. These benefits include a reduced risk of heart disease, stroke, and certain cancers. Research by Wilcox et al. focused on the traditional Okinawan diet and its influence on the remarkable longevity of Okinawans born between 1915 and 1925, often regarded as the longest-living population in the world. Their findings revealed that their diet was low in calories but high in nutrient density. Up until the 1960s, these Okinawans maintained a negative energy balance and a stable low body mass index (BMI) of 21.

The researchers suggest that the low caloric intake of the traditional Okinawan diet contributes to health benefits such as reduced mortality from age-related diseases and extended lifespans. The diet is characterized by a high intake of vegetables and legumes, with minimal consumption of meat, dairy, sugar, and grains. Sweet potatoes and soy served as primary protein sources, with sweet potatoes accounting for approximately 69 percent of caloric intake. On average, individuals consumed around 849 grams of sweet potatoes daily. Dietary fats primarily came from fish and soybeans.

When compared with the diets of mainland Japanese and Americans, the traditional Okinawan diet offered a survival advantage, likely due to its earlier nutritional patterns. However, the researchers note that recent dietary shifts away from this low-calorie, nutrient-rich approach may explain why younger generations in Okinawa do not experience the same longevity benefits (Wilcox et al. 2007).

The adverse effects of a Western-style diet have become increasingly apparent, particularly through the rise of metabolic syndromes among younger generations in Japan. After the Second World War, Japan underwent rapid Westernization, marked by a shift toward a diet rich in protein- and calorie-dense foods such as meat, dairy, and processed products. This dietary transformation contributed to a significant increase in metabolic diseases, including obesity and diabetes. In response, the Japanese government implemented dietary guidelines and actively promoted healthier eating habits, measures that have proven effective in curbing these trends (Nakamura 2011).

One of the government's major efforts to address these issues is the "Healthy Japan 21" program, which aims to enhance public health by encouraging better nutrition and lifestyle choices. This initiative focuses on reducing the prevalence of lifestyle-related diseases and promoting balanced eating habits among the population (Nakamura 2011).

At the heart of these efforts are the "Dietary Guidelines for Japanese," a comprehensive ten-point framework designed to encourage healthier eating. The guidelines highlight the importance of enjoying meals, maintaining regular mealtimes, achieving a proper body weight, and consuming a balanced diet that includes staple foods and side dishes. They recommend sufficient intake of grains, vegetables, fruits, dairy products, beans, and fish, while advocating for reduced salt consumption. Moreover, the guidelines emphasize embracing traditional Japanese dietary culture, preserving local dishes, minimizing food waste, and fostering a deeper understanding of food and nutrition.

Together, these initiatives aim not only to create a healthier population but also to preserve Japan's rich culinary heritage. By blending modern health strategies with traditional values, Japan continues to address the challenges posed by dietary shifts while promoting a sustainable and culturally meaningful approach to nutrition.

Authorities in Japan introduced the "Japanese Food Guide Spinning Top (JFG-ST)" as a visual tool to promote balanced eating habits. Designed to be accessible and practical, this guide recommends a daily intake of 1,800–2,200 calories, adjusted based on age, gender, and activity level. It emphasizes five primary food groups—grains, vegetables, fish and meat, milk and dairy products, and fruits—while offering clear guidance on appropriate portion sizes.

Complementing the JFG-ST is the concept of dietary education, or *Shokuiku*, which plays a central role in Japan's efforts to instill healthy eating habits. Officially adopted as a public health policy in 2005, *Shokuiku* aims to educate citizens about the value of a balanced diet while preserving Japan's rich culinary heritage (MAFF 2005).

In 2011, Japan further reinforced the importance of *Shokuiku* by integrating it into school curriculums and public health initiatives. These programs focus on reducing diet-related diseases, promoting traditional Japanese eating habits, and addressing the issue of solitary dining, particularly among the elderly. Recognizing the psychological and social benefits of shared meals, the guidelines prioritize reducing lonely dining, emphasizing the role of social interaction during meals in enhancing mental and physical well-being.

The Japanese school lunch system, or *kyūshoku*, exemplifies the nation's commitment to dietary education and serves as a cornerstone of its strategy to encourage healthy eating habits. Unlike in the United States, where school lunches are often treated as a break from academics, *kyūshoku* is an integral part of the educational process. These meals, freshly prepared and nutritionally balanced, are often made with local ingredients, teaching children the value of a wholesome diet from an early age.

A typical *kyūshoku* meal includes rice, soup, a main dish (such as fish or meat), a side of vegetables, and milk. Students eat together in their classrooms rather than in a cafeteria, creating a quiet and orderly environment where everyone shares the same experience. This system not only promotes good nutrition but also fosters social bonding and a sense of shared responsibility, aligning with Japan's broader goals of reducing solitary dining and reinforcing the communal aspect of meals (Korteman 2022).

In contrast, American school lunches often vary in quality and frequently include more processed and convenience foods. However, the Japanese school lunch system is not without its critics. Some argue that its emphasis on uniformity may limit students' exposure to a broader range of international cuisines and dietary choices (Korteman 2022).

A unique aspect of Japanese dining that complements its focus on nutrition is the use of chopsticks instead of forks and spoons. While chopsticks may be less efficient, they encourage slower eating, giving the brain more time to recognize fullness, believed to be a simple yet effective way to promote mindful eating (Kisaki 2023). This practice aligns with the broader Japanese approach to food, which emphasizes balance, mindfulness, and intentionality.

Japan's dietary practices and policies serve as an inspiring model for promoting health and longevity. From the nutrient-rich Okinawan diet to national initiatives like *Shokuiku* and the *kyūshoku* school lunch program, Japan seamlessly integrates nutrition, culture, and education into everyday life. Its core principles of moderation, mindfulness, and community provide valuable options for fostering healthier lifestyles.

Further Reading

Arafa, Ahmed, Yoshihiro Kokubo, Rena Kashima, Masayuki Teramoto, Yukie Sakai, Saya Nosaka, Youko M. Nakao, and Emi Watanabe. 2022. "The Lifelong Health Support 10: A Japanese Prescription for a Long and Healthy Life." *Environmental Health and Preventive Medicine, 27*: 23. doi: https://doi.org/10.1265/ehpm.22-00085.

Centers for Disease Control and Prevention (CDC). 2022. "Mortality in the United States, 2022." https://www.cdc.gov/nchs/data/databriefs/db492.pdf.

Japan Cabinet Office. 2021. "Annual Report on the Ageing Society (Summary)." https://www8.cao.go.jp/kourei/english/annualreport/2021/pdf/2021.pdf.

Kisaki, Yukiko. 2023. "Japanese Eating Habits and Dietary Guide." *Wawaza*. https://wawaza.com/blogs/japanese-eating-habits-and-dietary-guide/?srsltid=AfmBOoq0AQxiTOr_oIWC5Mqn1wj_yqwk6cwWTbPO7kL6QnK15INUi8iA. Accessed September 2, 2024.

Korteman, Jessica. 2022. "Japanese School Lunch: Why It's Awesome and One Reason It's Not." *Japanese Food Guide*. https://www.japanesefoodguide.com/japanese-school-lunch/. Accessed September 2, 2024.

Ministry of Agriculture, Forestry and Fisheries (MAFF). 2016. https://www.maff.go.jp/e/policies/tech_res/shokuiku.html.

Ministry of Agriculture, Forestry and Fisheries (MAFF). "Japanese Food Guide Spinning Top." https://www.maff.go.jp/e/policies/tech_res/shokuiku.html.

Ministry of Agriculture, Forestry and Fisheries (MAFF). 2015. "Basic Act on Shokuiku." https://www.maff.go.jp/e/policies/tech_res/attach/pdf/shokuiku-19.pdf.

Nakamura, Teiji. 2011. "Nutritional Policies and Dietary Guidelines in Japan." *Asia Pacific Journal of Clinical Nutrition, 20*(3): 452–4. https://pubmed.ncbi.nlm.nih.gov/21859666/.

Willcox, B. J., D. C. Willcox, H. Todoriki, A. Fujiyoshi, K. Yano, Q. He, J. D. Curb, and M. Suzuki 2007. "Caloric Restriction, the Traditional Okinawan Diet, and Healthy Aging: The Diet of the World's Longest-Lived People and Its Potential Impact on Morbidity and Life Span." *Annals of the New York Academy of Sciences, 1114*(1): 434–55. doi: https://doi.org/10.1196/annals.1396.037.

Overwork-Related Health Consequences in Japan and Korea

Scientific research confirms the harmful effects of long working hours on workers' health, a concern observed globally. Prolonged hours raise risks of cardiovascular diseases, chronic fatigue, stress, mental health issues, sleep disorders, and unhealthy habits like smoking and alcohol use. These impacts can lead to physical injuries and even fatalities.

A review by Pega et al., published by the World Health Organization (WHO) and International Labor Organization (ILO), analyzed the risks of ischemic heart disease and stroke among individuals working over 55 hours per week compared to those working 35–40 hours per week. The study found that working 55+ hours significantly increases the risk of these conditions. In 2016, an estimated 745,194 deaths and 23.3 million disability-adjusted life years (DALYs) were attributed to long working hours globally. Ischemic heart disease accounted for 3.7 percent of these deaths, and stroke accounted for 6.9 percent.

The study found that approximately 488 million people worldwide, or 8.9 percent of the global population, were exposed to long working hours, with middle-aged men most affected. Regional analysis showed the highest prevalence in South-East Asia and the lowest in Europe, while East Asia experienced the greatest disease burden from long working hours (Pega et al. 2021).

Japan and South Korea are two East Asian countries known for their long working hours and associated health consequences.

Japan is known for its culture of *karoshi*, or "death by overwork," rooted in an intense work culture characterized by long hours. The phenomenon drew attention in the 1980s when cases of sudden deaths from heart attacks or strokes among overworked employees became more frequent. A high-pressure environment, combined with societal expectations of loyalty and dedication to employers, has resulted in widespread overwork, mental health issues, and, in severe cases, *karoshi*.

In 2017, the Japanese Ministry of Health, Labor and Welfare released a White Paper on mortality linked to overwork. The report revealed that 22.7 percent of companies surveyed between December 2015 and January 2016 had employees working over eighty hours of overtime per month—a threshold where the risk of death from overwork becomes critical. It also highlighted that 21.3 percent of Japanese employees worked forty-nine or more hours per week on average, compared to 16.4 percent in the United States, 12.5 percent in the UK, and 10.4 percent in France. Mental and cardiovascular diseases were particularly prevalent in industries such as transportation, retail, postal services, and manufacturing. The White Paper also indicated that 20 percent of Japan's workforce was at risk of work-related mortality (JMHLW 2017).

In 2015, Matsuri Takahashi, a 24-year-old employee at the advertising giant Dentsu, tragically took her own life due to overwork. Weeks before her death, she posted on social media about feeling physically and mentally shattered, citing long working hours and getting less than ten hours of sleep per week. After joining Dentsu, she routinely worked over 100 hours of overtime per month, including weekends. Another notable case was that of Tocnang, an immigrant worker who died of heart failure. Before his death, he was working between 78.5 and 122.5 hours of overtime per month at a metal casting factory (McCurry 2016).

Overwork being a widespread issue in Japan is driven by several factors. Culturally, Japanese society places a high value on hard work and long hours, with workers who leave early often perceived as lacking dedication and loyalty. Managers commonly use time spent at work as a measure of performance. Japan has also faced a prolonged labor shortage. Following the economic bubble burst in the 1990s, the economy entered a recession, leading companies to downsize their workforce. The problem persists as Japan's population rapidly declines, further shrinking the labor pool (Dickinson 2023).

Another contributing factor is the cultural respect for seniority. In many workplaces, younger employees are expected to stay at work until their senior colleagues leave, as a sign of respect (Santillanes 2022).

To address these issues, Japan passed the "Work Style Reform Law" in 2018. This legislation limits overtime to forty-five hours per month, with an annual cap of 350 hours. It also mandates stricter enforcement of annual leave requirements.

In South Korea, death from overwork – known as *gwarosa* – is linked to morbidity and mortality rates comparable to those in Japan. This phenomenon has led to increased cases of cardiovascular diseases, mental health issues, suicides, and sudden deaths. South Korean culture places a strong emphasis on hard work, and when combined with economic pressures, it has fostered an environment where long working hours are standard (Kwon et al. 2018).

In South Korea, standard working hours are set at forty hours per week, with an eight-hour workday. However, these limits are often exceeded due to formal and informal expectations for overtime work. Prior to recent policy reforms, it was common for workers to log 50–60 hours per week, often without adequate compensation or regard for their health (Republic of Korea Ministry of Employment and Labor 2024).

A 2019 study by Kim et al. found that, despite reductions in weekly working hours and the prevalence of long workdays, employees in small companies with fewer than five workers and those in the service sector continue to work excessively long hours. Managerial roles showed the highest age-standardized mortality rates from cardiovascular diseases and suicide. In 2017, 589 cases of cardiovascular disease and 104 cases of mental disorders or suicide were officially recognized and compensated as occupational diseases. Of the fifty-nine suicides compensated between 2016 and 2017, 61 percent were directly linked to overwork.

Several factors contribute to the prevalence of overwork in South Korea. Similar to Japan, there is a strong cultural belief in the value of hard work, where dedication to one's job is considered virtuous. Staying late at the office is often viewed positively by employers and can even influence promotion decisions (Lee and Park 2020).

Economically, the competitive job market pressures employees to work longer hours to secure their positions and advance their careers. Many workers fear being seen as uncommitted or lazy, prompting them to stay late at work even when their workload does not demand it (Shin 2014).

Additionally, some argue that the lingering shadow of the ongoing conflict with North Korea, despite the armistice dating back to 1953, has contributed to the culture of overwork, fostering a sense of urgency and resilience (Kwon et al. 2018).

The South Korean government has introduced various policies to reduce working hours. In 2018, the Labor Standards Act was revised to lower the maximum weekly working hours from sixty-eight to fifty-two, including both regular hours and overtime. This reform was part of a broader effort to promote work-life balance and address the issue of *gwarosa* (death from overwork). Under the new law, employees are limited to forty regular working hours and a maximum of twelve hours of overtime per week, marking a significant step toward curbing excessive work (Republic of Korea Ministry of Employment and Labor 2024).

The Japanese term *karoshi* ("death from overwork") and the Korean term *gwarosa* share roots with the Chinese term *guolaosi*, reflecting a common cultural emphasis on relentless dedication to work across East Asia. This shared cultural attitude, while deeply ingrained, contributes to overwork-related deaths in the region, including in China, where *guolaosi* is a significant concern. Addressing this issue requires not only policy changes but also a shift in cultural attitudes toward work-life balance and employee well-being.

Further Reading

Dickinson, Kevin. 2023. "The World Must Learn from 'Karoshi,' Japan's Overwork Epidemic—Before It's Too Late." *Big Think*. https://bigthink.com/the-learning-curve/karoshi/.

Japanese Ministry of Health, Labour and Welfare (JMHLW). 2017. "White Paper on Measures to Prevent Karoshi, etc." https://fpcj.jp/wp/wp-content/uploads/2017/11/8f513ff4e9662ac515de9e646f63d8b5.pdf.

Kim, Inah, Min Ji Koo, Hye-Eun Lee, Yong Lim Won, and Jaechul Song. 2019. "Overwork-Related Disorders and Recent Improvement of National Policy in South Korea." *Journal of Occupational Health*, 61(4): 288–96. doi: https://www.ncbi.nlm.nih.gov/pmc/articles/PMC6620743/.

Kwon, Jake, and Alexandra Field. 2018. "South Koreans Are Working Themselves to Death. Can They Get Their Lives Back?" *CNN*. November 5. https://www.cnn.com/2018/11/04/asia/korea-working-hours-intl/index.html.

Lee, Juyeon, and Kyunghee Park. 2020. "Cultural and Economic Determinants of Overtime Work in South Korea." *Asian Journal of Social Psychology*, 23(4): 263–75.

Lee, Sangheon, Deirdre McCann, and Jon C. Messenger. 2007. *Working Time around the World: Trends in Working Hours, Laws, and Policies in a Global Comparative Perspective*. Geneva: International Labour Office. https://www.ilo.org/sites/default/files/wcmsp5/groups/public/@dgreports/@dcomm/@publ/documents/publication/wcms_104895.pdf.

McCurry, Justin. 2016. "Death from overwork: Japan's 'karoshi' culture blamed for young man's heart failure." *The Guardian*. https://www.theguardian.com/world/2016/oct/18/death-from-overwork-japans-karoshi-culture-blamed-young-mans-heart-failure.

Pega, Frank, Bálint Náfrádi, Natalie C. Momen, et al. 2021. "Global, Regional, and National Burdens of Ischemic Heart Disease and Stroke Attributable to Exposure to Long Working Hours for 194 Countries, 2000–2016: A Systematic Analysis from the WHO/ILO Joint Estimates of the Work-Related Burden of Disease and Injury." *Environment International, 154*: 106595. https://doi.org/10.1016/j.envint.2021.106595.

Republic of Korea Ministry of Employment and Labor. "Revision of the Labor Standards Act." Accessed August 29, 2024. https://www.moel.go.kr/english/policy/laborStandards.do.

Santillanes, Marcus. 2022. "Karoshi: A Deep Look into Japan's Unforgiving Working Culture." *Pulitzer Center*. https://pulitzercenter.org/stories/karoshi-deep-look-japans-unforgiving-working-culture.

Shin, Dongyup. 2014. "Long Working Hours and Health in Korea: Evidence from Time-Use Data and the Korean Labor & Income Panel Study." *Journal of Korean Medical Science*, *29*(3): 323–30.

Traditional Chinese Medicine and Its Contribution to Treatment and Prevention of Disease

Traditional Chinese Medicine (TCM) originates from ancient China and has a history spanning over 2,500 years. It is founded on the concept of *Qi* (life force) and the *Five Elements*—Wood, Fire, Earth, Metal, and Water—which represent various body functions and organs. TCM diagnosis involves techniques such as pulse and tongue examination, aiming to identify imbalances in the body. Treatments typically include acupuncture, herbal remedies, and lifestyle modifications. In contrast, Western medicine emphasizes evidence-based practices, where treatments are rigorously tested through scientific research and clinical trials to ensure effectiveness, primarily focusing on symptom relief using pharmaceuticals and surgery.

The differences in diagnosing and treating Covid-19 illustrate the contrasting approaches of TCM and Western medicine. TCM experts often categorize Covid-19 as a "cold-dampness plague," a term broadly covers symptoms such as fever and the disease's infectious nature (Zhao et al. 2021). According to TCM, "dampness poison" enters the body through the skin, nose, or mouth, disrupting the function of the lungs and spleen. This results in symptoms such as cough, chest tightness, shortness of breath, fatigue, and loss of appetite. In severe cases, the depletion of *Qi* and *Yin* can lead to life-threatening conditions as the disease progressively impacts deeper bodily systems.

For diseases attributed to cold-dampness, TCM emphasizes the importance of consuming warming foods as part of the treatment. Ingredients such as

Antibiotic Use in China: A Cultural and Political Perspective

Cultural shifts have profoundly shaped antibiotic use in China. In an article titled "Antibiotic Culture: A History of Antibiotic Use in the Second Half of the Twentieth and Early Twenty-first Century in the People's Republic of China" (Zhou 2023), the researcher examines how political efforts to improve public health, limited health care access, socioeconomic changes, and a culture of self-medication fueled widespread reliance on antibiotics.

Initially introduced in the 1940s as U.S. wartime aid, antibiotics like penicillin were rare and costly, benefiting mainly urban elites. By the 1950s, the new Communist government made antibiotics central to public health campaigns, promoting them to combat diseases and replace traditional remedies. State-controlled distribution enabled mass production of drugs such as penicillin and tetracycline.

In the 1960s, the "Barefoot Doctors" program brought antibiotics to rural areas, often with inadequate oversight. Promoted as a socialist "cure-all," indiscriminate use led to dependency. Economic reforms in the 1980s introduced privatization, making over-the-counter antibiotics widely available but poorly regulated, worsening misuse.

Urbanization in the 1990s drove rural migrants to cities, where limited health care access made antibiotics an affordable option. Despite stricter regulations in the 2000s, cultural dependence on antibiotics as quick fixes persisted, exacerbating the threat of antimicrobial resistance. Today, antibiotic-resistant illnesses pose a serious challenge to public health in China and beyond.

Further Reading

Centers for Disease Control and Prevention (CDC). 2024. "Antimicrobial Resistance Facts." https://www.cdc.gov/narms/resistance/index.html.

Zhou, Xun. 2023. "Antibiotic Culture: A History of Antibiotic Use in the Second Half of the 20th and Early 21st Century in the People's Republic of China." *Antibiotics*, 12(3): 510. https://doi.org/10.3390/antibiotics12030510.

---

ginger, garlic, and scallions are particularly recommended. For example, a diet featuring scallion, ginger, and jujube soup is thought to warm the stomach and improve circulation. For individuals with weak *Yang Qi*, Danggui ginger mutton soup is suggested. Ginger, in particular, is considered a cornerstone remedy due to its ability to warm the lungs, alleviate coughing, and potentially inhibit the

SARS-CoV-2 virus. TCM posits that ginger's properties can block viral entry, making it an essential dietary component in both the prevention and treatment of Covid-19.

In addition to dietary recommendations, TCM employs external treatments to combat cold-dampness, including herbal sachets, moxibustion, and sun exposure. Sachets filled with herbs such as *Atractylodes* and *Artemisia* are used to dispel cold and dampness. Moxibustion, a technique involving the burning of moxa sticks, stimulates acupoints such as Shenque and Guanyuan to balance *Yin* and *Yang* while strengthening *Yuan Qi* (foundation of health). Sun exposure, particularly directed at the Du Meridian on the back, is considered a natural way to enhance the body's *Yang Qi*, serving as a "battery" to fend off cold-damp pathogens and prevent illness (Zhao et al. 2021).

Western medicine is rooted in scientific principles and relies on a deep understanding of anatomy, physiology, and biochemistry. This foundation supports the analysis provided by organizations such as the Centers for Disease Control and Prevention (CDC) and the World Health Organization (WHO). From this perspective, SARS-CoV-2—referred to as "dampness poison" in TCM—is an RNA virus belonging to the coronavirus family. It is characterized by crown-like spike proteins on its surface that bind to ACE2 receptors on cells in the lungs, heart, and kidneys, enabling the virus to enter and replicate within host cells. Once inside, the virus hijacks the host's cellular machinery to replicate and spread to other cells.

The body's immune response is activated to combat the virus, involving immune cells and the release of cytokines. In severe cases, this response can become overactive, leading to a phenomenon known as a "cytokine storm." This excessive immune reaction causes widespread inflammation, which can result in lung damage, respiratory failure, and multi-organ failure—key features of severe Covid-19 disease.

Covid-19 presents a wide spectrum of symptoms, ranging from mild cases with fever, cough, and fatigue to severe respiratory distress requiring intensive care. Treatment approaches include vaccines to prevent infection, antiviral drugs to combat the virus, and supportive care such as oxygen therapy and mechanical ventilation for critically ill patients (CDC; Harrison et al. 2020).

A defining feature of Western medicine is its reliance on scientific evidence and targeted interventions. Its ability to quickly address acute illnesses, perform life-saving surgeries, and treat diseases using clinically tested medicines has solidified its role as the cornerstone of health care systems worldwide. Even in China, less than 30 percent of the population relies on Traditional Chinese Medicine (TCM) as a primary form of treatment. When TCM is used, it is often as a complement to Western medicine, influenced by factors such as age, the type of illness, and access to health care facilities (Fu et al. 2021).

Despite its complementary role, TCM offers invaluable contributions to health care, particularly in holistic, preventive care and chronic disease management. Cultural beliefs play a significant role in shaping medical decisions, with many people turning to practices they have grown up with or that are deeply rooted in their communities. TCM's personalized approach focuses on restoring balance in the body and strengthening natural defenses through acupuncture, herbal remedies, and dietary therapy. For example, many patients trust TCM for addressing milder illnesses like coughs and colds or as a means to enhance recovery after receiving Western medical treatments. Some believe that while Western medicine provides quick relief, TCM can "clear the root of the disease," "completely cure" it, or "cut the tail off" of an illness, reflecting its perceived role in providing a more thorough resolution of health issues (Lam 2001).

Traditional Chinese Medicine (TCM) has not only emphasized prevention but also contributed to the treatment of diseases, including those with acute symptoms. A prominent example is *Artemisia annua*, a plant used to treat malaria, which earned global recognition when the Nobel Prize was awarded in 2015 for its effectiveness in eliminating malaria-causing parasites. The use of *Artemisia annua* for malaria-like symptoms was first recorded in the fourth century CE. In the 1970s, researchers isolated arteannuin, a precursor to artemisinin, which became the foundation of modern anti-malarial drugs. The World Health Organization now recommends artemisinin-based combination therapies as the first-line treatment for uncomplicated malaria. Artemisinin derivatives, including dihydroartemisinin, artemether, and artesunate, have demonstrated proven efficacy in combating malaria (Fu et al. 2021).

TCM has also been reported effective in managing type-2 diabetes through personalized treatments tailored to the patient's specific condition. Remedies such as Tianqi Capsule, Jinlida Granule, and Gegen Qinlian Decoction are recognized for their ability to lower blood glucose levels and improve insulin sensitivity. Furthermore, integrating TCM with Western medicine has yielded promising results; for instance, combining Jinlida Granule with metformin has been reported to help blood sugar control and overall disease management (Fu et al. 2021).

The integrative approach reflects TCM's priority in prevention through lifestyle adjustments, dietary practices, and natural remedies, offering patients a holistic path to health. The World Health Organization supports further exploration of TCM's contributions to disease prevention, treatment, health maintenance, and health promotion (WHO 2013).

Further Reading

Centers for Disease Control and Prevention (CDC). "Covid-19." https://www.cdc.gov/covid/index.html.

Fu, Rao, Jie Li, Huatao Yu, Yang Zhang, Zhihong Xu, and Cathie Martin. 2021. "The Yin and Yang of Traditional Chinese and Western Medicine." *Medicinal Research Reviews*, 41(6): 3182–200. https://doi.org/10.1002/med.21793.

Harrison, Andrew, Tao Lin, and Penghua Wang. 2020. "Mechanisms of SARS-CoV-2 Transmission and Pathogenesis." *Trends in Immunology*, 41(12): 1100–15. doi: 10.1016/j.it.2020.10.004.

Lam, T. P. 2001. "Strengths and Weaknesses of Traditional Chinese Medicine and Western Medicine in the Eyes of Some Hong Kong Chinese." *Journal of Epidemiology and Community Health*, 55(10): 762–5. doi: 10.1136/jech.55.10.762.

World Health Organization (WHO). 2013. "WHO Traditional Medicine Strategy 2014-2023." https://www.who.int/publications/i/item/9789241506096.

Xu, Yufan. 2024. "Boundaries and Classification: the Cultural Logic of Treating Foreign Medicine." *Humanities and Social Sciences Communications*, 11: 79. doi: https://doi.org/10.1057/s41599-023-02484-2.

Zhao, Fangfang, Zhenghong Yang, Ningqun Wang, Kunlin Jin, and Yumin Luo. 2021. "Traditional Chinese Medicine and Western Medicine Share Similar Philosophical Approaches to Fight Covid-19." *Aging and Disease*, 12(5): 1162–8. doi: 10.14336/AD.2021.0512.

3

Social Determinants of and Policy Impacts on Health

Ill-planned public health policies, socioeconomic disparities, and conflicts or wars are formidable obstacles to public health. They hinder efforts to control and prevent disease and, in many cases, actively contribute to its spread. These factors do not operate in isolation but often intertwine, creating complex challenges that demand comprehensive and coordinated solutions. Exploring specific cases sheds light on how these dynamics play out globally, influencing health outcomes and shaping public health strategies.

China's Zero-Covid policy, initially lauded for containing the virus through strict lockdowns, mass testing, and mobility restrictions, provides a striking example of how policy can both succeed and falter. While early measures curbed the spread of Alpha and Delta variants associated with higher mortality and more severe disease, the highly transmissible Omicron variant rendered the approach unsustainable. Economic strain, social unrest, impact on mental health, and reliance on less effective domestic vaccines ultimately forced an abrupt shift in late 2022. On the other hand, beyond medical measures, communities across different cultures have historically turned to religious figures, folklore, and ritual as psychological and social responses to epidemic disease. From Japan's revival of the yōkai Amabie during Covid-19 to India's worship of cholera goddess Ola Bibi, AIDS Amma, and Corona Mata, and from the veneration of plague saints in Renaissance Italy to the Aztec god Xipe Totec during the smallpox epidemic, these cultural practices helped people cope with fear and uncertainty. Rather than opposing science, such beliefs function as meaningful frameworks that offer emotional resilience and collective hope, reminding us that effective public health strategies often rely as much on cultural understanding as on medical intervention.

Likewise, Covid handling in the United States was divided. The U.S. response to Covid-19 revealed the influence of political and cultural divides on public health. While some states embraced expert-driven measures like masking and vaccination, others resisted, prioritizing individual freedoms over collective action. Political affiliation became a stronger predictor of health behaviors than demographics, leading to uneven vaccination rates and outcomes. Media polarization further deepened divisions, complicating the nation's ability to mount a unified response. This fragmentation highlights the challenges of managing public health crises in politically divided societies.

The eradication of smallpox in 1980, in contrast, demonstrates the transformative power of coordinated global action. Through mass vaccination campaigns and containment strategies, smallpox, once a devastating scourge, was eliminated. This success relied on the simplicity of smallpox's human-only transmission and Edward Jenner's pioneering vaccine. However, it also serves as a reminder that progress in public health can be undermined by modern challenges such as vaccine hesitancy and misinformation.

Diseases eradicated in some contexts can resurface when conditions shift. Syphilis, eliminated in China in the 1960s, reemerged after economic reforms in the late twentieth century. Factors such as rural-to-urban migration, changes in societal norms, and health care inaccessibility fueled its resurgence, particularly in urban and coastal regions. Additionally, decades without infection led to a lack of immunity in the population, creating an unexpected vulnerability that made them more susceptible to rapid infection.

Socioeconomic disparities often exacerbate public health issues, as seen in the rising rates of depression and anxiety among U.S. college students. Financial pressures, academic stress, and the isolation of the Covid-19 pandemic have left nearly half of students grappling with depression and over a third with anxiety. Similarly, malnutrition in the United States, driven by food insecurity and reliance on calorie-dense but nutrient-poor diets, reflects deeper structural inequities. Low-income communities, particularly in the "Poverty Belt," face overlapping crises of obesity, diabetes, and cardiovascular diseases. These examples highlight how economic disparities can shape health outcomes in profound ways.

Vaccination efforts offer a powerful counter to many public health challenges. China's success in combating hepatitis B through universal newborn vaccination programs reduced prevalence among children under five to just 0.3 percent by 2021. This achievement attests to the potential of vaccination campaigns, though challenges such as regional disparities and older population prevalence remain. However, diseases like diphtheria, tetanus, and pertussis persist in areas with poor health care access, necessitating continued vigilance and expansion of vaccination coverage.

Foodborne illnesses like *Salmonella* and *E. coli* further illustrate how gaps in public health infrastructure can lead to widespread harm. High-profile outbreaks linked to global food chains demonstrate the need for robust safety protocols and international cooperation. Similarly, the opioid crisis in the United States, driven by synthetic drugs like fentanyl, reveals the interplay between socioeconomic factors and health. Poverty and unemployment have intensified addiction rates, particularly in regions like Appalachia, where overdose deaths far exceed national averages.

War and migration compound these challenges. The Syrian conflict displaced millions, destroying health care systems and exacerbating outbreaks of diseases such as tuberculosis and leishmaniasis. Refugees faced malnutrition, overcrowding, and poor sanitation, straining host countries like Lebanon, where refugees accounted for 30 percent of the population. Women bore particular hardships, including high maternal mortality, forced marriages, and limited access to reproductive health care.

The war in Ukraine has similarly devastated public health. Destroyed infrastructure and overcrowded shelters have driven surges in Covid-19, tuberculosis, HIV, and polio. Vaccine-preventable diseases such as polio and measles have reemerged due to low immunization rates and poor sanitation. Non-communicable diseases, including diabetes and cardiovascular conditions, have worsened amid disrupted medical supplies. International aid and collaborative efforts are critical to addressing these overlapping crises.

Migration further amplifies health vulnerabilities. Migrants often face hazardous transit conditions, overcrowded shelters, and limited health care access, heightening their risks for infectious diseases including HIV, tuberculosis, and malaria. Post-migration challenges, such as discrimination and economic exploitation, compound their struggles. Louse-borne diseases like typhus and relapsing fever, once nearly eradicated, have resurfaced among displaced populations and refugees living in unsanitary conditions. These examples demonstrate how migration and displacement can propagate diseases and strain public health systems.

The historical precedent of the 1918 flu pandemic offers further insight into the interplay between war and disease. The First World War's overcrowded camps and poor sanitation enabled the H1N1 virus to infect one-third of the global population, killing over 50 million people. This pandemic underscores the importance of transparency and preparedness in managing global health crises during periods of instability.

Efforts to mitigate these challenges must integrate public health into broader strategies addressing socioeconomic disparities, conflict resolution, and migration management. Legal pathways for migration, international collaboration on vaccination campaigns, and culturally competent health care delivery are critical. Public health policies must prioritize equitable access to care, recognizing the interconnected nature of these challenges.

Through examining these cases, it becomes clear that public health is not only about addressing immediate crises but also about tackling the structural inequities and systemic vulnerabilities that allow diseases to thrive. Coordinated global responses, informed by past and present lessons, are essential to building resilient systems capable of withstanding future public health challenges.

Public Policies' Impact on Public Health

China's Zero-Covid Policy and Its Abrupt Ending

When Serenitie Wang, a CNN journalist, arrived in Shanghai in early March 2022, she initially spent three weeks in government-mandated quarantine for inbound travelers. What she didn't expect was to spend the next forty-nine days, first in a sealed-off apartment, and later at the National Exhibition and Conference Center, which had been converted into an isolation facility with 50,000 beds. There, she stayed alongside 3,000 other Shanghai residents who had tested positive (Wang 2022). From April 1 to June 1, the Omicron variant swept through Shanghai, a city of 25 million, with infections reaching over 28,000 daily. This prompted authorities to enforce a full lockdown for two months. Schools and non-essential businesses were closed, streets emptied, and residents were only allowed out for rolling PCR screenings, a procedure to detect existence of the viral RNA. Even grocery deliveries were occasionally disrupted due to truck drivers being placed in quarantine. There were also reports of parents being separated from their young children and violent clashes between residents and law enforcement.

Meanwhile, Beijing began implementing a strategy known as "dynamic zeroing," where residents were required to undergo daily PCR screenings. When a positive case was detected, the affected neighborhood would be quarantined until the outbreak was eliminated, rather than maintaining constant lockdowns across a much larger area. A common sight in cities across China was the long lines outside testing booths. Mobile technology was effectively deployed for contact-tracing, with test results sent directly to individuals' mobile devices. If someone's health code turned red, they would be denied access to public places such as university campuses and public transportation.

In a sense, Shanghai's lockdown was not as unthinkable as it might seem, given that dozens of Chinese cities had experienced full or partial lockdowns. In 2020, Wuhan, a city of 11 million, was the first to be locked down for nearly three months. Since then, cities like Wenzhou (9 million), Shijiazhuang (11 million), Xi'an (8.5 million), and Shenzhen (17 million) had also faced closing, ranging from one week (Shenzhen) to twenty-six days (Xi'an). China stood firm as the only country in the world adhering to the Zero-Covid policy, relying on severe restrictions on people's mobility, while the rest of the world had adopted a "living with Covid" approach through widespread vaccination.

However, China's stringent measures came with steep social and economic costs. The government argued that these costs could have been much higher, claiming that "Zero-Covid" was a policy of "great benevolence with long-term benefits." Critics of China's Zero-Covid strategy were accused of "harboring ill-intentions towards our party and government" (Wang Xingping 2022). Disagreements, such as WHO Director-General Tedros Adhanom Ghebreyesus' statement that China's Zero-Covid strategy was unsustainable, had been censored. Shanghai's authority reported 500,000 Covid infections and a low death toll of just 285, which raised more questions, however, than admiration (Liang 2022).

China's economy suffered significant losses. A group of Chinese economists estimated that the Shanghai lockdown alone could reduce the country's GDP by approximately 4 percent during that period (Chen et al. 2022). The government spent roughly 11.5 billion yuan on PCR tests in the first quarter of 2022. When cash-strapped local governments tried to shift the cost of testing to residents, people angrily refused (Watanabe 2022). The lockdowns triggered food shortages, mental distress, and drained medical resources needed for patients with other illnesses. The scale and harshness of the restrictions, reminiscent of the Mao era, severely damaged public trust in the leadership (Huang 2022).

A deteriorating economy carries the risk of jeopardizing stability and solidarity, something the Chinese government maintains at all costs. But why did China stick to the highly impacting Zero-Covid policy? The answer lies in it being a familiar and possibly the default tool in the government's playbook. Historically, China has used mass campaigns to eliminate infectious diseases. These efforts helped China eradicate syphilis in the early 1960s, stop the spread of SARS in 2003, and control early Covid-19 outbreaks in Wuhan in 2020. As of

June 2022, China's strategy seemed to have paid off, with fewer than 15,000 total Covid-related deaths compared to over one million in the United States (Johns Hopkins Coronavirus Resource Center). However, the Omicron variant, which is twice as transmissible as the Alpha and Delta variants but poses 60 percent less in mortality and 80 percent less risk of hospitalization (HKUMed 2021), presented a serious challenge. It made the Zero-Covid strategy increasingly costly and ineffective.

A more compelling reason for China's adoption of the Zero-Covid policy may have been tied to the country's health care infrastructure. First, primary care was relatively new and severely lacking in China. When people became ill, whether it be the flu or chest pain, their first stop was the hospital. This meant that a fast-spreading pandemic could have quickly overwhelmed hospitals, limiting access to treatment for other health conditions. Second, vaccines remained a sensitive topic, and China had been hesitant to rely on or import vaccines produced in the West. The two available homegrown vaccines, CoronaVac and Sinopharm, both used inactivated SARS-CoV-2 virus, but they offered lower protection against Covid symptoms compared to the mRNA vaccines from Moderna and Pfizer-BioNTech (Smriti 2021). Third, China's growing elderly population had one of the lowest vaccination rates. Surveys indicated that fewer than 60 percent of people aged eighty and older, compared to over 90 percent in the United States, had received even the first dose, mainly due to concerns about side effects.

As Zero-Covid enforcement prolonged, questions grew on whether Zero-Covid policy was really effective in saving lives. One study argued that, since Omicron's rate of infection was extremely high and its average case fatality was lower than that of the common flu, intervention could focus on treating the disease and preventing deaths rather than avoiding infections. Hence, if the government would use its resources to raise the vaccination rate of the elderly and other vulnerable groups, it could do better in saving GDP and people's lives than locking down cities (Feng 2022). A more straightforward proposal by Zhong Nanshan, a well-known Chinese virologist, called for reopening the country and normalizing socioeconomic development. To make this happen, he proposed the following steps: combining homegrown inactivated vaccines with mRNA-based vaccines such as products of Pfizer-BioNTech, adopting and researching on drugs such as paxlovid and molnupiravir to reduce illness progression; promoting antigen testing (such as home test kits) and reduce reliance of PCR; and adjusting policies according to epidemic characters of the disease through performing pilot investigation in designated cities and regions (Guan et al. 2022). Opinions like these were scrubbed from Chinese media.

End of Zero-Covid

China's exit from Zero-Covid has been widely reported as lack of preparation and poorly coordinated (Li 2023).For example, on November 11, 2022, the government pledged to firmly uphold the "dynamic zero-COVID" policy through its portal the Xinhua News Agency:

> Currently, the situation of pandemic prevention and control remains complex and severe. The COVID-19 virus continues to mutate, the global pandemic is still widespread, new outbreaks are emerging domestically, and the spread is accelerating in some areas, increasing the risk of resurgence. The more challenging and complex the situation becomes, the more we must maintain strategic focus, unwaveringly uphold the principles of putting people and lives first, steadfastly implement the overarching strategy of "preventing imported cases and domestic resurgence," and consistently follow the "dynamic zero-COVID" policy. This approach aims to maximize the protection of people's lives and health while minimizing the impact of the pandemic on economic and social development. (Xinhua November 11 2022)

In the meantime, however, a major shift was quietly taking place. On December 7, 2022, the Chinese government issued a "10-point" directive to "optimize" the Covid response. According to this circular, negative test results and health code checks were no longer required to access most public venues or for travel, except in high-risk places like nursing homes, hospitals, and schools. Infected individuals were to be treated based on the severity of their infection, with asymptomatic or mild cases allowed to quarantine at home if possible (Xinhua December 12, 2022).

Studies show that the government's policy of gradual relaxation led to confusion at the provincial level. Local officials interpreted the signals as a sign that Beijing planned to end the Zero-Covid policy abruptly rather than gradually. In response, they rushed to reopen, fearing they might fall behind. As a result, the central government lost control of the process and ultimately followed the pace set by local authorities. A study described the situation as follows:

> Facing the sudden opening at the local level, Beijing realized that "the horse has already left the barn"; all it could do was accept the reality. On December 26, the State Council issued a new circular that codified opening at the local level. The circular deleted requirements for drawing high-risk areas and quarantine enforcement. It also reaffirmed the end of mandatory mass COVID-19 testing. Overall, Beijing adopted and legitimized local governments' quick opening

rather than trying to reassert control over localities and enforce incremental opening. (Li 2023)

On January 8, 2023, the Chinese government officially ended its Zero-Covid policy. Covid-19 management was downgraded, in terms of severity of infection and prevention priority, from Class A to Class B under the country's infectious disease prevention laws. Centralized quarantine, close-contact tracing, and mass nucleic acid testing were discontinued, and testing booths were swiftly removed from city streets. China entered a new phase in its Covid-19 response, shifting focus to managing the pandemic's impacts (Lancet Editorial 2023).

The sudden exit from Zero-Covid left many people unprepared and lacking medicine to manage fever and inflammation due to omicron infection. Analysts believe that mounting and unsustainable economic costs, psychological strain, and rising protests were among the factors that forced the abrupt end of the Zero-Covid policy (Pei 2023; Li 2023). According to some estimates, the short notice may have overwhelmed hospitals and resulted in deaths of over a million in China (Lancet 2023; Glanz et al. 2023).

In evaluating China's Zero-Covid strategy, an editorial in the renowned *Lancet* medical journal highlighted several drawbacks, including low natural immunity due to limited infections, widespread vaccine hesitancy, and disrupted international cooperation caused by strict border controls. Additionally, frequent mass testing, quarantines, and sudden lockdowns strained public life, increased government costs, and diverted resources from other health care needs. Abrupt lockdowns, particularly during omicron outbreaks, revealed further issues such as family separations, food shortages, and restricted access to medical care. On the positive side, the editorial noted:

> Beyond all doubts, the dynamic zero-COVID-19 policy has protected the most vulnerable populations from five global COVID-19 waves and avoided widespread infections with the original strain and the delta variant. Its border closure policy blocked, or at least postponed, the entry of variants from abroad. It also won precious time for the whole society to be better prepared for high infection rates in the population. (Lance 2023)

Lancet's estimate of the death toll was also supported by Du et al.'s study (2023) which placed the death toll to be above 1.4 million (Du et al. 2023).

In the years to come, epidemiologists will revisit China's Zero-Covid policy with keen interest. All things considered, China's Covid response will likely be remembered as a culturally distinctive approach to one of the deadliest pandemics in history.

Further Reading

Chen, Jingjing, Wei Chen, Ernest Liu, Jie Luo, and Zheng (Michael) Song. 2022. "The Economic Cost of Lockdown in China: Evidence from City-to-City Truck Flows." https://michaelzsong.weebly.com/uploads/4/8/1/4/48141215/truck_flow_and_covid19_220315.pdf. Accessed June 22, 2022.

Du, Zhanwei, Yuchen Wang, Yuan Bai, Lin Wang, Benjamin John Cowling, and Lauren Ancel Meyers. 2023. "Estimate of COVID-19 Deaths, China, December 2022–February 2023." *Emerging Infectious Diseases, 29*: 10. https://wwwnc.cdc.gov/eid/article/29/10/23-0585.

Feng, Zhenghu. 2022. "从抗疫转向防疫的政策"(A Policy Transition from Strict Epidemic Control to Epidemic Prevention and Mitigation). *Citizen Oversight*. https://gmjd.org/?p=2033. Accessed June 3, 2025.

Glanz, James, Mara Hvistendahl, and Agnes Chang. 2023. "How Deadly Was China's Covid Wave." *The New York Times*. https://www.nytimes.com/interactive/2023/02/15/world/asia/china-covid-death-estimates.html.

Guan, Wei-jia, and Zhong Nanshan. 2022. "Strategies for Reopening in the Forthcoming COVID-19 Era in China." *National Science Review, 9*(3). https://doi.org/10.1093/nsr/nwac054. Accessed June 24, 2022.

HKUMed. 2021. "HKUMed Finds Omicron SARS-CoV-2 Can Infect Faster and Better than Delta in Human Bronchus But with Less Severe Infection in Lung." *HKUMED*. December 15. https://www.med.hku.hk/en/news/press/20211215-omicron-sars-cov-2-infection. Accessed June 24, 2022.

Huang, Tianlei. 2022. "Zero-Covid in Shanghai Comes at High Social and Economic Costs." *Peterson Institute for International Economics*. April 15. https://www.piie.com/blogs/realtime-economic-issues-watch/zero-covid-shanghai-comes-high-social-and-economic-costs#_ftn8.

Lancet Regional Health—Western Pacific (Lancet). 2023. "The End of Zero-Covid-19 Policy Is Not End of COVID-19 for China," *30*: 100702. https://www.thelancet.com/journals/lanwpc/article/PIIS2666-6065(23)00020-2/fulltext.

Li, Zhuoran. 2023. "How Beijing Accidentally Ended the Zero COVID Policy." *The Diplomat*. https://thediplomat.com/2023/01/how-beijing-accidentally-ended-the-zero-covid-policy/.

Liang, Rachel. 2022. "China Censors WHO Chief's Call to End Covid-19 Strategy Dubbed Unsustainable." *WSJ*. May 11. https://www.wsj.com/articles/china-censors-who-chiefs-call-to-end-unsustainable-covid-19-strategy-11652270048. Accessed June 23, 2022.

Mallapaty, Smriti. 2021. "China's Covid Vaccines Have Been Crucial: Now Immunity Is Waning." *Nature*. doi: https://doi.org/10.1038/d41586-021-02796-w.

McDonald, Joe. 2022. "China Fights Economic Slump, Sticks to Costly Zero Covid." *AP News*. May 12. https://apnews.com/article/covid-health-xi-jinping-shanghai-06c212f9ab9f58fbeb5922ee0c00e83c. Accessed June 22, 2022.

Pei, Meixin. 2023. "The Sudden End of Zero-Covid: An Investigation." *CLM*. https://www.prcleader.org/post/the-sudden-end-of-zero-covid-an-investigation.

Stanway, David. "Explainer: Shanghai Death Numbers Raise Questions over Its Covid Accounting." *Reuters*. April 28. Accessed June 27, 2022.

Wang, Serenitie. 2022. "Shanghai Surprise: How I Survived 70 Days Confinement in the World's Strictest Covid Lockdown." *CNN*. June 17. https://www.cnn.com/2022/06/17/asia/shanghai-covid-quarantine-lockdown-experience-dst-intl-hnk/index.html. Accessed June 20, 2022.

Wang, Xingping. 2022. "Dynamic Zeroing Is a Grand Policy of Benevolence with Comprehensive and Prolonged Impacts." *China Office of Central Cyber Affairs Commission*. http://www.cac.gov.cn/2022-06/15/c_1656911989056747.htm. Accessed June 17, 2022.

Watanabe, Shin. 2022. "Cost of China's Zero-COVID Push Stocks Growing Frustration." *NIKKI Asia*. https://asia.nikkei.com/Spotlight/Coronavirus.

Xinhua News Agency (Xinhua). December 7, 2022. "China Focus: Covid-19 Response Further Optimized with 10 New Measures." *EnglishNews.cn*. https://english.news.cn/20221207/ca014c043bf24728b8dcbc0198565fdf/c.html. AccessedOctober 25, 2024.

Xinhua News Agency (Xinhua). 2022. "Xinhua Commentator: Stay Firmly Committed to the 'Three Unwavering Principles' (original text in Chinese)." November 19. www.gov.cn.https://www.gov.cn/xinwen/2022-11/19/content_5727810.htm. Accessed October 25, 2024.

Covid-19 and Politics in the United States—It's More Than Fighting the Virus

One key takeaway from the Covid-19 pandemic is that a purely biological perspective is insufficient for fully understanding disease. While a virus infects human cells in a consistent way across state boarders, the rates of mortality and morbidity can vary drastically depending on how communities respond. The spread of Covid-19 in early stage offers a telling example. When the Covid-related death toll in China was below 15,000 by mid-2022, according to Johns Hopkins Coronavirus Resource Center, the number of deaths in the United States had surpassed one million. Cultural variations significantly influenced the extent to which the pandemic's impact was either mitigated or intensified across different countries.

When Covid-19 first emerged in late 2019, China's immediate response was to lock down the epicenter, Wuhan, a city of 11 million residents, for nearly four months. The government then expanded the Zero-Covid policy, which

> ## How Moderna's Spikevax Was Developed in Record Time
>
> Moderna's Covid-19 vaccine, Spikevax, was developed rapidly thanks to prior research by the NIH on a prototype coronavirus vaccine. This prototype, based on mRNA technology, allowed quick adaptation to target SARS-CoV-2 after Chinese scientists published its genome in January 2020.
>
> Unlike traditional vaccines, mRNA vaccines deliver genetic instructions for human cells to produce the virus's spike protein, prompting an immune response without exposure to an active virus. By February 2020, the vaccine candidate mRNA-1273 was ready and entered Phase 1 trials in March. Larger trials followed, and the vaccine received FDA emergency use authorization on December 18, 2020.
>
> This collaboration between NIH and Moderna exemplifies a groundbreaking achievement in vaccine science, enabling the swift rollout of a life-saving vaccine.
>
> **Further Reading**
>
> Garnett, Carla. 2020. "Fast, Reliable, Universal: Corbett Recounts Quest for Covid Vaccine." *NIH Record*. https://nihrecord.nih.gov/2020/12/11/corbett-recounts-quest-covid-vaccine.
>
> Neergaard, Lauran. 2020. "Behind the Scenes, Scientists Prep for Covid-19 Vaccine Test." *PBS.org*. https://www.pbs.org/newshour/health/behind-the-scenes-scientists-prep-for-covid-19-vaccine-test.

involved mass quarantines and mandatory antigen testing nationwide, despite the significant economic costs and human suffering these measures caused (Li 2022). The underlying cultural tradition encouraged people to endure constraints to the individual for the greater good, namely, to fight Covid-19. A similar cultural ethos is seen prevalent in the value systems of several Asian countries as well.

In the medical research arena, there is ongoing examination of whether collectivist-based societies have advantages in mitigating pandemics like Covid-19. The hypothesis is that collectivist cultures, which emphasize group harmony, cooperation, and prioritizing the well-being of the community over individual interests, may be better equipped to implement and adhere to public health measures, ultimately resulting in more lives being saved.

For example, one study published in *Humanities and Social Sciences Communications* analyzed the spread of Covid-19 from a cross-cultural perspective. The researchers found that countries and regions with collectivistic, Confucian, or tight (restrictive) cultures experienced lower Covid-19 spread rates. Specifically, a one standard deviation increase in the collectivism score was associated with a 1.38 percent reduction in the weekly growth rate of Covid-19 cases. The effect was even more pronounced during lockdown periods, suggesting that collectivist cultures may enhance the effectiveness of stringent public health measures (Liu et al. 2023). Another study published in *Frontiers in Public Health* explored the relationship between cultural orientations and Covid-19 outcomes. The researchers found that more individualistic countries had higher numbers of Covid-19 cases and deaths. They argue that individualism, which emphasizes personal freedom and autonomy, may hinder collective action and compliance with public health measures, leading to more severe disease impact (Maaravi et al. 2021). These studies offer an interesting perspective on the study of pandemics and contribute to our broader understanding of public health responses.

In the United States, the federal system of governance grants states and individuals significant power in public health decisions. As a result, the implementation of safety and preventive measures, such as vaccination, mask-wearing, and compliance with stay-at-home orders, became the subject of debate, often influenced by polarized political views. Partisan divides notably amplified the impact of Covid-19. Generally, the Democratic Party emphasized unity in combating the virus by following the guidance of scientists and health experts, while the Republican Party often downplayed the disease's severity, comparing it to the common flu. The fight against Covid thus became a political battleground (Albrecht 2022).

Studies have shown that Americans' reactions to Covid-19 were sharply divided along party lines. From the outset of the pandemic in the United States, Republicans and Democrats held differing views and understandings of the virus.

Studies have further shown that political views and party affiliation became a powerful predictor of Americans' decisions regarding vaccination and safety measures. A study by Rothwell and colleagues (2020) found that political affiliation was a more significant predictor of people's likelihood to practice safety measures than factors such as age, gender, race, education level, or even preexisting medical conditions. The study revealed that behaviors such as workplace visits, social distancing, and mask-wearing were driven more by party identification than by local public health conditions, state economic circumstances, or state public health policies.

Throughout the pandemic, particularly in its early stages, news media were deeply divided. A study by Sol Hart et al. (2020) found that both newspaper and network news coverage were highly polarized and politicized, with newspapers showing even more politicization than network news. The researchers suggest that when the media amplify partisan voices, they can shape public opinion and encourage individuals to follow political elites rather than experts. A poll by the University of New Hampshire (Hamilton and Safford 2020) found that only half of the residents who frequently consumed media with a conservative viewpoint reported wearing a mask in public. Furthermore, only 12 percent of these individuals believed that containing the virus should be the country's top priority, compared to 81 percent of residents who did not regularly engage with such media sources. A study by Abrecht (2022) on how political views shaped people's attitudes toward the Covid-19 vaccine offers particularly notable findings. The study found that counties with lower vaccination rates tended to experience significantly higher Covid-19 cases and deaths per 100,000 residents. This inverse relationship was associated with the prevalence of political ideologies that were less supportive of public health measures such as vaccination. In contrast, counties with higher levels of educational attainment generally showed higher vaccination rates and lower mortality. The study also identified an important exception: communities with higher poverty levels, regardless of political orientation, were more likely to have lower vaccination rates and higher Covid-19 death rates. This included some historically underserved Black neighborhoods in the South, where crowded housing and limited access to healthcare contributed to increased vulnerability. Moreover the structure of the American federal system grants states considerable authority in setting and enforcing public health regulations. As a result, state-level policies on vaccine and mask mandates often reflected differing policy approaches. Following the federal announcement of vaccine and mask mandates in 2021 (The White House 2021), some states expressed strong opposition. Several states enacted legislation limiting the ability of state and local agencies to require vaccination or mask-wearing for public employees, educators, health care workers, and certain businesses. In states such as Alabama and Florida, laws provided broad exemptions for workplaces from federal requirements. In Florida, executive orders were issued prohibiting local governments and schools from enforcing mask mandates. In contrast, some states implemented policies requiring government employees, health care workers, and employees in various sectors to provide proof of full Covid-19 vaccination or undergo regular testing (Routh and Markowitz 2022). The variation in state-level vaccination rates became so pronounced that Dr. Anthony Fauci warned of the potential emergence of "two Americas"—one with high vaccination coverage and another where lower vaccination rates could lead to localized surges in cases (Elamroussi and Vera 2021).

The pandemic revealed deep societal divisions in the United States, with political perspectives influencing many aspects of public life, including public health responses. Some commentators have described Covid-19 as a "partisan pandemic," reflecting the degree to which differing political views shaped public attitudes and behaviors. Others, however, argue that addressing major public health crises requires a unified approach, emphasizing cooperation over division to achieve more effective outcomes (Oberland 2024).

Further Reading

Albrecht, Don. 2022. "Vaccination Politics and Covid-19 Impacts." *BMC Public Health*, 22. January 14: 96. doi: https://doi.org/10.1186/s12889-021-12432-x.

Elamroussi, Aya and Amir Vera. 2021. "The Delta Variant Has Now Been Detected in All 50 States and Washington, DC." *CNN*. https://www.cnn.com/2021/06/30/health/us-coronavirus-wednesday/index.html.

Hamilton, Lawrence C. and Thomas G. Safford. 2020. "Conservative Media Consumers Less Likely to Wear Masks and Less Worried about COVID-19." *Carsey Perspectives*. Carsey School of Public Policy, University of New Hampshire September 1. https://scholars.unh.edu/carsey/415/.

Li, Zhuoran. 2022. "What Keeps China's Zero-COVID Policy Going." *The Diplomat*. https://thediplomat.com/2022/03/what-keeps-chinas-zero-covid-policy-going/. Accessed July 19, 2022.

Liu, Ming, Wu Haomin, Lin Bingxuan, and Zhang Jingxia. 2023. "A Small Global Village: The Effects of Collectivist, Tight and Confucian Cultures on the Spread of COVID-19." *Humanities and Social Sciences Communications, 10*: 789. https://doi.org/10.1057/s41599-023-02289-3.

Maaravi, Yossi, Aharon Levy, Tamar Gur, Dan Confino, and Sandra Segal. 2021. "The Tragedy of the Commons: How Individualism and Collectivism Affected the Spread of the COVID-19 Pandemic." *Frontiers in Public Health, 9*: 627559. https://doi.org/10.3389/fpubh.2021.627559.

Oberland, Jonathan. 2024. "Polarization, Partisanship, and Health in the United States." *Journal of Health Politics, Policy and Law, 49*(3). June 2024: 329–50. doi: 10.1215/03616878-11075609.

Rothwell, Jonathan, and Christos Makridis. 2020. "The Real Cost of Political Polarisation: Evidence from the COVID-19 Pandemic." *VoxEU.org. Centre for Economic Policy Research*. https://cepr.org/voxeu/columns/real-cost-political-polarisation-evidence-covid-19-pandemic.

Routh and Markowitz. 2022. "List of Corona-Virus Related Restrictions in Every State." Updated July 14. https://www.aarp.org/politics-society/government-elections/info-2020/coronavirus-state-restrictions.html.

Sol Hart, P., Sedona Chinn, and Stuart Seroka. 2020. "Politicization and Polarization in Covid-19 News Coverage." *Science Communication, 42*(5): 679–97. doi: 10.1177/1075547020950735.

The White House. 2021. "Fact Sheet: Biden Administration Announces Details of Two Major Vaccination Policies." https://www.whitehouse.gov/briefing-room/statements-releases/2021/11/04/fact-sheet-biden-administration-announces-details-of-two-major-vaccination-policies/.

Eradication of Smallpox—The First Major Milestone of Modern Vaccination

Smallpox, a highly contagious and deadly disease caused by the Variola virus, holds a prominent place in human history due to its devastating impact and the extraordinary achievement of its eradication. This success, officially declared by the World Health Organization (WHO) in 1980, serves as an early testament to the effectiveness of coordinated global health efforts and the vital role of vaccination.

The journey from the ancient scourge of smallpox to its eradication was grounded in a scientific approach rooted in observation and experimentation. Edward Jenner's use of cowpox to provide immunity against smallpox was instrumental in the development of the smallpox vaccine in the late eighteenth century. The term "vaccine" itself originates from the Latin word vacca, meaning cow, in recognition of Jenner's use of cowpox to confer immunity in human body (Hopkins 2002). Edward Jenner's pioneering work laid the foundation for the development of vaccination and contributed significantly to the emergence of immunology as a scientific field. His contributions have had a profound and lasting impact on medical science and public health, securing his place as a central figure in the history of immunological research. The Variola virus, a member of the *Orthopoxvirus* genus, is the causative agent of smallpox. It is exclusively a human pathogen, meaning it does not naturally infect other species, which is a key factor in the success of the eradication campaign. Smallpox has two primary variants: Variola major, which is more severe and can have a mortality rate of up to 30 percent, and Variola minor, which is a less severe form of the smallpox with a much lower mortality rate typically around 1 percent, according to the Centers for Disease Control and Prevention (CDC).

The Variola virus is primarily transmitted through respiratory droplets, making close contact with infected individuals the most common route of spread. It can also be transmitted through contaminated objects, such as bedding or clothing, though this method of transmission is less frequent. The disease typically begins with a prodromal phase marked by high fever, malaise, and body aches, followed by the development of a characteristic rash. This rash progresses through multiple stages—macules, papules, vesicles, pustules, and finally scabs (CDC).

Historically, smallpox had a high mortality rate, especially in cases of Variola major. Mortality rates for Variola major ranged from 20 percent to 30 percent, with even higher rates reported in certain populations and during specific outbreaks, as detailed in "History of the Smallpox Vaccine" (WHO-b). Survivors of smallpox often carried deep, permanent scars, and some suffered blindness if their eyes were affected.

Beyond its physical toll, smallpox caused widespread social and economic upheaval. Epidemics instilled fear and paralyzed communities, with quarantines and travel restrictions severely disrupting trade and daily life. The combination of high mortality and severe morbidity made smallpox one of the most feared diseases in human history.

The origin of smallpox is unknown; the earliest traces were found on mummified Egyptian corpses. Smallpox was introduced to the Americas in the early sixteenth century, primarily through European colonization and the transatlantic slave trade. Historical records indicate that the disease first appeared in the Caribbean around 1507, likely brought by Spanish settlers and enslaved Africans. By 1518, an outbreak occurred on the island of Hispaniola and decimated the Indigenous population. The virus subsequently spread to other Caribbean islands, including Cuba and Puerto Rico, before reaching the mainland. In 1520, smallpox arrived in Mexico, with the Spanish conquest of the Aztec Empire. The epidemic devastated the Aztec population, contributing to the fall of Tenochtitlán. The introduction of smallpox and other Old World diseases had catastrophic effects on Indigenous populations, who lacked immunity, resulting in mortality rates as high as 90 percent in some communities (CDC).

Before the advent of the modern smallpox vaccine, ancient methods of inoculation, known as variolation, were practiced in various parts of the world. Variolation involved deliberately introducing material from smallpox pustules—typically from a mild case—into the skin of a healthy individual. The goal was to induce a mild infection that would confer immunity to the disease. This practice was carried out in China, India, and Africa long before it was introduced to Europe. In China, variolation dates back to the tenth century and involved blowing dried smallpox scabs into the nostrils. In India and Africa, it was more common to insert the material through a small incision in the skin. While variolation was effective in providing immunity, it carried substantial risks, including the possibility of severe disease and death (CDC).

Edward Jenner, born in 1749, was an English physician credited with developing the first successful smallpox vaccine. His groundbreaking work began with the observation that milkmaids who had contracted cowpox—a related, but far less severe, disease—appeared immune to smallpox. This observation led him to hypothesize that exposure to cowpox could protect against smallpox, later termed "cross-immunization."

In 1796, Jenner tested his hypothesis by inoculating an eight-year-old boy, James Phipps, with material taken from a cowpox lesion on the hand of a milkmaid named Sarah Nelmes. Phipps developed a mild case of cowpox but remained free of smallpox even when later exposed to the virus. Jenner's subsequent experiments confirmed that cowpox inoculation provided immunity to smallpox, leading to the creation of the first smallpox vaccine.

Jenner's work represented a significant advancement over the earlier practice of variolation, which involved transferring material from smallpox sores to healthy individuals. Unlike the traditional variolation which carried considerable risks of infection and death, Jenner's cowpox-based vaccine was safer and more effective, establishing the foundation for modern vaccination (WHO-b; Riedel 2005).

The impact of Jenner's vaccine was transformative. It led to the widespread adoption of vaccination and ultimately the eradication of smallpox. The global eradication campaign, initiated by the WHO in 1967, employed mass vaccination, surveillance, and containment strategies. The last naturally occurring case of smallpox was reported in Somalia in 1977, and the disease was officially declared eradicated in 1980 (WHO-a).

In the United States, routine smallpox vaccination ended in 1972. However, smallpox vaccines are still stockpiled as a precaution against potential use of the virus as a bioterrorism agent (CDC).

Vaccination remains a cornerstone of public health, saving millions of lives each year by preventing diseases like measles, polio, and influenza. The creation of RNA vaccines against Covid-19 represents giant step in timely public health response backed by modern science (Poland et al. 2011).

The eradication of smallpox remains a monumental achievement in medical history, demonstrating the power of scientific innovation and global collaboration. Edward Jenner's pioneering work laid the foundation for modern vaccination, saving countless lives and alleviating immense suffering. As we navigate contemporary public health challenges, the lessons of smallpox eradication serve as a vital reminder: vaccination is one of the most powerful tools humanity has for protecting public health and preventing disease.

Further Reading

Centers for Disease Control and Prevention. 2024. "About Smallpox." *Centers for Disease Control and Prevention*. Last reviewed October 22, 2024. https://www.cdc.gov/smallpox/about/index.html.

Henderson, Donald A. 2009. *Smallpox: The Death of a Disease*. Amherst, NY: Prometheus Books.

Hopkins, Donald R. 2002. *The Greatest Killer: Smallpox in History*. Chicago, IL: University of Chicago Press.

Pertwee, Edward, Clarissa Simas, and Heidi J. Larson. "An Epidemic of Uncertainty: Rumors Conspiracy Theories and Vaccine Hesitancy." *Nature Medicine, 28*: 456–9. https://www.nature.com/articles/s41591-022-01728-z.

Poland, Gregory A. and Robert M. Jacobson. 2011. "The Age-Old Struggle against the Antivaccinationists." *New England Journal of Medicine, 364*(2): 97–9. doi: 10.1056/NEJMp1010594.

Riedel, Stefan. 2005. "Edward Jenner and the History of Smallpox and Vaccination." *Proc (Bayl Univ Med Cent), 18*(1): 21–5. https://pmc.ncbi.nlm.nih.gov/articles/PMC1200696/.

World Health Organization (WHO)-a. "Smallpox." https://www.who.int/health-topics/smallpox#tab=tab_1.

World Health Organization (WHO)-b. "History of the Smallpox Vaccine." https://www.who.int/news-room/spotlight/history-of-vaccination/history-of-smallpox-vaccination.

Resurgence of Syphilis in China

Syphilis is a sexually transmitted disease (STD) with a long history of human infection. Its origin remains disputed today. In Europe, syphilis was known to have caused horrendous mortality to military personnel during the fifteenth and sixteenth centuries, and eventually became endemic affecting people of all classes, from monarchs to the pauper. Effective treatment was unavailable until the discovery of penicillin in 1943.

Historical records indicate that syphilis was introduced in China by Portuguese traders in the 1500s. By the 1940s, syphilis had infected 5 percent of China's urban dwellers, 3 percent of rural peasants, and over 50 percent of prostitutes across the country (Hesketh et al. 2008). After Communist China was founded in 1949, the government labeled STDs an evil from the West, and made wiping out STDs a patriotic movement. The government closed brothels, incarcerated prostitutes, banned pre-marital sex, and trained health workers to conduct surveillance, treatment, and propaganda in large cities such as Guangzhou and Shanghai (Cohen et al. 1996). By 1964, China proclaimed syphilis eradicated (Hu et al. 1965). The achievement was hailed a miracle in world history (Hesketh et al. 2008).

However, in 1979 several syphilis cases were reported (Gong et al. 2001). In the following two decades syphilis returned in a grand scale. The open-door policy in the early 1980s that welcomed Westerners to visit China was allegedly a source of infection (Cohen et al. 1996). By early 2000s, the *Infectious Disease Prevention Act of China* ranked syphilis a Class B notifiable disease, after Class A diseases such as the plague and cholera (NPC 2004). In 2010, the government issued *National Program for Prevention and Control of Syphilis in China (2010–2020)* (MOH 2010). Once again, China is faced with eliminating syphilis, and this time the challenge proves to be much greater.

Elusive Symptoms

Syphilis is a multi-stage STD caused by the bacterium *Treponema pallidum*. The infection undergoes primary, secondary, and tertiary stages, with primary and secondary being the most infectious. At the primary and secondary stages, sores, known as "chancres," and rash develop in infected areas such as the genitals and the mouth. The patient may also experience flu-like symptoms. At early stages syphilis can be relatively easily diagnosed and treated. However, because these symptoms usually do not cause pain and can recede without treatment, the patient may unwittingly believe to have healed while the infection goes into a latent phase without symptoms that may last months or years. At the onset of the tertiary stage, the disease can flare up and attack the heart, brain, bone structure, nerves system, and even cause insanity and paralysis. Without aggressive treatment the patient may die, and certain damages can be irreversible. Syphilis can be passed along by a mother to her child during pregnancy, resulting in congenital syphilis. Congenital syphilis may cause abortion or early death of the child (CDC 2018; Tapley et al. 1989; Chen et al. 2007).

Prevalence

After the new cases were reported in 1979, the Chinese government undertook intensive intervention measures. The Ministry of Health (MOH) established the Chinese National Center for STD Control in 1986 and launched the National STD Surveillance System in 1987 with twenty-six sentinel sites throughout the country. Hospitals and clinics are required by law to report new cases within twelve hours in cities and twenty-hour hours in rural areas (Zhang et al. 2016). Physicians who detect an infection must submit a report card with the patient's demographic profile, lab results, and route of transmission (Chen et al. 2007). The data collected showed syphilis in rapid spread. In 1993, the total rate of syphilis infection in China was 0.2 cases per 100,000 individuals; by 2005, primary and secondary syphilis alone represented 5.7 cases per 100,000. The rate of congenital syphilis increased greatly with an average yearly rise from 0.01 cases per 100,000 livebirths in 1991 to 19.68 cases per 100,000 livebirths in 2005. More than 70 percent of reported cases were 20–49 years of age with the mean age being 37.6. In 2005, the highest rates of total syphilis cases were reported in major cities and provinces along the east coast such as Shanghai (55.3/100,000), Zhejiang (35/100,000), Fujian (26.8/100,000), and Jiangsu (13/100,000). Beijing had a high infection rate of 24.9 per 100,000 population, which was higher than the Pearl River Delta Region known as China's most densely populated urban region and where the infection rate was 14–21 cases per 100,000. Northeastern provinces and western provinces such as Qinghai and Xinjiang reported 5–12 cases per 100,000. Comparatively, incidence of primary and secondary syphilis in China in 2005 (5.67/100,000) substantially surpassed that of the United States (2.7/100,000). Researchers cautioned that the statistics may be underreported, since between 27 percent and 40 percent of patients sought initial care at non-government-run sites or private caregivers who likely failed to report the cases (Chen et al. 2007).

In a 2016 study, Zhang and colleagues used time series analysis to model the trend at all stages including congenital syphilis between 2005 and 2012. A steady rising trend can be clearly observed—cases per 100,000 individuals were 9.73 in 2005, 12.80 in 2006, 15.88 in 2007, 19.49 in 2008, 23.07 in 2009, 26.86 in 2010, 29.47 in 2011, and 30.44 in 2012. Latent syphilis was the most common type, accounting for over 55 percent of the total number of syphilis cases in 2012. Primary syphilis (first stage of infection, typically within the first 3 weeks of exposure) ranked the second, accounting for 26.02 percent, followed by secondary syphilis 15.92 percent, congenital syphilis 2.68 percent, and tertiary 0.74 percent. Additionally, their study reveals a strong seasonal variation—reporting rates in all stages of syphilis trended higher in May–August and declined in December–February. The researchers suggest that the seasonality may be associated with peak months of rural-to-urban migration for work and ramp-up of surveillance by agencies on high-risk populations during peak months. Low reporting rates in January and February could be attributable to the New Year and Spring Festival when clinical visits are low (Zhang et al. 2016).

Reasons for the Resurgence

1. Rural-to-urban Migration

    Researchers generally agree that since the late 1970s the massive rural-to-urban migration had prepared a hotbed for sexually transmitted infection (STI). By 2014, China's migrant population reached 250 million, compared to 160 million in 2010, and 50 million in 1990 (China Statistical Yearbook 2018). Surplus rural labors migrate seasonally to urban areas with preference for first line cities, such as Beijing, Shanghai, and Guangzhou. Because migrants are primarily male, a market for sex work is in demand. A 2006 sexuality survey in China revealed that among men 15–49 years of age, the estimated urban prevalence of having commercial sex (paid sex) in a year was 7.2 percent, which was higher than the world median and exceeded by only four countries (Cambodia, Zambia, Mozambique, and Tanzania). As such, migrant population is highly exposed to syphilis, HIV, and other STIs (Chen et al. 2007; Tucker et al. 2005). Additionally, employed with low-paying jobs, most immigrants can't afford medical services (Lu et al. 2016); privatization of China's health care facilities had jacked up charges of drugs and office visits further discouraging patients to seek help (Chen et al. 2019; Wong et al. 2017).

    Experts believe, in addition to massive migration, increase in STI was also assisted by changes in sociocultural environment. In particular, traditional monogamous imperative is in decline (Hesketh et al. 2008; Chen B et al. 2005; Buckley 2016), and various other modes of relationships such as homosexuality, a traditionally rejected behavior, have risen noticeably. It is estimated that China's MSM population could be as large as 5 to 10 million (Wang et al. 2019). Moreover, having multiple partners appears to be an acceptable practice, which puts the group at higher risk of STI (Ruan et al. 2007; MOH 2010; Das et al. 2015). A survey by China CDC among MSM

in sixty-one cities showed MSM to have the highest rate of HIV-syphilis co-infection (Liu et al. 2015).
2. Did Eradication Help Resurgence?

Experts suspect that the eradication of syphilis in the 1960s may have produced adversary effects (Chen et al. 2007; Hesketh et al. 2008). A study by Grassly and colleagues on syphilis epidemics in U.S. cities confirmed that in both treated and untreated syphilis partial immunity to reinfection does occur (Grassly et al. 2005). Hence, the absence of syphilis in China for twenty years (1960–80) had likely deprived the population of protective immunity, and set stage for massive infection.

3. Challenges Ahead

Studies show, as of 2025, syphilis remains a growing public health concern in China. In 2023, 616,933 cases were reported—a nearly 40 percent increase from 2022. The epidemic shows regional clustering, particularly in the northwest, southeastern coast, and southwest. Latent syphilis has shown a rising trend as well, highlighting the importance of early detection. High-risk groups, including men who have sex with men and migrant populations, face disproportionately high rates. Though mortality is low, mother-to-child transmission and late-stage complications remain concerns. China's 2010–2020 national plan emphasized comprehensive interventions and targeted screening, but sustained efforts are still needed (Yuan 2024; China CDC 2024).

Today, rather than pursuing drastic measures to eradicate syphilis, the Chinese government has adopted a comprehensive approach focused on controlling its spread. This strategy includes advancing scientific solutions, strengthening STD prevention and education, and expanding access to health care for at-risk groups, including migrant populations. Through coordinated public health efforts, China aims to reduce transmission while addressing social and systemic barriers to care.

Further Reading

Buckley, Sarah. 2016. "China's High-Speed Sexual Revolution." *BBC News*. https://www.bbc.com/news/magazine-35525566. Accessed August 13, 2019.

Centers for Disease Control and Prevention (CDC). 2025. "Syphilis—CDC Fact Sheet." https://www.cdc.gov/syphilis/about/?CDC_AAref_Val=https://www.cdc.gov/std/syphilis/stdfact-syphilis.htm. Accessed July 25, 2019.

Chen, Bin, Lu-ping Wang, Hong-xiang Wang, Yin-fa Han, et al. 2005. "Survey of Reproductive Health Status of Shanghai College Students." *Zhonghua Han Ke Xue*, *11*(10): 744–7. https://pubmed.ncbi.nlm.nih.gov/16281506/.

Chen, Xinlong, Guigang Li, Yanling Gan, Tongshen Chu, and Dianchang Liu. 2019. "Availability of Benzathine Penicillin G for Syphilis Treatment in Shandong Province, Eastern China." *BMC Health Services Research*, *19*: 188. https://bmchealthservres.biomedcentral.com/articles/10.1186/s12913-019-4006-4.

Chen, Zhi-qiang, Guo-cheng Zhang, Xiang-dong Gong, Charles Lin, Xing Gao, Guo-jun Liang, Xiang-sheng Chen, and Myron S. Cohen. 2007. "Syphilis in China: Results of a National Surveillance Program." *Lancet*, *369*(9556): 132–8. doi: 10.1016/S0140-6736(07)60074-9.

China Bureau of Statistics. 2019. *China Statistical Yearbook 2018*. http://www.stats.gov.cn/tjsj/ndsj/2018/indexeh.htm. Accessed July 30, 2019.

China Center of Disease Control and Prevention (China CDC). 2018. "2018 Survey of Legally Defined Infectious Diseases." http://www.nhc.gov.cn/jkj/s3578/201904/050427ff32704a5db64f4ae1f6d57c6c.shtml?from=groupmessage. Accessed July 23, 2019.

China Ministry of Health (MOH). 2010. "Notice of the Ministry of Health on Issuing National Program for Prevention and Control of Syphilis in China (2010–2020)." http://m.chinacdc.cn/jkzt/crb/yl/md/jszl_8939/201810/P020181010472391637444.pdf (in Chinese Language). Accessed July 31, 2019.

Cohen, M. S., G. E. Henderson, P. Aiello, and H. Zheng. 1996. "Successful Eradication of Sexually Transmitted Diseases in the People's Republic of China: Implications for the 21st Century." *Journal of Infectious Diseases*, *174*(Suppl 2): S223–S229. https://doi.org/10.1093/infdis/174.supplement_2.s223.

Das, Aritra, Jianjun Li, Fei Zhong, Lin Ouyang, Tanmay Mahapatra, Weiming Tang, Gengfeng Fu, Jinlou Zhao, and Roger Detels. 2015. "Factors Associated with HIV and Syphilis Co-infection among Men Who Have Sex with Men in Seven Chinese Cities." *International Journal of STD & AIDS*, *26*(3): 145–55. doi: 10.1177/0956462414531560.

DBTS/MOH. 1996. *National Standard of the People's Republic of China: Diagnostic Criteria and Management of Syphilis*. Beijing: Standard Press of China. https://unece.org/sites/default/files/2022-03/Attachment%201%20GB14622-2016_EN_0.pdf.

Fu, Rong, Jinkou Zhao, Dan Wu, Xiayan Zhang, Joseph D. Tucker, Meiwen Zhang, and Weijing Tang. 2018. "A Spatiotemporal Meta-Analysis of HIV/Syphilis Epidemic among Men Who Have Sex with Men Living in Mainland China." *BMC Infectious Diseases*, *18*(1): 652. https://doi.org/10.1186/s12879-018-3532-8.

Gao, L., L. Zhang, Q. Jin. 2009. "Meta-analysis: Prevalence of HIV Infection and Syphilis among MSM in China." *Sexually Transmitted Infections Journal*, *85*(5): 354–8.

Gong, X. D., G. C. Zhang, and S. Z. Ye, et al. 2001. "Epidemiological Analysis of Syphilis in China from 1985 to 2000."*Chinese Journal of Sexually Transmitted Infections* (1): 1–6.

Gong, Xiangdong, Yue Xiaoli, teng Feign, Jiang Ning, and Men Peixuan. 2014. "Syphilis in China from 2000 to 2013: Epidemiological Trends and Characteristics." *China Journal of Dermatology*, *47*(5): 310–15 (in Chinese).

Grassly, Nicholas C., Christophe Fraser, and Geoffrey P. Garnett. 2005. "Host Immunity and Synchronized Epidemics of Syphilis across the United States." *Nature*, *433*: 417–21. https://www.nature.com/articles/nature03072.

Guangxi CDC. 2014. *Prevention: Analysis of HIV/STD Epidemic in 2014*. Nanning, China.

Han, Pengyu, Yanxia Teng, Xiuxin bi, Jinge Li, and Dianxing Sun. 2019. "Epidemiology Survey of Infectious Diseases in North Korean Travelers, 2015–2017." *BMC Infectious Diseases*, 19(1): 13. https://doi.org/10.1186/s12879-018-3664-x.

Hesketh, T. 2003. "Getting Married Chinese Style: Pass the Medical First." *BMJ*, 326(7383): 277–9. doi: 10.1136/bmj.326.7383.277.

Hesketh, T., XJ Ye, and WX Zhu. 2008. "Syphilis in China: The Great Comeback." *Emerging Health Threats Journal*, 1: e6. doi: 10.31334/ehtj.08.006.

Hu, Chuankui, Zhong Qianyun, and Chen Xitang. 1965. "Eradication and Control of Syphilis in Our Country" (in Chinese). *Bulletin of Science (Ke Xue Tong Bao)*, 16(6): 503–10.

Li, Dongliang, Xueying Yang, Zheng Zhang, Zinxin Wang, Xiao Qi, Yuhua Ruan, Yunhua Zhou, Chunrong Li, Fengji Luo, and Joseph FT.F. Lau. 2016. "Incidence of Co-infections of HIV, Herpes Simplex Virus Type 2 and Syphilis in a Large Cohort of Men Who Have Sex with Men in Beijing, China." *PLoS ONE*, 11(1): e0147422. doi:10.1371/journal.pone.0147422.

Liang, Yongxuan. n.d. "Names of Syphilis in Historical Chinese Documents." http://square.umin.ac.jp/mayanagi/visit.sch/meiduGB.htm. Accessed August 6, 2019.

Lin, Charles, Xing Gao, Xiang-Sheng Chen, Qiang Chen, and Myron S. Cohen. 2006. "China's Syphilis Epidemic: A Systematic Review of Seroprevalence Studies." *Journal of the American Sexually Transmitted Diseases Association*, 33(12): 726–36. https://pubmed.ncbi.nlm.nih.gov/16755273/.

Liu, Guowu, Lu Hongyan, Wang Juan, Xia Ddongyan, Sun Yanming, Mi Guodong, and Wang Liming. 2015. "Incidence of HIV and Syphilis among Men Who Have Sex with Men (MSM) In Beijing: An Open Cohort Study." *PLoS One*, 10(10): e0138232. doi: 10.1371/journal.pone.0138232.

Lu, Ming, and Yiran Xia. 2016. *Migration in the People's Republic of China*. Asian Development Bank Institute. https://www.adb.org/sites/default/files/publication/191876/adbi-wp593.pdf. Accessed August 8, 2019.

National Bureau of Statistics of China. 2018. *China Statistical Yearbook 2018*. China statistics Press. https://www.stats.gov.cn/sj/ndsj/2018/indexeh.htm.

National Health Commission of the People's Republic of China. 2024. "The National Syphilis Prevention and Control Plan of China (2010–2020)" (in Chinese). https://www.chinacdc.cn/jkyj/crb2/yl/md/jswj_md/202409/P020240909360298141832.pdf.

National People's Congress (NPC). 2004. *The Infectious Disease Prevention Act (The 17th Presidential Decree of the People's Republic of China*.

Pan, Suiming, William L. Parish, and Yingying Huang. 2011. "Clients of Female Sex Workers: A Population-based Survey of China." *J Infect Dis*, 204 (Suppl 5): 1211–17.

Ruan, Yuhua, Dongliang Li, Xinxu Li, et al. 2007. "Relationship between Syphilis and HIV Infections among Men Who Have Sex with Men in Beijing, China." *Sexually Transmitted Diseases*, 34(8): 592–7. doi:10.1097/01.olq.0000253336.64324.ef.

Tapley, Donald F. Thomas Q. Morris, Lewis P. Rowland, Robert J. Weiss, Genell J. Subak-sharpe, and Diane M. Goetz, eds. 1989. *Complete Home Medical Guide*, pp. 469–70. New York: Crown Publishers.

Tucker, Joseph D., Gail E. Henderson, Tian F. Wang, Y. Ying, William Parish, Sui M. Pan, S. Xiang, and Myron S. Cohen. 2005. "Surplus Men, Sex Work, and the Spread of HIV in China." *AIDS, 19*(6): 539–47.

Wang, Liming, Dylan Podsan, Zihuang Chen, Hongyan Lu, Vania Wang, Colin Shepard, John K. Williams, and Guodong Mi. 2019. "Using Social Media to Increase HIV Testing among Men Who Have Sex with Men—Beijing, China, 2013–2017." *MMWR Morb Mortal Wkly Rep 2019, 68*(21): 478–82. doi: http://dx.doi.org/10.15585/mmwr.mm6821a3.

Wong, Ngai Sze, Shujie Huang, Heping Zheng, Lei Chen, Peizhen Zhao, Joseph D. Tucker, Li Gang Yang, Beng Tin Goh, and Bin Yang. 2017. "Stages of Syphilis in South China—A Multilevel Analysis of Early Diagnosis. *BMC Public Health, 17*: 135. doi: 10.1186/s12889-016-4004-y.

Yuan, Jun. 2024. "Analysis of Syphilis Incidence, Mortality, and Transmission Routes in China: In 2023, the Number of Reported Syphilis Cases Nationwide Reached 616,933, Representing a 39.84% Increase Compared to 2022" (In Chinese). *AIDS Care.* https://www.chyxx.com/industry/1197257.html.

Zhang, K., D. Li, H. Li, and E. J. Beck. 1999. "Changing Sexual Attitudes and Behaviour in China: Implications for the Spread of HIV and Other Sexually Transmitted Diseases." *AIDS Care, 11*(5): 581–9. doi: 10.1080/09540129947730.

Zhang, Xingyu, Tao Zhang, Jiao Pei, Yuanyuan Liu, Xiaosong Li, and Pau Medrano-Gracia. 2016. "Time Series Modelling of Syphilis Incidence in China from 2005 to 2012." *PLoS ONE, 11*(2): e0149401. doi: https://doi.org/10.1371/journal.pone.0149401.

The Healing Power of Belief: Worship as a Societal Antibiotic

Despite advances in modern medical science, epidemiological research and intervention cannot succeed without cultural context. Epidemics often reveal deep epistemological tensions between biomedical science and local or historical knowledge systems. Yet these systems can coexist and even complement each other when approached with cultural sensitivity. The examples below demonstrate how culture functions as an immune system, not in the biological sense, but socially and psychologically. Whether embodied in a yōkai, a saint, or a ritual, cultural responses to disease help communities regain a sense of agency, coherence, and hope. Recognizing this, many public health programs today integrate anthropologists into epidemic response teams—not just to translate language, but to translate meaning.

Amabie—A Legendary Guardian

A remarkable recent example of cultural anthropology intersecting with epidemiology in Japan is the revival of the Amabie, a legendary *yōkai* (supernatural creature) from the Edo period. During the Covid-19 pandemic, this ancient folklore figure became a living, breathing part of contemporary public health response—and a fascinating case of cultural epidemiology in action.

The earliest known depiction of Amabie dates back to the mid-1800s, in an illustrated woodblock print (kawaraban) describing the appearance of a three-legged, fish-scaled creature off the coast of Higo (modern-day Kumamoto). The creature prophesied six years of good harvest and promised protection from disease, instructing people to share its image. In early 2020, Japanese Twitter saw a resurgence of Amabie imagery, appearing in artworks, pastries, stickers, and masks, often accompanied by messages like "#AmabieChallenge" as talismanic expressions of hope. As one scholar noted, the figure re-emerged "as an icon of protection … an art effigy of our pandemic present" (Merli 2020).

In early 2020, manga artist Hide Shigeoka tweeted an illustration of Amabie with the caption "A new Coronavirus countermeasure," accompanied by the Japanese hashtag #Amabie. Other artists quickly joined in, creating their own versions of the creature, ranging from the sensual to the playfully cute. By early March, many of these Amabie images had been retweeted tens of thousands of times, including by newly engaged fans outside Japan. The creature's centuries-old directive to share its image had found new relevance in the age of social media. While no one expected an image to stop a virus, Amabie provided psychological comfort and a sense of collective action. As one artist remarked, "Art is powerless against a virus … but by drawing Amabie, we can take solace in having made our own little contribution" (Alt 2020).

Ola Bibi, AIDS Amma, and Corona Mata

In India, people often turn to deities for protection against pestilence. Ola Bibi, a goddess associated with cholera, embodies the syncretic character of Indian religious tradition. Prominent in the oral folklore of Bengal, she is venerated at numerous shrines throughout the region. When the first cholera pandemic emerged in Bengal in the early nineteenth century and spread across India by 1820, claiming hundreds of thousands of Indian lives and tens of thousands of British soldiers, the crisis extended as far as China. During this period, Ola Bibi was widely invoked, and regular prayers were offered at her shrines in hopes of healing and protection.

While many well-known deities have historical origins, new ones continue to emerge in response to contemporary crises. In the mid-1990s, as fear and misinformation about AIDS spread across India, a schoolteacher in the village of Menasi Kyathanahalli in Mysore district marked World AIDS Day (December 1, 1997) by painting a silhouette of a boy and girl, turned away from each other, on a roadside pillar. What began as a simple public awareness message gradually took on spiritual significance, eventually leading to the creation of a temple dedicated to "AIDS Amma"—a maternal deity who warns against unprotected sex. Over time, this public health gesture evolved into a sacred space where those living with the disease now pray for healing and protection. Inscribed in both English and Kannada, the site reflects how public health messaging merged with local religious traditions, transforming fear into ritualized hope.

As the Covid-19 pandemic swept across the globe, claiming countless lives, communities in India responded by creating a deity known as Corona Mata. Although temples and places of worship were closed to prevent the spread of the virus, people continued to offer prayers to this newly imagined goddess. Devotees presented ghee-laden sweets, incense, flowers, and cloves in hopes of appeasing her and stopping the spread of the disease. These offerings were often buried as part of the ritual, based on the belief that such acts would protect their families from the wrath of the virus and shield them from infection (Sen 2020).

Saint Sebastian and Saint Roch

During waves of bubonic plague in Renaissance Italy, communities turned to spiritual figures like Saint Sebastian and Saint Roch for protection against the relentless scourge. Their intercession was not merely an act of devotion but became deeply woven into the fabric of communal resilience.

Saint Sebastian, an early Christian martyr who was pierced with arrows, came to symbolize collective suffering. Towns afflicted by plague commissioned frescoes and altarpieces depicting Sebastian as miraculously shielding the sick. In San Gimignano, for instance, the local government commissioned Benozzo Gozzoli to paint an image of Sebastian in 1464. According to chroniclers, the plague ceased miraculously the very next day, reinforcing popular belief in the saint's protective power (Cranfield 2021).

Similarly, Saint Roch emerged as a "pandemic pilgrim," revered during the fifteenth-century plague in northern Italy. Hagiographies recount how he personally cared for the sick and survived the disease himself. His cult spread rapidly, leading to the construction of chapels and frescoes in his honor. Entire city-states sought his protection by commissioning altarpieces, erecting statues, and organizing public processions, often carrying relics, to invoke divine favor. These efforts reflected a profound psychological need and served to sanctify communal fear, transforming helplessness into ritualized hope.

Xipe Totec—God of Skin and Disease

The sudden emergence of smallpox, which killed an estimated 90 percent of Indigenous populations, was not merely a biological catastrophe but a profound cultural trauma. In response, people turned to existing religious frameworks, particularly deities associated with skin, pestilence, and death, to make sense of what seemed like divine or supernatural devastation. Among the Aztecs, Xipe Totec was revered as the god of skin diseases and was believed to punish individuals with afflictions such as scabies, abscesses, and rashes. During festivals, those suffering from such conditions would march in hopes of appeasing him and securing a cure. After the Spanish arrival and the onset of the smallpox epidemic, Xipe Totec became specifically associated with smallpox. Other deities were also linked to disease: Tezcatlipoca was believed to inflict venereal diseases, particularly syphilis, as punishment for immoral behavior; Xochiquetzal, the goddess of love, was thought to cause rashes and skin infections; and Nanahuatl (or Nanahuatzin) was worshipped as the god of leprosy (Marchán-Martínez et al. 2024).

From an anthropological perspective, these practices are not distractions from science but essential tools for making meaning. In the absence of biomedical solutions, spiritual intercessors helped fill emotional and explanatory voids, grounding entire communities in ritualized faith during times of crisis. Their enduring legacy reminds us that effective responses to epidemics often depend not only on medicine, but also on cultural coherence and shared symbols of hope.

Further Reading

Alt, Matt. 2020. "From Japan, A Mascot for the Pandemic." *The New Yorker*. https://www.newyorker.com/culture/cultural-comment/from-japan-a-mascot-for-the-pandemic.

Cranfield, Nicholas. 2021. "St Sebastian: Arrow Prayers for a Time of Pestilence." *Church Times*. https://www.churchtimes.co.uk/articles/2021/15-january/books-arts/visual-arts/st-sebastian-arrow-prayers-for-a-time-of-pestilence.

Marcchan-Martinez, Melissa, Eiana Bonilla, and Chinenye Onejeme. 2024. "Exploring the Origins of Dermatology in the Aztec Empire. *Medtigo Journal of Medicine, 2*: 4. https://doi.org/10.63096/medtigo30622450.

Merli, Claudia. 2020. "A Chimeric Being from Kyushu, Japan: Amabie's Revival during Covid-19." *Anthropol Today*, 36(5): 6–10. doi:10.1111/1467-8322.12602.

Museu de São Roque. "Saint Roch: the Plague, the Cult and the Image—A Brief Journey through the Saint's Iconography and the Works of the Museu de São Roque Dedicated to Him." *Museu de São Roque*. https://artsandculture.google.com/story/sAUxRLvGRYOWLw.

Sen, Nandini C. 2020. "Corona Mata and the Pandemic Goddesses." *The Wire*. https://thewire.in/culture/corona-mata-and-the-pandemic-goddesses.

Socioeconomic Divide and Health

China's Blueprint for Hepatitis B Control—An Extraordinary Public Health Success Story

Hepatitis B virus (HBV), a global health concern known for causing acute and chronic liver diseases, spreads through direct contact with infectious body fluids, including blood, semen, and vaginal secretions. Major transmission routes include perinatal transmission, sexual contact, and sharing of needles. However, HBV is not spread through casual contact, such as hugging or sharing food (CDC 2023). Misunderstanding these pathways has led to widespread stigmatization of individuals living with HBV.

According to the World Health Organization (WHO), an estimated 296 million people globally were living with chronic hepatitis B in 2019, and the virus causes approximately 820,000 deaths annually due to complications such as cirrhosis and hepatocellular carcinoma, a type of liver cancer. The burden of HBV is particularly severe in East Asia and Africa, where prevalence rates can exceed 8 percent in endemic regions, making it a leading cause of chronic liver disease and an elevated cancer risk (WHO 2022). In the United States, around 2.4 million people are estimated to be living with chronic HBV infection (CDC 2023).

The discovery of HBV and the subsequent development of a vaccine represent a milestone in medical history. The virus was first identified in 1967 by Dr. Baruch Blumberg, an American scientist who discovered the Australia antigen, later recognized as the hepatitis B surface antigen (HBsAg), in the blood of an Australian Aboriginal patient. This breakthrough enabled the detection of HBV and provided crucial insights into its transmission. In 1969, Blumberg co-developed the HBV vaccine, a significant achievement that earned him the Nobel Prize in Physiology or Medicine in 1976. The identification of HBsAg revolutionized diagnostic and preventive approaches, with the HBV vaccine playing a critical role in reducing the incidence of hepatitis B, particularly in countries implementing universal vaccination programs (Blumberg 2002).

Hepatitis B is closely associated with globalization, forced migration, and socioeconomic challenges characteristic of the twentieth and twenty-first centuries. The global movement of people, driven by conflict, economic opportunities, and environmental changes, has facilitated the cross-border spread of HBV. Migrants from regions with high HBV prevalence, such as sub-Saharan Africa and Southeast Asia, often relocate to areas with lower prevalence, potentially introducing the virus to new populations. In countries with inadequate health care systems for screening and treating HBV among immigrant populations, the disease could spread and remain undetected, posing significant public health challenges.

Socioeconomic factors play a crucial role in the persistence and spread of HBV. In low- and middle-income countries, where health care infrastructure is weak, the virus continues to spread. Limited access to health care services, including vaccination, diagnostic testing, and treatment, increases the vulnerability of affected communities. In these settings, perinatal transmission poses a significant challenge due to the lack of routine screening for pregnant women and the absence of timely immunization for newborns. Additionally, poor living conditions and inadequate education about the virus contribute to its continued transmission. In the early 1990s, HBV was endemic in China, with 120 million infections out of a total population of 1.16 billion, as reported in a 1992 sero-epidemiology survey (Yan et al. 2014).

China's HBV outbreaks had significant economic underpinnings. During the 1970s and the 1980s, China underwent drastic economic reforms under the leadership of Deng Xiaoping. The nation was encouraged to pursue wealth, and people sought various ways to make money. Blood donation became a source of income, particularly in rural areas where poverty was widespread. However, unsafe practices, such as needle reuse, caused rapid HBV transmission. By the late 1980s, it was estimated that nearly one out of nine in the total population were infected with hepatitis B, which the media described as "the nation's number 1 disease"(An Zi 2020). By the early 2000s, the prevalence was halved due to the introduction of vaccines and strict regulation of medical practices (Yan et al. 2014).

Unsafe medical practices have also contributed to HBV outbreaks in developed countries. In the United States, a significant HBV outbreak occurred in 2008 among patients undergoing dialysis treatment at multiple facilities. The CDC determined that the outbreak resulted from breaches in infection control practices, including the reuse of multidose vials and improper sterilization of equipment. This incident highlighted the critical importance of strict adherence to infection control protocols in medical settings to protect vulnerable patients from HBV exposure (CDC 2008–2019).

China achieved remarkable success in controlling hepatitis B virus (HBV) through a multifaceted approach combining vaccination, education, and health care access. The cornerstone of its strategy has been the universal newborn hepatitis B vaccination program, initiated in 1992 and expanded in 2002 to include free vaccines for all newborns. By ensuring timely birth doses and comprehensive prenatal screening, China significantly reduced mother-to-child transmission, with HBV prevalence among children under five dropping to just 0.3 percent by 2021. Public awareness campaigns, coupled with efforts to reduce stigma, encouraged testing and treatment, while robust surveillance systems monitored progress. Access to affordable antiviral treatments further improved outcomes for those with chronic infections. These efforts have collectively lowered HBV prevalence in the general population to 3 percent, down from much higher levels in previous decades, making China a global model for HBV control (Liu et al. 2023).

Despite these achievements, challenges remain, especially among older age groups. For instance, individuals aged 19–59 years have an HBsAg prevalence of 4.7 percent, and those aged sixty years and above have a prevalence of 5.6 percent. Additionally, regional disparities persist, with prevalence rates ranging from less than 1.5 percent in North China to over 6 percent in Taiwan and Hong Kong (Liu et al. 2023).

To achieve the World Health Organization's goal of eliminating hepatitis B as a public health threat by 2030, China continues to enhance its strategies, focusing on increasing diagnostic coverage, expanding antiviral treatment, and improving vaccination efforts among susceptible adult populations (Li et al. 2023).

China's success in HBV control highlights the power of universal vaccination and public health reforms. In 2015, the WHO lauded China for reducing hepatitis B infections among children under 15 to less than 1 percent, calling it an "extraordinary public health success story" (WHO 2015). With a strategy combining vaccination, education, and treatment, China demonstrates that eliminating hepatitis B is achievable. As the world targets the WHO's 2030 elimination goal, China's approach serves as a valuable model for similar challenges globally.

Further Reading

An Zi. 2020. "The Illness That Has Afflicted 120 Million Chinese People for Half a Century, Known as 'China's No. 1 Disease,' Has Finally Become a Thing of the Past" (in Chinese). *Jian Kang Jie (CN Healthcare)*. https://www.peopleapp.com/rmharticle/30018235942.

Blumberg, Baruch S. *Hepatitis B: The Hunt for a Killer Virus*. Princeton, NJ: Princeton University Press, 2002.

Centers for Disease Control and Prevention (CDC). 2008–2019. "Health Care-Associated Hepatitis B and C Outbreaks (≥ 2 cases) Reported to the Centers for Disease Control and Prevention (CDC) 2008–2019." *CDC Archive*. https://archive.cdc.gov/#/details?url=https://www.cdc.gov/hepatitis/statistics/healthcareoutbreaktable.htm.

Centers for Disease Control and Prevention (CDC). 2023. "Hepatitis B Information." July 28, 2023. https://www.cdc.gov/hepatitis/hbv/index.htm.

Li, Rui, Mingwang Shen, Jason J. Ong, et al. 2023. "Blueprint to Hepatitis B Elimination in China: A Modelling Analysis of Clinical Strategies." *JHEP Reports, 5*(10). doi: https://doi.org/10.1016/j.jhepr.2023.100833.

Liang, T. Jake. 2009. "Hepatitis B: The Virus and Disease." *Hepatology, 49*(S5): S13–S21. doi: 10.1002/hep.22881.

Liu, Zhenqiu, Chunqing Lin, Xianhua Mao, Chengnan Guo, Chen Suo, Dongliang Zhu, Wei Jiang, Yi Li, Jiahui Fan, Ci Song, Tiejun Zhang, Li Jin, Catherine De Martel, Gary M Clifford, and Xingdong Chen. 2023. "Changing Prevalence of Chronic Hepatitis B Virus Infection in China between 1973 and 2021: A Systematic Literature Review and Meta-Analysis of 3740 Studies and 231 Million People." *GUT*. doi: 10.1136/gutjnl-2023-330691.

Schweitzer, Aparna, Johannes Horn, Rafael T. Mikolajczyk, Gérard Krause, and Jördis J. Ott. 2015. "Estimations of Worldwide Prevalence of Chronic Hepatitis B Virus Infection: A Systematic Review of Data Published between 1965 and 2013." *The Lancet, 386*(10003): 1546–55. doi: 10.1016/S0140-6736(15)61412-X.

World Health Organization. 2022. "Hepatitis B." World Health Organization. June 24. https://www.who.int/news-room/fact-sheets/detail/hepatitis-b.

World Health Organization (WHO). 2015. "World Hepatitis Day: WHO Praises China's Vaccination Success, but Calls for More Progress on Improving Access to Treatment."

Yan, Yong-ping, Hai-xia Su, Zhao-Hua Ji, Zhong-Jun Shao, and Zhong-shu Pu. 2014. "Epidemiology of Hepatitis B Virus Infection in China: Current Status and Challenges." *J Clin Transl Hepatol.* doi: 10.14218/JCTH.2013.00030.

Depression and Anxiety in College Population in the United States

Major depression is characterized by distinct episodes lasting at least two weeks, though many episodes persist much longer. During these periods, individuals experience sadness, emptiness, irritability, and difficulties with cognitive functioning. These symptoms can severely impact a person's ability to manage daily activities. Anxiety, on the other hand, is a mental disorder marked by excessive and persistent fear and nervousness (APA 2013). While distinct, depression and anxiety frequently occur together, research indicates that nearly half of individuals diagnosed with major depression also experience severe and persistent anxiety (Tjornehoj 2017).

Both anxiety and depression are increasingly common in the U.S. population. Among Americans, individuals aged 18–24 years who have completed some college education are at the highest risk for major depressive disorders, with a prevalence rate of 21 percent. This means approximately one in five people in this group has been diagnosed with a major depressive disorder (Lee et al. 2020).

The prevalence of anxiety and depression is notably higher among college students compared to the general population. A comprehensive survey conducted by the Healthy Minds Network in 2021–2, which examined the mental health of college students in the United States, found that 44 percent of students experienced moderate to major depression, 37 percent reported having an anxiety disorder, and 15 percent had suicidal thoughts in the past year (Eisenberg et al. 2022).

Another study conducted in 2020 reported that 71 percent of students experienced symptoms of both depression and anxiety, with increased stress due to the Covid-19 pandemic identified as a major contributing factor (Son et al. 2020). However, research has shown that rates of anxiety and depression were already rising before the onset of Covid-19, indicating that the causes are multifaceted and not solely pandemic-related (Goodwin et al. 2022).

The alarming state of mental health on college campuses suggests an urgent need for effective and accessible therapeutic interventions.

Anxiety and depression can have numerous adverse effects on students' academic performance and physical health. Research shows that students struggling with anxiety and depression are more vulnerable to substance abuse, including alcohol addiction and the use of marijuana and other drugs. Additionally, depression is a major risk factor for suicidal tendencies among young individuals (Kerr 2017).

According to a 2022 survey by the American College Health Association, 64.8 percent of students reported that anxiety and depression had the greatest impact on their academic performance. The survey also identified other significant stressors, including concerns about future careers, financial issues, intimate relationships, and procrastination. Notably, procrastination was highly prevalent, with three out of four college students acknowledging its negative impact on their academic performance (ACHA 2022).

Research has demonstrated that procrastination is a common manifestation of depression. Depressed individuals often experience a loss of interest and energy, making it difficult for them to engage in activities they usually enjoy. Moreover, students with higher levels of anxiety and depression are more likely to engage in negative repetitive thoughts, which can exacerbate procrastination (Constantin et al. 2018).

To develop effective measures for mitigating anxiety and depression among students, researchers have been working to identify emerging factors that significantly affect students' mental health. One such factor is financial concerns. In the United States, student loan debt remains at alarmingly high levels, fluctuating around $1.7 trillion for several years. As of the second quarter of 2024, the total federal and private student loan debt stood at $1.74 trillion, only slightly lower than $1.76 trillion during the same period in 2023, according to LendingTree. This range has been consistent since 2021 (Schulz et al. 2024).

Delinquent student loans make up a substantial portion of severely overdue debt in the country, contributing to significant financial stress for borrowers. The pressure to secure a well-paying job and repay these loans has become a growing concern for students. The anticipation of having to repay a considerable amount of money in the future often negatively impacts the mental health of borrowers in their daily lives.

Some students choose to work multiple jobs to minimize their borrowing, but this choice often compromises their ability to meet academic expectations. A 2019 survey by Student Loan Planner found that 53 percent of borrowers with substantial student loan debt reported experiencing depression due to their financial burden. Additionally, 90 percent of borrowers reported significant anxiety related to their loan obligations, and some even contemplated suicide because of their student loans (Lockert 2024).

Another emerging factor contributing to psychological pressure is the shift of social values. A survey conducted by researcher at Boston University, which included nearly 33,000 college students nationwide, revealed that students today are increasingly driven by extrinsic motivation." This means that achieving a successful career, making more money, and getting more followers and likes on social media have become a higher priority in their life pursuits. In contrast, previous generations were more inclined to be driven by "intrinsic motivations," such as striving to be a valuable member of the community. Consequently, students today tend to be more self-critical and demanding of themselves, according to a 2021 survey by Boston University (McAlpine 2021).

The Covid-19 pandemic has profoundly impacted the mental well-being of students, contributing to rising levels of anxiety and depression. A significant factor is the lifestyle changes brought about by measures such as social distancing, the transition to online learning, and periods of quarantine. Studies have consistently shown that the pandemic has increased feelings of loneliness, stress, anxiety, and depression among a majority of college students in the United States (Lee et al. 2021).

The decline in mental health among college students in the United States is attributed to a combination of factors, as research has shown. These include the physical and psychological challenges associated with this age group, socioeconomic pressures, shifts in social values, and other factors that are not yet fully understood. Experts in education and health care emphasize the importance of expanding mental health education, enhancing student support systems, and strengthening academic assistance. Addressing anxiety and depression among students requires a comprehensive, community-wide effort that involves educators, health care providers, families, and policymakers working together to create supportive environments.

Further Reading

American College Health Association. 2022. "National College Health Assessment: Undergraduate Student Reference Group Executive Summary—Spring 2022." https://www.acha.org/documents/ncha/NCHA-III_SPRING_2022_UNDERGRAD_REFERENCE_GROUP_EXECUTIVE_SUMMARY.pdf.

American Psychiatric Association (APA). 2013. *Diagnostic and Statistical Manual of Mental Disorders.* https://doi.org/10.1176/appi.books.9780890425596.

Constantin, Kaytlin, Megan M. English, and Dwight Mazmanian. 2018. "Anxiety, Depression, and Procrastination among Students: Rumination Plays a Larger Mediating Role Than Worry." *APA PsycNet*. https://doi.org/10.1007/s10942-017-0271-5.

Eisenberg, Daniel, Sarah K. Lipson, Justin Heinze, and Sasha Zhou. 2022. "Healthy Minds Study—2021–2022 Data Report." *The Healthy Minds Network*. https://healthymindsnetwork.org/wp-content/uploads/2023/03/HMS_national_print-6-1.pdf.

Goodwin, Renee D., Lisa C. Dieker, Melody Wu, Sandro Galea, Christina Hoven, and Andrea Weinberger. 2022. "Trends in U.S. Depression Prevalence from 2015 to 2020: The Widening Treatment Gap." *American Journal of Preventive Medicine*, 63(5): 726–33. doi: https://www.ncbi.nlm.nih.gov/pmc/articles/PMC9483000/.

Kerr, Michael. 2017. "Depression and College Students." *Healthline*. https://www.healthline.com/health/depression/college-students.

Lee, Benjamin, Yan Wang, Susan A. Carlson, et al. 2020. "National, State-Level, and County-Level Prevalence Estimates of Adults Aged ≥18 Years Self-Reporting a Lifetime Diagnosis of Depression—United States, 2020." *MMWR*. doi: 10.15585/mmwr.mm7224a1.

Lee, Jungmin, Hyun Ju Jeong, and Sujin Kim. 2021. "Stress, Anxiety, and Depression among Undergraduate Students during the Covid-19 Pandemic and Their Use of Mental Health Services." *Innov High Educ*, 46(5): 519–38. doi: 10.1007/s10755-021-09552-y.

Lockert, Melanie. 2024. "2024 Student Debt and Mental Health Survey Reveals Borrowers Are Still Hurting." *Student Planner.com*. https://www.studentloanplanner.com/mental-health-awareness-survey/.

McAlpine, Kat J. 2021. "Depression, Anxiety, Loneliness Are Peaking in College Students." *The Brink*. https://www.bu.edu/articles/2021/depression-anxiety-loneliness-are-peaking-in-college-students/.

National Institute of Mental Health. "Major Depression." https://www.nimh.nih.gov/health/statistics/major-depression.

Schultz, Matt, and Dan Shepard. 2024. "Student Loan Debt Statistics." *Lendingtree*. https://www.lendingtree.com/student/student-loan-debt-statistics/.

Son, Changwon, Sudeep Hegde, Alec Smith, Xiaomei Wang, and Farzan Sasangohar. 2020. "Effects of Covid-19 on College Students' Mental Health in the United States: Interview Survey Study." *Journal of Medical Internet Research*, 22(9): e21279. https://www.ncbi.nlm.nih.gov/pmc/articles/PMC7473764/.

Tang, Xinfeng, Susin Tang, Zhihong Ren, and Daniel Fu Keung Wong. 2019. "Prevalence of Depressive Symptoms among Adolescents in Secondary School in Mainland China: A Systematic Review and Meta-analysis." *Journal of Affective Disorders*, 245: 498–507. doi: https://doi.org/10.1016/j.jad.2018.11.043.

Tjornehoj, Thomas. 2017. "The Relationship between Anxiety and Depression." *Hartgrove*. https://hartgrovehospital.com/relationship-anxiety-depression/.

World Economic Forum. 2019. "America's Student Debt Crisis Explained." https://www.weforum.org/agenda/2019/09/us-student-debt-crisis-explained-america-education/.

Preventable Diseases in an Unequal World—Addressing Diphtheria, Tetanus, and Pertussis

Diphtheria, tetanus, and pertussis are three bacterial infections that have posed major public health challenges for centuries. While vaccines have significantly reduced their prevalence, these diseases remain a threat, particularly in impoverished regions with limited health care infrastructure.

Diphtheria is caused by the bacterium *Corynebacterium diphtheriae*, which produces a toxin that can lead to severe respiratory distress. This occurs when a thick gray membrane forms in the throat, potentially obstructing breathing. Additional symptoms include fever, sore throat, and swollen glands. In severe cases, the toxin can spread to other parts of the body, causing complications such as myocarditis (inflammation of the heart muscles) and neuritis (inflammation of the nerves) (WHO 2023).

Diphtheria has a long history, with descriptions dating back to the fifth century BCE. However, it was not until the 1880s that *Corynebacterium diphtheriae* was identified as the cause. A major medical breakthrough came in the 1890s with Emil von Behring's development of the diphtheria antitoxin. The introduction of the diphtheria toxoid vaccine (an inactivated toxin) in the 1920s led to a dramatic reduction in cases (Plotkin et al. 2017).

Tetanus is caused by *Clostridium tetani*, a bacterium commonly found in soil, dust, and animal feces. It enters the body through wounds and produces a powerful neurotoxin called tetanospasmin, which disrupts nerve signals. This disruption results in muscle stiffness and painful spasms, often starting with the jaw muscles—a condition known as lockjaw. Without treatment, tetanus can be fatal, especially when it affects the respiratory muscles (CDC 2021).

Tetanus has been known since ancient times, it wasn't until the late nineteenth century that *Clostridium tetani* was identified as its cause. The tetanus toxoid vaccine, developed in the 1920s, became widely used during the Second World War to protect soldiers, dramatically reducing tetanus cases among the wounded (Rappuoli et al. 2011).

Pertussis, commonly known as whooping cough, is caused by *Bordetella pertussis*. These bacteria attach to the upper respiratory tract, releasing toxins that cause inflammation and impair the clearance of mucus. The disease is marked by severe coughing fits, often followed by a distinctive "whooping" sound during inhalation. Pertussis is particularly dangerous for infants, as it can lead to complications such as pneumonia, seizures, and, in some cases, death (CDC 2019).

Pertussis was first described in the sixteenth century, with *Bordetella pertussis* identified as its cause in the early twentieth century. The first pertussis vaccine was developed in the 1940s and was later combined with diphtheria and tetanus vaccines to create the DTP (diphtheria, tetanus, and pertussis) vaccine. This combination vaccine has become a cornerstone of childhood immunization programs worldwide (Cherry 2016).

The introduction of vaccines has dramatically reduced the incidence of these diseases, particularly in developed countries like the United States. However, they continue to pose significant risks globally, especially in impoverished communities with limited access to health care. Diphtheria is now rare in the United States, thanks to effective vaccination programs. However, it remains a concern in regions with low vaccination coverage, including parts of Africa, Asia, and Eastern Europe. Without prompt treatment, diphtheria can have a case fatality rate of up to 10 percent (CDC 2021).

Likewise, tetanus has become rare in the United States, but it remains widespread in low-income countries, particularly in rural areas where injuries are more common, and access to health care is limited. Neonatal tetanus, often caused by unsanitary childbirth practices, continues to be a major cause of infant mortality in these regions (WHO 2023).

Pertussis remains a public health concern even in the United States, with periodic outbreaks often attributed to waning immunity or gaps in vaccination coverage. Infants are particularly vulnerable, and the disease can be fatal in this age group (California Department of Public Health 2010).

In various cultures, these diseases are known by names that describe their symptoms. In China, for example, diphtheria is called "white throat," referring to the grayish membrane that forms in the throat. Tetanus is known as "wound wind," stemming from the traditional belief that it is caused by wind entering a wound. Pertussis is referred to as the "hundred-day cough," emphasizing the prolonged coughing fits characteristic of the disease (Yuan 2008).

Socioeconomic conditions heavily influence disease spread. In low-income regions with poor health care and low vaccination rates, communities face higher risks. For instance, tetanus is prevalent in rural regions where injuries are common, and access to vaccines and wound care is limited (Rappuoli et al. 2011). Poor hygiene during childbirth can cause neonatal tetanus, while unsanitary and crowded conditions heighten the risk of diphtheria and pertussis. Both diseases spread easily in densely populated areas, such as refugee camps or urban centers (WHO 2023; CDC 2019).

Multiple diphtheria outbreaks in Yemen since 2023, driven by conflict and the collapse of health care infrastructure, affected thousands of people. A recent study by Shedaiwah and colleagues (2024) found that, while low vaccination rates and population displacement accelerated the spread of the disease, females of childbearing age in Yemen face an even higher risk of diphtheria despite expected vaccination, revealing gender-based disparities in healthcare access. Cultural norms, limited mobility, and conflict contribute to these gaps, underscoring the need for targeted public health interventions for women (WHO "Tetanus").

Without adequate vaccination, outbreaks could happen in developed countries as well. A 2010 pertussis outbreak in California resulted in over 9,000 cases, fueled by low vaccination rates in certain communities and waning immunity among older children and adults. The outbreak was particularly fatal for infants, leading to multiple deaths (California Department of Public Health 2010). These incidents highlight the critical importance of vaccinations. One key benefit of globalization is its ability to improve access to vaccines and health care resources, helping to control and prevent infections in communities worldwide (Plotkin et al. 2017).

Past lessons teach us that global control of diphtheria, tetanus, and pertussis depends on broad vaccination, improved healthcare access, and community education to reduce transmission and vulnerability. Stronger surveillance and rapid response systems are also essential to containing future outbreaks, reinforcing the need for sustained global coordination.

Further Reading

Centers for Disease Control and Prevention (CDC). "Pertussis (Whooping Cough)." Last reviewed October 7, 2019. https://www.cdc.gov/pertussis/index.html.

Centers for Disease Control and Prevention (CDC). "Tetanus." Last reviewed January 22, 2021. https://www.cdc.gov/tetanus/.

California Department of Public Health. "Pertussis Report—December 2010." https://www.cdph.ca.gov.

Cherry, James D. 2016. "The Epidemiology of Pertussis: A Comparison of the Epidemiology of the Disease Pertussis with the Epidemiology of Bordetella Pertussis Infection." *Pediatric Infectious Disease Journal*, 35(1): 22–7.

Plotkin, Stanley A., Walter Orenstein, Paul A. Offit, and Kathryn M. Edwards. 2017. *Vaccines*. 7th ed. Philadelphia: Elsevier.

Rappuoli, Rino, Michel Nussenzweig, and Stanley Plotkin. 2011. "Challenges and Opportunities for the World's Newest Vaccine: The Conjugate Vaccine against Meningococcal Group A Disease." *Vaccine*, *29*(3): 15–20.

Shedaiwah, Sameer, Hamood Alsharabi, Labiba Anam, and Mohammed Abdullah Al Amad. 2024. "Risk Factors of Diphtheria Outbreak in Damt District of Al Dhalea Governorate, 2023 -Yemen: A Case–Control Study." *BMC Infectious Diseases*, *24*:1034. https://doi.org/10.1186/s12879-024-09932-7.

World Health Organization (WHO). "Diphtheria." https://www.who.int/health-topics/diphtheria.

World Health Organization (WHO). "Tetanus." Last reviewed March 22, 2023. https://www.who.int/news-room/fact-sheets/detail/tetanus.

Yuan, Jing. 2008. "A Study on Chinese Medical Terms." *Journal of Chinese Linguistics*, *36*(2): 302–21.

Malnutrition in the United States—A Socioeconomic Challenge

Despite technological advancements and overall improvements in global living conditions, food insecurity and malnutrition remain pressing challenges. According to the United Nations' latest assessment of the state of food and nutrition, approximately one-third of the global population, around 2.3 billion people, experience moderate to severe food insecurity. Alarmingly, one in twelve individuals globally faces severe food insecurity (Lederer 2022).

However, food insecurity and malnutrition are not confined to developing economies; studies reveal that developed nations are also affected. A 2021 survey by the U.S. Department of Agriculture (USDA) found that 10.2 percent of US households (13.5 million) experienced food insecurity at some point during the year, a figure that has remained largely unchanged over the past three years. Among these households, 40 percent experience "very low food security," meaning disruptions in eating patterns and food intake occur throughout the year. The remaining 60 percent manage to maintain regular meals, often by consuming less varied diets, relying on federal assistance programs, or seeking help from community food pantries. Furthermore, the survey shows that children are among the groups most impacted by food insecurity. As many as 5 million children live in food-insecure households, demonstrating the far-reaching consequences of this issue.

Food insecurity extends beyond logistical challenges and is closely tied to socioeconomic disparities. Lower socioeconomic status, both regionally and individually, is strongly associated with malnutrition and related health issues. In the United States, food insecurity is disproportionately concentrated in southern states such as West Virginia, Kentucky, Tennessee, Alabama, Mississippi, Arkansas, Louisiana, Oklahoma, New Mexico, and Texas. These states, often referred to as "America's Poverty Belt" (Florida 2011), have many residents whose incomes fall below the thresholds set by the U.S. federal Poverty Guidelines. Survey data indicate that Black non-Hispanic and Hispanic populations make up a significant proportion of low-income and food-insecure households, revealing socioeconomic and racial inequities in access to sufficient and nutritious food (USDA 2021).

Food insecurity presents a unique challenge in the United States compared to developing economies due to its association with health issues. While hunger, starvation, and physical symptoms like wasting, stunting, and being underweight are relatively rare in the United States, the primary issue is overweight and obesity caused by unhealthy and limited diets. Low-income households often rely on calorically dense but nutrient-poor foods, leading to what is known as the "dual burden"—the coexistence of malnutrition and overweight (Bowers et al. 2018).

In adults, overweight is defined as a body mass index (BMI) of 25 or higher, while obesity is classified as a BMI over 30. According to the Centers for Disease Control and Prevention (CDC) 2017–18 survey, 31.1 percent of American adults are overweight, 42.2 percent are obese (Freyar et al. 2020), and 1 in 6 children in the U.S. is obese (CDC 2024). Overweight and obesity are especially common in areas grappling with poverty and unemployment. The five states with the highest obesity rates—West Virginia, Mississippi, Alabama, Arkansas, and Louisiana—are all situated in the "Poverty Belt," where more than one-third of adults are classified as obese, based on CDC's data.

Obesity is linked to increased mortality and the severity of a wide range of non-communicable diseases (NCDs). Over sixty NCDs, including diabetes, cardiovascular disease, stroke, asthma, and cancer, are among the most prevalent conditions associated with obesity. In many ways, malnutrition carries more severe consequences than hunger or underweight, scientists believe. Given the intrinsic connection between poverty, malnutrition, and obesity, it is unsurprising that the states comprising America's "Poverty Belt," "Diabetes Belt," and "Stroke Belt" largely overlap. These shared regions highlight the interplay between socioeconomic disparities and health outcomes.

Studies have identified several pathways linking malnutrition to NCDs. First, malnutrition disproportionately affects economically disadvantaged groups. In the 1980s, the American Heart, Lung, and Blood Institute identified a group of southern states with stroke mortality rates at least 10 percent higher than the national average, designating the region as the "Stroke Belt." These states include Alabama, Arkansas, Georgia, Indiana, Kentucky, Louisiana, Mississippi, North Carolina, South Carolina, Tennessee, and Virginia. The region's elevated stroke prevalence has historical roots dating back to the 1940s and remains two to four times higher than other areas, according to CDC (Howard et al. 2020).

Second, demographic and economic data reveal that these states have a significant proportion of Black residents living in low-income conditions. A notable disadvantage in history in the region is the lower per-capita availability of physicians and medical facilities compared to the national average, making health care access more challenging.

Third, behavioral risk studies further indicate that sedentary lifestyles, unhealthy diets, and obesity are so widespread in these states that they may account for up to 30 percent of the excess NCD risk. Additionally, a study by Barker (2011) found that 37 percent of diabetes cases are attributable to nonmodifiable factors such as age, gender, and race/ethnicity, underscoring the role of demographics in shaping health outcomes.

The overall situation suggests that addressing malnutrition and encouraging healthier lifestyles are key to reducing obesity and its associated diseases. However, eradicating malnutrition requires more than simply resolving food insecurity.

Logistically, ensuring consistent access to fresh, nutrient-dense foods in underserved areas requires substantial infrastructure, such as reliable transportation networks, cold storage facilities, and local distribution centers. Financially, the costs of sourcing high-quality food, maintaining supply chains, and covering operational expenses are immense, especially as demand often exceeds available funding. Nonprofits rely heavily on donations and grants, which can be inconsistent, while government programs must navigate budget constraints and competing priorities. Additionally, the challenge of reaching remote or marginalized communities, where limited awareness and cultural barriers may hinder the adoption of healthier dietary practices.

Providing calorically dense but nutrient-poor meals can have unintended negative effects. Instead of merely alleviating hunger in poverty-stricken households, nonprofit organizations must focus on offering nutritionally balanced, health-sustaining meals, studies indicate. Tackling malnutrition is an economically challenging task for a developed country like the United States, but the long-term costs of inaction could be even higher (Food Research and

Action Center 2017). Clearly, investing in solutions now can help prevent the escalating health care expenses and societal impacts associated with obesity and related diseases.

Further Reading

Barker, Lawrence E. 2011. "Geographic Distribution of Diagnosed Diabetes in the U.S.: A Diabetes Belt." *American Journal of Preventive Medicine*, *40*(4): 434–9.

Bowers, Kara Shifler, Erica Francis, and Jennifer L. Kraschnewski. 2018. "The Dual Burden of Malnutrition in the United States and the Role of Non-profit Organizations." *Preventive Medicine Reports, 12*: 294–7. https://doi.org/10.1016/j.pmedr.2018.10.002.

Centers for Disease Control and Prevention (CDC). 2024. "Childhood Obesity Facts." *CDC*. https://www.cdc.gov/obesity/childhood-obesity-facts/childhood-obesity-facts.html.

Centers for Disease Control and Prevention (CDC). 2020. "Stroke Death Rates, 2018–2020 Adults, Ages 35+, by County." https://www.cdc.gov/dhdsp/maps/images/stroke_all.jpg.

Florida, Richard. 2011. "Map of the Day: America's Poverty Belt." *Bloomberg News*, December 8. https://www.bloomberg.com/news/articles/2011-12-08/map-of-the-day-america-s-poverty-belt.

Food and Agriculture Organization of the United States. 2022. *The State of Food Security and Nutrition in the World 2022*. https://doi.org/10.4060/cc0639en.

Food Research & Action Center. December 2017. *Hunger & Health: The Impact of Poverty, Food Insecurity, and Poor Nutrition on Health and Well-Being*. Washington, DC: Food Research & Action Center. https://frac.org/wp-content/uploads/hunger-health-impact-poverty-food-insecurity-health-well-being.pdf.

Fryar, Cheryl D., Margaret D. Carroll, M. S. P. H., and Joseph Afful. 2020. "Prevalence of Overweight, Obesity, and Severe Obesity among Adults Aged 20 and Over: United States, 1960–1962 through 2017–2018." *CDC*. https://www.cdc.gov/nchs/data/hestat/obesity-adult-17-18/overweight-obesity-adults-H.pdf.

Howard, George, and Virginia J. Howard. 2020. "Twenty Years of Progress toward Understanding the Stroke Belt." *American Heart Association Journals, 51*(3). https://www.ahajournals.org/doi/10.1161/STROKEAHA.119.024155.

Lederer, Edith. 2022. "U.N. Says 2.3 Billion People Severely or Moderately Hungry in 2021." *PBS News*. https://www.pbs.org/newshour/world/u-n-says-2-3-billion-people-severely-or-moderately-hungry-in-2021.

USDA. 2021. "Food Security Status of U.S. Households in 2021." https://www.ers.usda.gov/topics/food-nutrition-assistance/food-security-in-the-u-s/key-statistics-graphics/.

Beyond Outbreaks: The Global Rise of *Salmonella* and *E. coli* Infections

Salmonella and *Escherichia coli* (*E. coli*) are among the most common bacterial pathogens causing foodborne illnesses worldwide. A large proportion of food recalls by companies is linked to contamination with these bacteria. Despite belonging to the same *Enterobacteriaceae* family, *Salmonella* and *E. coli* differ in their pathogenic mechanisms, modes of transmission, and the types of illnesses they cause. While vaccines for animals are available to help reduce the spread of these pathogens, vaccines for human use are still under development, according to the Centers for Disease Control and Prevention (CDC).

Salmonella is a rod-shaped, gram-negative bacteria (GNB) that includes over 2,600 serotypes, with *Salmonella enterica* being the most common cause of human infections, according to the CDC. GNB can be highly resistant to antibiotics due to their cell wall structure and the enzymes they carry. Infections often require patients to receive intensive care, and patients are at risk of high morbidity and mortality. These bacteria primarily infect the gastrointestinal tract, leading to illnesses such as salmonellosis (Winfield et al. 2003). *E. coli*, another GNB, naturally resides in the intestines of humans and animals. While most *E. coli* strains are harmless, certain pathogenic strains like "O157:H7" can cause severe foodborne illnesses. Both *Salmonella* and pathogenic *E. coli* are primarily transmitted through the consumption of contaminated food or water, making them significant public health concerns (Johns Hopkins Medicine).

The potential for these bacteria to co-infect arises from their similar transmission routes and ability to survive in various environments. For instance, agricultural practices that involve using contaminated water for irrigation can introduce both pathogens into the food supply, leading to co-infections in humans (Winfield et al. 2003).

Salmonella and *E. coli* have evolved to survive under various environmental conditions, enhancing their potential to cause contamination. *Salmonella* can persist in low-moisture environments, such as dried foods, for extended periods. It can also form biofilms, which are complex communities of bacteria that adhere to surfaces and resist disinfection, making it particularly challenging to eradicate in food processing environments. *E. coli* strains are notable for their ability to survive in water and on fresh produce. Moreover, the O157:H7 strain can cause outbreaks even at a small quantity of bacterial cells. Both *Salmonella* and *E. coli* form biofilms on surfaces, which are often resistant to cleaning

Notable Outbreaks of Foodborne Diseases in Fast-food Chains

McDonald's *E. coli* Outbreak

In September and October 2024, an *E. coli* outbreak linked to McDonald's Quarter Pounders caused 104 illnesses across 14 states, with 34 hospitalizations, and 1 death in Colorado. While Colorado reported the most cases, others occurred in Midwestern and Mountain states. The CDC traced the likely source to uncooked slivered onions supplied by Taylor Farms. In response, Taylor Farms recalled its yellow onions, and McDonald's pulled the Quarter Pounder from menus in affected areas.

Chipotle's Multiple Outbreaks

Between 2015 and 2018, over 1,100 people fell ill from food contamination at Chipotle, leading to a $25 million criminal fine in 2020 and mandated safety measures. The U.S. Justice Department charged Chipotle with food adulteration after outbreaks of *E. coli*, *Salmonella*, and norovirus in 2015, a norovirus outbreak in Virginia in 2017, and a *Clostridium perfringens* outbreak in Ohio in 2018. In Boston in 2015, 141 people were sickened after a sick employee was forced to work. In Ohio in 2018, nearly 650 cases were linked to improper food temperature controls. Contributing factors included poor training, understaffing, and pressure on ill employees to work.

Jack in the Box's *E. coli* Crisis

In 1993, an *E. coli* O157:H7 outbreak traced to Jack in the Box hamburgers caused 700 illnesses and four deaths across four states. Prompted by a Seattle pediatrician's report of children with bloody diarrhea, the investigation revealed contaminated meat. The crisis cost the company $160 million in lost sales, recalls, and legal settlements, including a $15 million payment for a child's brain injury.

The outbreak spurred stricter federal regulations, including higher cooking temperatures for hamburgers, mandatory safe-handling labels, and increased *E. coli* testing in raw beef. Affected families founded the advocacy group STOP, and the beef industry invested in detection and prevention strategies. The National Cattlemen's Beef Association later established the Beef Industry Food Safety Council to combat pathogens across the sector.

> **Further Reading**
>
> Centers for Disease Control and Prevention. 2024. *Outbreak of E. coli O157:H7 Infections Linked to Slivered Onions Served at McDonald's (Final Update)*. Atlanta, GA: U.S. Department of Health and Human Services. December 3. https://www.cdc.gov/ecoli/outbreaks/e-coli-O157.html.
>
> Food Safety News. 2020. "Chipotle Agrees to Pay $25 Million Federal Fine for Role in Some Outbreaks." https://www.foodsafetynews.com/2020/04/chipotle-agrees-to-pay-25-million-federal-fine-for-role-in-some-outbreaks/.
>
> Golan, Elise, Tanya Roberts, Elisabete Salay, Julie Caswell, Michael Olliger, and Danna Moore. 2004. "Food Safety Innovation in the United States: Evidence from the Meat Industry." *USDA*. https://www.ers.usda.gov/publications/pub-details/?pubid=41636.
>
> Office of Public Affairs, U.S. Department of Justice. 2020. "Chipotle Mexican Grill Agrees to Pay $25 Million Fine and Enter a Deferred Prosecution Agreement to Resolve Charges Related to Foodborne Illness Outbreaks." *DOJ*. Press Release Number: 20–394.

detergents, complicating efforts to control their spread in food processing plants (Winfield et al. 2003).

Salmonella and *E. coli* infections are top public health concerns globally. The CDC estimates that Salmonella alone causes over one million infections annually in the United States; nearly one-third of patients require hospitalizations, and hundreds die of the infections annually (CDC 2021). With respect to *E. coli*-related infections, the CDC reports about 73,000 infections annually in the United States, leading to approximately 2,168 hospitalizations and 61 deaths (CDC 2005). Globally, non-typhoidal *Salmonella* is responsible for approximately 78 million cases of foodborne illness each year, with 59,000 associated deaths, making it a leading food poisoning pathogen worldwide (WHO 2015).

Salmonella infection, or salmonellosis, typically presents with symptoms such as diarrhea, fever, and abdominal cramps within 6–72 hours after exposure. Most people recover without specific treatment, though severe cases may require hospitalization, especially among vulnerable groups such as young children, the elderly, and immunocompromised individuals (Mead et al. 1999). In some cases, the infection can become systemic, leading to life-threatening conditions like septicemia, an infection of the blood.

E. coli infections, particularly those caused by the O157:H7 strain, due to the Shiga toxin it produces, often result in severe abdominal pain, bloody diarrhea, and vomiting. A critical complication of *E. coli* infection is hemolytic uremic syndrome (HUS), a condition that can lead to kidney failure, especially in children and the elderly. Tarr and colleagues reported that about 15% of children younger than 10 years with E. coli O157:H7 infection develop HUS. (Tarr et al. 2005).

Treatment for *Salmonella* and *E. coli* infections generally involves supportive care, such as hydration and rest. Antibiotics are usually not recommended for these infections. However, patients are strongly recommended to check with their physicians for proper procedures to follow (Scallan et al. 2011). Preventive measures are crucial in reducing the incidence of *Salmonella* and *E. coli* infections. Public health initiatives emphasize proper food handling, cooking, and storage practices to prevent contamination. For example, cooking meat and poultry thoroughly, washing hands and surfaces regularly, and avoiding cross-contamination in the kitchen are essential steps in preventing these infections (CDC 2021).

The spread of *Salmonella* and *E. coli* is often influenced by social, environmental, and economic factors. Contamination is more prevalent in areas with inadequate sanitation, limited access to clean water, and poor food safety practices—conditions often found in low-income communities in both developed and developing countries (Mead et al. 1999). Several foodborne illness outbreaks have occurred in fast-food chains across the United States, raising public awareness about the high contamination risk of these pathogens. Communities with limited health care access, low education levels, and poor living conditions are particularly vulnerable to foodborne illnesses. Furthermore, a lack of awareness about safe food handling practices can lead to significantly higher infection rates in these populations (Scallan et al. 2011).

Cultural practices, such as consuming raw or undercooked foods, can also play a role in the spread of *Salmonella* and *E. coli*. In some cultures, raw meat or eggs are considered delicacies, which increases the risk of exposure to these bacteria. Furthermore, the use of untreated manure in agriculture and reliance on contaminated water sources can introduce these pathogens into the food supply, potentially causing outbreaks (Winfield et al. 2003).

Agricultural practices, particularly those associated with livestock farming, can contribute to the spread of *Salmonella* and *E. coli*. The mass production of poultry and cattle often involves the routine use of antibiotics, which can facilitate the emergence of antibiotic-resistant strains of these bacteria. This resistance complicates treatment options and can lead to more severe infections (Manyi-Loh et al. 2018; Mead et al. 1999).

The global food supply chain presents significant risks of contamination. Food processing, packaging, and distribution practices must follow stringent safety protocols to prevent the spread of bacteria such as *Salmonella* and *E. coli*.

However, lapses in these processes can result in widespread contamination, as demonstrated by numerous outbreaks linked to processed foods. Globalization has further complicated food safety, with food products often traveling long distances before reaching consumers. This interconnected distribution network means that a contamination event in one country can trigger outbreaks in multiple regions, making it challenging to trace and control the source of infection. The complexity of the global food supply chain underscores the critical need for international collaboration in food safety measures and outbreak response efforts (FAO 2004).

Climate change presents additional challenges to food safety, studies show. Rising temperatures and shifting weather patterns can influence the survival and proliferation of *Salmonella* and *E. coli* in the environment. For instance, warmer temperatures can accelerate bacterial growth in food and water, increasing the risk of contamination. Extreme weather events, such as floods, can also introduce these bacteria into water supplies and agricultural fields, potentially triggering outbreaks (Milho et al. 2019; Winfield et al. 2003).

The following two notable outbreak cases highlight the devastating impact of *Salmonella* and *E. coli* contamination.

In the United States, the 1993 Jack in the Box *E. coli* O157:H7 outbreak remains one of the most notorious foodborne illness incidents. The outbreak was linked to undercooked hamburgers served at the fast-food chain, infecting over 700 people across four states: Washington, Idaho, California, and Nevada. Tragically, the outbreak resulted in four deaths, primarily among children, and prompted significant regulatory changes, including the implementation of the Hazard Analysis and Critical Control Points (HACCP) system in the U.S. meat processing industry (CDC 1993).

In December 2017, an outbreak of *Salmonella* Agona infections was identified among infants in France, traced to contaminated infant milk products manufactured at a single facility. The outbreak was first detected in late November 2017, when the French National Reference Centre (NRC) for *Salmonella* observed an unusual increase in *Salmonella* Agona cases among infants. A total of thirty-seven confirmed cases were reported, with the affected infants having a median age of four months. Symptoms included diarrhea, fever, and vomiting, with most cases occurring between mid-August and early December 2017.

The outbreak was linked to five different infant milk products produced at the facility, with one product accounting for the majority of cases. Notably, the same facility had been implicated in a *Salmonella* Agona outbreak in 2005. The contaminated products were distributed to sixty-six countries, prompting international alerts through the European Rapid Alert System for Food and Feed (RASFF) and the World Health Organization's INFOSAN network.

This event highlights the challenges of managing foodborne illnesses in vulnerable populations and underscores the importance of rigorous food safety protocols and rapid public health responses (Jourdan-da Silva et al. 2018).

Salmonella and *E. coli* contamination remain significant public health challenges due to their ability to persist in diverse environments. The prevalence of these bacteria is shaped by various social, environmental, and economic factors. With globalization and climate change adding to the complexity of controlling these pathogens, public health systems must remain vigilant and prepared to mitigate the associated risks.

Further Reading

Centers for Disease Control and Prevention (CDC). 2024. "About Escherichia coli Infection." https://www.cdc.gov/ecoli/about/index.html.

Centers for Disease Control and Prevention (CDC). 2025. "Estimates of Foodborne Illness in the United States." https://www.cdc.gov/foodborneburden/2011-foodborne-estimates.html. Accessed August 19, 2024.

Centers for Disease Control and Prevention (CDC). 1993. "Infections Linked to Ground Beef, 1993." https://www.cdc.gov/mmwr/preview/mmwrhtml/00020219.htm#:~:text=of%20e%2Dmail.-

Centers for Disease Control and Prevention (CDC). 2005. "Outbreaks of Escherichia coli O157:H7 Associated with Petting Zoos—North Carolina, Florida, and Arizona, 2004 and 2005." *MMWR*. https://www.cdc.gov/mmwr/preview/mmwrhtml/mm5450a1.htm.

Centers for Disease Control and Prevention (CDC). "Salmonella." https://www.cdc.gov/salmonella/index.html.

Food and Agriculture Organization of the United Nations. 2004. "Globalization of Food Systems in Developing Countries: Impact on Food Security and Nutrition." *FAO Food and Nutrition Paper 83*. https://openknowledge.fao.org/server/api/core/bitstreams/08bb8465-e0ae-40e7-971d-c695b58e534e/content. Accessed August 20, 2024.

Johns Hopkins Medicine. "Health: Escherichia coli O157:H7." https://www.hopkinsmedicine.org/health/conditions-and-diseases/escherichia-coli-o157-h7.

Jourdan-da Silva, Nathalie, Laetitia Fabre, Eve Robinson, et al. 2018. "Ongoing Nationwide Outbreak of Salmonella Agona Associated with Internationally Distributed Infant Milk Products, France, December 2017." *Euro Surveillance*, 23(2): 17-00852. doi: 10.2807/1560-7917.ES.2018.23.2.17-00852.

Manyi-Loh, Christy, Sampson Mamphweli, Edson Meyer, and Anthony Okoh. 2018. "Antibiotic Use in Agriculture and Its Consequential Resistance in Environmental Sources: Potential Public Health Implications." *Molecules, 23*(4): 795. doi: 10.3390/molecules23040795. Accessed August 20, 2024.

Mead, Paul S., Laurence Slutsker, Vance Dietz, Linda F. McCaig, Joseph S. Bresee, Craig Shapiro, Patricia M. Griffin, and Robert V. Tauxe. 1999. "Food-Related Illness and Death in the United States." *Emerging Infectious Diseases 5*(5): 607–25. https://doi.org/10.3201/eid0505.990502.

Milho, C., M. D. Silva, D. Alves, H. Oliveira, C. Sousa, L. M. Pastrana, J. Azeredo, and S. Sillankorva. 2019. "Escherichia Coli and Salmonella Enteritidis Dual-Species Biofilms: Interspecies Interactions and Antibiofilm Efficacy of Phages." *Science Reports*. doi: 10.1038/s41598-019-54847-y.

Scallan, Elaine, Robert M. Hoekstra, Frederick J. Angulo, Robert V. Tauxe, Mar-Alain Widdowson, Sharon L. Roy, Jeffery L. Jones, and Patricia M. Griffin. 2011. "Foodborne Illness Acquired in the United States—Major Pathogens." *Emerging Infectious Diseases*, *17*(1): 7–15. doi: https://doi.org/10.3201/eid1701.P11101.

Tarr, Phillip I, Carrie A Gordan, and Wayne L. Chandler. 2005. "Shiga-toxin-producing Escherichia Coli and Haemolytic Uraemic Syndrome." *The Lancet, 365*(9464): 1073–86. https://doi.org/10.1016/S0140-6736(05)71144-2.

Winfield, Mollie D., and Eduardo a Groisman. 2003. "Role of Nonhost Environments in the Lifestyles of Salmonella and Escherichia coli." *Applied and Environmental Microbiology*, *69*(7): 3687–94. doi: 10.1128/AEM.69.7.3687-3694.2003.

World Health Organization (WHO). 2015. "WHO Estimates of the Global Burden of Foodborne Diseases." https://iris.who.int/bitstream/handle/10665/199350/9789241565165_eng.pdf. Accessed August 20, 2024.

Synthetic Opioids and Methamphetamine Addiction: Escalating Crises in American Public Health

Synthetic opioids and methamphetamine (meth) are extremely addictive and rank among the deadliest drugs. They are extensively misused in the United States, resulting in tens of thousands of annual deaths due to overdose. Data of the Centers for Disease Control and Prevention (CDC) shows that there were 91,799 deaths from drug overdose in 2020, marking a 30 percent surge compared to 2019. This rise was predominantly attributed to fentanyl and its combined use with cocaine and methamphetamine (Mattson et al. 2022).

Synthetic opioids constitute a category of drugs including fentanyl, carfentanil (commonly employed as a veterinary tranquilizer), and other synthetic opioids with chemical resemblance to morphine, but produced within laboratory settings. Notably, fentanyl, a potent synthetic opioid, surpasses heroin's strength by a factor of 50 and morphine's by 100, according to the CDC.

Due to fentanyl's extremely high potency in small quantity and cheap prices, fentanyl has become a favorite money maker for drug traffickers. According to CDC's data, in recent years, fentanyl-involved deaths have accounted for the majority of overdose-related deaths. A factor that makes illicit fentanyl particularly lethal is that the drug is often laced with heroin, cocaine, and methamphetamine. These combinations are often shaped into pills resembling prescription opioids. The CDC's "Fentanyl Facts" indicate that over 150 individuals die of overdoses linked to synthetic opioids like fentanyl on a daily basis.

The addictive nature of opioids derives from their ability to activate the reward centers within the human brain. Opioids induce the release of endorphins, which dampen the mind's perception of pain and amplify sensations of pleasure. Once the effects of an opioid dose diminish, individuals often consume more of the substance to sustain the desired effect, a pattern that fosters addictive behavior. Moreover, prolonged opioid use disrupts the body's natural production of endorphins and leads to the development of drug tolerance. As the same dosage of opioids no longer triggers a desired surge of positive feelings, individuals tend to escalate their doses. The risk of addiction can be further intensified by factors such as poverty, unemployment, severe depression, anxiety, and overall stressful circumstances, according to Mayo Clinic.

Methamphetamine represents one of the most extensively misused stimulant drugs within the United States, as indicated by the National Institute on Drug Abuse (NIDA). In 2021, a total of 16.8 million Americans aged 12 or older (accounting for 6.0 percent of the population) had experimented with methamphetamine at least once in their lives; approximately 2.5 million individuals disclosed using methamphetamine within the past twelve months, according to NIDA. A recent study illustrates a nearly fivefold increase in age-adjusted rates of drug overdose deaths involving methamphetamine in the United States between 2011 and 2018, which equates to a surge from 1.8 to 10.1 deaths per 100,000 men, and from 0.8 to 4.5 deaths per 100,000 women (Han et al. 2021). The bulk of methamphetamine available in the United States is manufactured by transnational criminal organizations in Mexico. Notably, this product boasts high purity levels, potency, and remains economically accessible, according to NIDA.

NIDA's "Drug Facts" indicates that methamphetamine use can lead to permanent bodily disfigurement, contributing to memory loss, aggression, psychotic behavior, cardiovascular system damage, malnutrition, and an increased risk of contracting hepatitis and HIV/AIDS. Unlike synthetic opioid overdoses that can be reversed using Narcan, there is currently no available counteracting medication for meth overdoses. Treatment primarily relies on behavioral therapy.

Addiction to synthetic opioids and meth in the United States stems from a variety of reasons. As broadly reported in studies by NDIA and the CDC, some people become addicted after being prescribed these drugs for pain management and then develop a dependence on them. Others may use these drugs recreationally to manage stress or emotional issues. Synthetic drugs are highly addictive and can cause physical dependence even after short-term use. Additionally, synthetic drugs are often mixed which can increase the risk of addiction and overdose.

However, association between socioeconomic status and drug abuse appears to be a more profound explanation attested by many studies. The risk of synthetic opioid addiction and death is higher among people who live in poverty or are unemployed. People who live in poverty or are unemployed may have less access to health care and addiction treatment services, which can make it more difficult to get help for drug use (Altekruse et al. 2020). An example of this association is the situation in the Appalachian region of the United States, where household incomes and educational attainment levels lag behind national averages. A report by the U.S. Department of Health and Human Services (HHS) indicates that this region is faced with an opioid overdose death rate that surpasses that of other states in the United States by 72 percent (HHS 2020).

Managing drug abuse is a complex challenge. While strong law enforcement is necessary to combat drug trafficking, reducing demand is equally important. This effort must also include expanding health care services, advancing education, and improving employment opportunities. Ultimately, addressing drug addiction requires a coordinated, society-wide response.

Further Reading

Altekruse, Sean F., Candace M. Cosgrove, William C. Altekruse, Richard A. Jenkins, and Carlos Blanco. 2020. "Socioeconomic Risk Factors for Fatal Opioid Overdoses in the United States: Findings from Morality Disparities in American Communities Study (MDAC)." *PLOS ONE*, *15*(1): e0227966. doi: https://doi.org/10.1371/journal.pone.0227966.

Centers of Disease Control and Prevention (CDC). "Fentanyl Facts." https://www.cdc.gov/stopoverdose/fentanyl/index.html.

Centers of Disease Control and Prevention (CDC). "Overdose Prevention." https://www.cdc.gov/overdose-prevention/index.html.

East Tennessee State University and NORC at the University of Chicago. 2019. "Creating A Culture of Health in Appalachia—Disparities and Bright Spots." *ARC.gov*. https://www.arc.gov/wp-content/uploads/2020/06/HealthDisparitiesRelatedtoOpioidMisuseinAppalachiaApr2019.pdf.

Han, Beth, Jessica Cotto, Kathleen Etz, Emily B. Einstein, Wilson M. Compton, and Nora D. Volkow. 2021. "Methamphetamine Overdose Deaths in the US by Sex and Race and Ethnicity." *JAMA Psychiatry,* 78(5): 564–7. doi: 10.1001/jamapsychiatry.2020.4321.

Mattson, Christine L., Sagar Kuma, Laren Tanz, Priyam Patel, Qingwei Luo, and Nicole Davis. 2022. "Drug Overdose Deaths in 28 States and the District of Columbia: 2020 Data from the State Unintentional Drug Overdose Reporting System." *SUDORS*. https://www.cdc.gov/overdose-prevention/media/pdfs/SUDORS-Data-Brief-1.pdf.

Mayo Clinic Staff. "How Opioid Addiction Occurs." https://www.mayoclinic.org/diseases-conditions/prescription-drug-abuse/in-depth/how-opioid-addiction-occurs/art-20360372.

National Center for Drug Abuse Statistics (NCDAS). "Drug Overdose Death Rates." https://drugabusestatistics.org/drug-overdose-deaths/.

National Institute on Drug Abuse (NIDA). 2024. "Methamphetamine Research Report." https://nida.nih.gov/publications/research-reports/methamphetamine/overview.

Oxford Treatment Center (OTC). 2023. "How Meth Is Made: Meth Cutting & Manufacturing." *OxfordTreatment.com*. https://oxfordtreatment.com/substance-abuse/crystal-meth/how-its-made/.

U.S. Department of Health and Human Services (HHS). 2020. "Opioids in Medicaid: Concerns about Opioid Use among Beneficiaries in Six Applachian States in 2018." *HHS.gov*. https://oig.hhs.gov/oei/reports/OEI-05-19-00410.pdf.

War and Forced Migration

Control and Prevention of Polio in Africa

The eradication of wild polio virus in Africa is one of the most remarkable achievements in medical science and global health. This monumental milestone, certified in 2020 by the World Health Organization (WHO), reflects decades of relentless effort, innovation, and collaboration among governments, international organizations, health care workers, and local communities. However, it's important to note that vaccine-derived poliovirus (VDPV) cases occasionally occur in areas with low immunization coverage. This happens when the weakened virus used in oral polio vaccines mutates and spreads in communities where too few people are immunized. Efforts to maintain high vaccination rates and strengthen health care systems continue to ensure polio does not return to Africa (WHO; CDC).

Poliomyelitis, commonly known as polio, has existed since prehistoric times, and have been given different descriptions in historical documents. Evidence of the disease can be seen in an ancient Egyptian stele from the second millennium BCE, depicting a patient with withered limbs walking with a cane—characteristic signs of polio (WHO).

The origin of the poliovirus remains poorly understood; however, scientists have confirmed that humans are the only natural hosts for the virus. Poliovirus consists of single-stranded RNA enclosed in a capsid and is classified into three serotypes: P1, P2, and P3. Once the virus enters the human body, it replicates in the gastrointestinal tract and can spread to other parts of the body, including skeletal muscles and the central nervous system. Paralysis or death may result if the virus damages the spinal cord or brain cells. In the twentieth century, polio became one of the most feared diseases. According to the Global Polio Eradication Initiative (GPEI), before widespread vaccination in the 1980s, polio paralyzed 1,000 children worldwide every day.

Polio is highly infectious due to a number of reasons, according to CDC and GPEI. First, the virus is shed from the body through fecal matters, making it capable of contaminating food and water in poor hygiene and sanitation conditions. As such, polio has had a long and devastating impact in poor countries of the world. Typically, young children under age five and who are not toilet trained are found to be the most vulnerable to disease transmitted through fecal-mouth route. Additionally, polio infections are mostly asymptomatic, some patients may experience only mild fever and fatigue, and less than 1 percent results in limb paralysis or death. As a result of asymptomatic transmission, polio infections can spread fast in a community before being detected.

There is no cure for polio; vaccination is the only way to control and ultimately eradicate the infection. In 1955, Dr. Jonas E. Salk developed the first injectable polio vaccine (IPV) made from inactivated polio virus, followed by Dr. Albert B. Sabin's oral polio vaccine (OPV) in 1961, which contains attenuated live virus.

According to Mayo Clinic, before the IPV was licensed in 1955, the United States experienced 16,000 cases of paralytic polio annually. Despite the effectiveness of IPV, the OPV, due to its ease of storage and lower cost, became the preferred choice in national vaccination programs in the United States and worldwide. However, a drawback of OPV is the slight risk of outbreaks caused by circulating vaccine-derived poliovirus (cVDPV) in communities with low immunity. According to the GPEI, out of 10 billion doses of OPV administered globally, fewer than 800 cases of infection resulted from cVDPV outbreaks. When compared to the estimated 6.5 million children saved from paralytic polio, the vaccine's benefits far outweigh its risks.

The most effective strategy to eliminate cVDPV includes broadening vaccination, achieving widespread herd immunity, and eventually phasing out OPV. In the United States, OPV has not been administered since 2000, according to the CDC.

Thanks to mass immunization efforts, polio infections have been drastically reduced worldwide. By 1979, the United States became one of the first countries to be declared polio-free. In the global campaign to eradicate polio, organizations such as the GPEI, the World Health Organization (WHO), Rotary International, U.S. Centers for Disease Control and Prevention (CDC), the Global Alliance for Vaccines and Immunization (GAVI), the Bill & Melinda Gates Foundation, and the United Nations International Children's Emergency Fund (UNICEF) have played pivotal roles.

In 2020, the WHO declared Africa free of wild poliovirus; 95 percent of the continent's population were immunized and no naturally occurring cases reported for four years, per standard measurement. However, polio remains endemic in Pakistan and Afghanistan, the last two countries where the virus continues to circulate, according to GPEI.

The presence of endemic sources of wild poliovirus and vaccine-derived polio highlights the ongoing risk of transmission through activities such as travel and tourism. For example, a case of paralytic polio reported in the United States in July 2022 was likely contracted during international travel, according to CDC. Genetic sequencing revealed that the virus was related to strains found in wastewater samples from Canada, the United Kingdom, and Israel, indicating a connection to poliovirus strains circulating internationally (Link-Gelles et al. 2022). The case stresses the importance of maintaining high vaccination rates and global vigilance to prevent the resurgence of polio.

While vaccinating the world against polio is widely acknowledged as the only way to eliminate the disease, the path to achieving this goal has been fraught with challenges. The efforts to administer polio vaccines in African countries exemplify the obstacles health organizations have faced. Despite these difficulties, the GPEI has played a crucial role in launching and sustaining vaccination campaigns across the continent.

Established in 1988, GPEI is a public-private partnership led by national governments in collaboration with five key partners: the World Health Organization, Rotary International, the U.S. CDC, the United Nations Children's

Fund (UNICEF), and the Bill & Melinda Gates Foundation. Its overarching mission is to eradicate polio worldwide.

According to the GPEI, instability and conflict present the most significant barriers to delivering vaccines to children. Conflicts between militant factions often disrupt routine immunization systems and cause mass displacement, rapidly lowering population immunity and increasing vulnerability to polio outbreaks. The success of polio eradication depends on vaccination workers consistently reaching and immunizing over 95 percent of children. However, conflict and violence have hindered these efforts and endangered the lives of health workers.

In addition to local conflicts, mistrust and misinformation have undermined public support for eradication efforts. In Nigeria, for example, some Muslim leaders claimed that polio vaccines were part of a plot to sterilize Muslims or infect them with HIV (Klobucista et al. 2022). In areas controlled by radical groups, the threat of polio is downplayed, education is limited, and even some local medical practitioners falsely believe polio can be cured.

Compounding these challenges is the rare but real occurrence of VDPV, which can cause outbreaks in areas with low immunization coverage. Outbreaks of VDPV have been reported in several African countries, including Nigeria, the Democratic Republic of Congo, the Central African Republic, Angola, Mozambique, and Malawi (Chinele et al. 2022). These outbreaks pose a serious threat to the progress achieved in Africa and necessitate ongoing surveillance and vaccination campaigns.

Despite these obstacles, GPEI has successfully collaborated with African governments to eradicate polio from the continent, maintaining Africa's polio-free status since 2020. GPEI continues its mission by supporting vaccination campaigns in Pakistan and Afghanistan—the only two countries where polio remains endemic—and closely monitoring "at-risk countries," particularly in Africa, to prevent the reintroduction of polio due to low immunity.

Further Reading

Adebisi, Yusuff Adebayo, Eliseo-Lucero Prisno D 3rd, and B. B. Nuga. 2020. "Last Fight of Wild Polio in Africa: Nigeria's Battle." *Public Health Pract (Oxf), 1*: 100043. doi: 10.1016/j.puhip.2020.100043.
Centers for Disease Control (CDC). "Polio." https://www.cdc.gov/polio/index.html.
Centers for Disease Control (CDC). "Why We Could Not Eradicate Polio from Pakistan and How Can We?" https://www.cdc.gov/vaccines/vpd/polio/hcp/vaccine-derived-poliovirus-faq.html.

Chinele, Josephine and Maya Prabhu. 2022. "Wild Polio Returns to Africa: How the GPEI Is Helping Stop an Outbreak from Becoming an Inferno." *Vaccines Work*. https://www.gavi.org/vaccineswork/wild-polio-returns-africa-how-gpei-helped-stop-outbreak-becoming-inferno.

Global Polio Eradication Initiative (GPEI). https://polioeradication.org/.

Kimbal, Spencer. 2022. "How Polio Came Back to New York for the First Time in Decades, Silently Spread and Left a Patient Paralyzed." *CNBC*. October 4. https://www.cnbc.com/2022/10/04/how-polio-silently-spread-in-new-york-and-left-a-person-paralyzed.html.

Klobucista, Claire, and Danielle Renwick. 2022. "Why Hasn't the World Eradicated Polio?" *Council on Foreign Relations*. https://www.cfr.org/backgrounder/why-hasnt-world-eradicated-polio.

Link-Gelles, Ruth, Emily Lutterloh, Patricia Schnabel Ruppert, P. Bryon Backenson, Kirsten St. George, Eli S. Rosenberg, Bridget J. Anderson, et al. 2022. "Public Health Response to a Case of Paralytic Poliomyelitis in an Unvaccinated Person and Detection of Poliovirus in Wastewater—New York, June–August 2022." *Morbidity and Mortality Weekly Report 71*(33): 1065–8. https://doi.org/10.15585/mmwr.mm7133e2.

Mayo Clinic. "Outbreaks and Vaccine Timeline." https://www.mayoclinic.org.

Nomoto, Akio. 2007. "Molecular Aspects of Poliovirus Pathogenesis." *Proceedings of the Japan Academy, Series B Physical and Biological Sciences*, 83(8): 266–75. doi: 10.2183/pjab/83.266.

World Health Organization. "Poliomyelitis." https://www.who.int/health-topics/poliomyelitis#tab=tab_1.

Impact of Migration on the Spread of HIV/AIDS

HIV/AIDS disproportionately affects economically underdeveloped communities, where poverty is a significant social issue. The underlying relationship suggests that poverty increases vulnerability to HIV while HIV exacerbates poverty (O'Farrell 2001). The disease is more prevalent in urban areas, particularly in metropolitan regions with populations of 500,000 or more, as noted by the Centers for Disease Control and Prevention (CDC). An estimated 1.2 million people in the United States were living with HIV at the end of 2022, which includes both diagnosed and undiagnosed cases. Notably, 87 percent of these individuals were aware of their HIV status, reflecting a slight increase from 86 percent in 2018, according to the CDC.

HIV (human immunodeficiency virus) is zoonotic in origin, meaning it originated in animals before crossing over to humans. However, it is now exclusively transmitted between humans. According to the CDC, HIV may have been present in the United States since the 1970s.

Resolving the Patient Zero Myth through Genetic Research

Today, approximately 1.2 million people in the United States are living with HIV. The first recognized cases of AIDS appeared in 1981, marking the beginning of public awareness of the HIV epidemic. Initially, Gaëtan Dugas, a French-Canadian flight attendant, was labeled "Patient Zero" who brought the HIV outbreak to North America. Dr. Michael Worobey of University of Arizona, Tucson, and colleagues were able to prove that the identification was a result of a labeling error. Their genetic and archival research showed that the mislabeling stemmed from early epidemiological studies, where Dugas was listed as "Patient O" (indicating he was "Outside California"). This "O" was later misinterpreted as the numeral zero, misleadingly suggesting he was the origin of the virus in North America.

The study by Worobey and colleagues used an advanced genetic analysis called "RNA jackhammering" to reexamine archival samples from the 1970s. By sequencing eight complete HIV genomes from samples in that period, the research team revealed extensive genetic diversity, suggesting that HIV had been circulating in the United States which included Dugas's strain. Phylogenetic analysis identified that HIV subtype B most likely originated in the Caribbean and entered North America around 1971, with New York City emerging as an early epicenter.

The insight brought by the study was significant for rigorously tracing HIV infection in North America. It debunked the "single-source" myth by showing that HIV transmission in the United States and North America likely had diverse sources from the start. Additionally, Worobey and colleagues' study cleared the status of "patient 0" for Gaëtan Dugas who died of AIDS-related complications in 1984.

Further Reading

CDC. 2024. "National HIV Surveillance System (NHSS)." *HIV Data*. https://www.cdc.gov/hiv-data/nhss/index.html.

HIV.gov. "Fast Facts." https://www.hiv.gov/hiv-basics/overview/data-and-trends/statistics.

Worobey, Michael, Thomas D. Watts, Richard A. McKay, et al. 2016. "1970s and 'Patient 0' HIV-1 Genomes Illuminate Early HIV/AIDS History in North America." *Nature*, 539: 98–101. https://doi.org/10.1038/nature19827.

A defining characteristic of HIV is its aggressive attack on the immune system. The virus targets and depletes CD4 cells, also known as T-cells, which are crucial for immune defense. If left untreated, this leads to the eventual collapse of the immune system. The most common modes of transmission are through sexual contact or needle sharing.

During the primary and secondary stages of infection, patients often experience flu-like symptoms. These early stages are particularly infectious due to the high viral load and subtle onset of symptoms. In the tertiary stage, the most advanced and severe phase, the patient develops acquired immunodeficiency syndrome (AIDS). At this point, the immune system is severely compromised, leaving the patient vulnerable to various opportunistic infections.

As of now, there is no cure or vaccine for HIV/AIDS. However, the good news is that HIV can be effectively managed with antiretroviral therapy (ART). Early treatment can reduce the viral load to undetectable levels, allowing patients to lead a normal life (CDC).

Impact of Migration on HIV Transmission

Globally, studies have shown that the spread of HIV strongly correlates with population mobility, and poorly managed migration can increase transmission rates. Studies have shown that migration and population movement can facilitate the transmission of HIV, particularly when combined with factors such as limited access to health care, socioeconomic instability, and increased exposure to high-risk behaviors. The International Organization for Migration (IOM) has highlighted that many of the underlying factors sustaining mobility, such as including unequal distribution of resources, unemployment, socioeconomic instability, and political unrest, are also determinants of increased risk of HIV. The global rise in migration presents unique challenges in ensuring access to HIV prevention, treatment, and care for mobile populations (IOM 2004).

Widespread migration is a defining characteristic of our era. In addition to seasonal migration for employment, climate change displaces millions of people annually. Understanding the epidemiological effects of population movement is becoming increasingly vital for developing effective policies to control the transmission of HIV and other sexually transmitted diseases (STDs). Below are a few ways migration was found to contribute to the spread of infections, according to various studies:

Behavioral Changes due to Disruption of Social Norms and Structures

Migration can disrupt established ethical codes and social obligations, leading to behavioral changes that increase the risk of HIV infection. Studies of several African societies highlighted this dynamic. For instance, research on seasonally migrating agrarian populations in Uganda revealed that the HIV seroprevalence rate among individuals who never migrated was 5.5 percent, while the rate among those migrating for work was twice as high. Among a cohort of migrants from various regions, the infection rate was three times higher.

A study shows that migrants make up a quarter of Côte d'Ivoire's population, making it one of the most mobile societies in West Africa; meanwhile the country also has the highest HIV infection rate in the region. Researchers believe that seasonal migration fosters environments where young male farm workers are temporarily free from the strict social norms of their home villages. Researchers also found that plantations often attract large numbers of sex workers, frequently brought in by employers on paydays. These conditions significantly heighten the risk of HIV transmission. Notably, more than 80 percent of sex workers in Abidjan, the capital of Côte d'Ivoire, were found to be HIV-positive (Decosas et al. 1995).

Economic Vulnerability in Host Society

Reports of migrants being subjected to abuse, kidnapping, and human trafficking are widespread globally. In host countries, migrants are often among the most vulnerable members of society (United Nations 2017). A recent study by Pannetier (2018) and colleagues on African migrant women living in France revealed that discrimination and abuse significantly increase their risk of HIV infection.

Notably, the study found that many migrant women from sub-Saharan Africa acquired HIV after migration, often as a result of forced sexual encounters. Sexual abuse was frequently associated with being hosted by family or friends and lacking legal residency status.

These findings point to the urgent need to address post-migration HIV infection, as an estimated 30 percent of sub-Saharan African women living with HIV in France are believed to have contracted the virus after migrating (Pannetier et al. 2018).

Magnifier Effect of Migration

Studies have shown that migration can exacerbate existing social problems, increasing vulnerability to HIV/AIDS. A recent study on the HIV/AIDS situation in China revealed a sharp rise in infections through heterosexual contact, growing from 44.9 percent in 2008 to 95.1 percent in 2017. Researchers attribute this trend to a combination of bachelorhood, commercial sex, and migration (Xiao et al. 2019).

The root cause, according to the study, is sex ratio imbalance resulting from three decades of family planning policies. Sex-selective abortions have led to disproportionately high female mortality, creating a "marriage squeeze." Rural males are particularly affected, with an estimated 51 million men entering the marriage market between 1983 and 2020, and one in ten aged 50 and over expected to remain unmarried.

The study highlights that never-married male migrants face particularly high risks of HIV/STD infection due to their engagement in commercial sex and inconsistent condom use. Conversely, while never-married nonmigrants may be less vulnerable due to limited access to commercial sex, inconsistent condom use can still expose them to infection. These findings emphasize the need for targeted interventions to address these vulnerabilities in both migrant and nonmigrant populations, the researchers suggest.

Together, these cases reveal how migration contributes to the dynamics of HIV transmission and emphasize the urgency of integrating mobility into public health strategies. As global migration continues to rise, a deeper understanding of its intersection with HIV vulnerability is not only necessary but essential for developing effective, inclusive responses that protect both migrants and the broader communities in which they live.

Further Reading

Centers for Disease Control and Prevention (CDC). "HIV." https://www.cdc.gov/hiv/default.html.

Decosas, J., F. Kane, J. K. Anarfi, K. D. R. Sodji, and H. U. Wagner. 1995. "Migration and AIDS." *Lancet*, 346(8978): 826–8. doi:10.1016/s0140-6736(95)91631-8.

O'Farrell, Nigel. 2001. "Poverty and HIV in Sub-Saharan Africa." *The Lancet*, 357(9256): 636–7. doi:10.1016/s0140-6736(95)91631-8.

International Organization for Migration (IOM). 2004. "Population Mobility and HIV/AIDS." https://publications.iom.int/system/files/pdf/pop_mobility_en.pdf.

Pannetier, Julie, Andrainolo Ravalihasy, Nathalie Lydié, France Lert, and Annabel Desgrées du Loû, on behalf of the Parours study group. 2018. "Prevalence and Circumstances of Forced Sex and Post-Migration HIV Acquisition in Sub-Saharan African Migrant Women in France: An Analysis of the ANRS-PARCOURS Retrospective Population-Based Study." *Lancet Public Health, 3*(1):e16–e23. doi: 10.1016/S2468-2667(17)30211-6.

United Nations. 2017. *International Migration Report 2017*. New York: United Nations.

Xiao, Quanying, Huijun Liu, and Bei Wu. 2019. "How Bachelorhood and Migration Increase the HIV Transmission Risk through Commercial Sex in China?" *AIDS and Behavior, 24*: 791–801. https://doi.org/10.1007/s10461-019-02640-3.

Resurgence of Louse-Borne Diseases due to Migration

Lice are host-specific parasites, and some species adapted exclusively to humans. Evidence of lice has been found on Egyptian mummies and in the remains of individuals from Pompeii. Scientists believe that the body louse (*Pediculus humanus*) that lives and multiplies only in layers of clothing could be an evidence that lice have evolved after humans started to wear clothing (Toup et al. 2010). Historically, louse-borne diseases, such as louse-borne relapsing fever (LBRF), trench fever, and endemic typhus, have been life-threatening in regions of poverty and poor hygienic conditions. With improvement of living conditions since the end of the Second World War, louse-borne diseases have been significantly reduced in most parts of the world, with exception of regions in East Africa, studies suggest. Since the early 2000s, on the heels of waves of migration of African refugees to European countries, cases of LBRF reemerged in Europe (Antinori 2016).

Among the many species of lice, three currently pose threat to public health worldwide, they are the head louse (*Pediculus humanus capitis*), body louse (*Pediculus humanus humanus*), and pubic louse (*Pthirus pubis*), among which the body louse is responsible for most transmissions of louse-borne diseases. Head-louse and pubic louse have not been confirmed to spread diseases. The highest prevalence of louse infestation today is found in places with precarious hygienic conditions and overcrowded living conditions. Countries in the region of Horn of Africa, such as Ethiopia, Somalia, and surrounding neighbors have witnessed outbreaks of louse-borne diseases in recent decades. What drives prevalence in this region is believed to be the colder temperature and economic distress. Poor people in highland areas wear multiple layers of clothing, but due to limited resources, they can hardly maintain cleanliness, such as by washing clothes in hot water of 135°F and frequent changes of clothing, resulting in a widespread lice infestation (Raoult et al. 1999).

In developed countries of the Western Hemisphere, body lice infestations are rare and have been decreasing since the Second World War. However, louse-borne diseases have been reported in homeless shelters. In the United States, a 1994 seroprevalence study of 192 residents in a low-income area of Seattle, Washington, found that 20 percent tested positive for *Bartonella quintana*, the bacterium responsible for trench fever primarily transmitted by lice. Among those who tested positive, half had a history of alcoholism or drug use (Jackson et al. 1996).

Similarly, a study of 930 homeless individuals in Marseille, France, found lice infestations in 22 percent of participants, with 5.3 percent testing positive for *B. quintana* (Brouqui et al. 2005). More recently, an outbreak of lice-borne trench fever was identified within the homeless population in Denver, Colorado (KJCT News 2020).

In contrast, head lice present a different scenario. Since head lice spread through direct person-to-person contact, they are common across all countries, including developed ones, regardless of hygiene standards. School-age children are particularly susceptible to head lice infestations. However, unlike body lice, head lice are not known to transmit diseases (Ouarti et al. 2023).

In the early 1900s, lice were identified as vectors for the transmission of infectious bacteria, with three species recognized as louse-borne: *Borrelia recurrentis*, *Bartonella quintana*, and *Rickettsia prowazekii*. These bacteria are responsible for relapsing fever, trench fever, and epidemic typhus, respectively.

In 1909, Charles Jules Henri Nicolle successfully demonstrated that body lice could transmit typhus fever to humans. For this groundbreaking work, he was awarded the Nobel Prize in Physiology or Medicine in 1928 (Raoult et al. 1999).

Historically, louse-borne diseases claimed the lives of tens of thousands of soldiers during the First World War. This was primarily due to the unsanitary conditions in crowded trenches, where there was little access to effective hygiene measures. Hot water above 133°F, which is capable of killing lice, according to the CDC, was often unavailable. These conditions gave rise to the terms "trench fever" and "war fever" (a reference to epidemic typhus) to describe the diseases.

During a typical process of infection, the lice first inject an anticoagulant protein into the human body to keep the blood flowing. This protein, in conjunction with other infectious materials such as the execration of the lice, causes pruritus (discomfort) and scratching by the victim of the infected area, or practicing "louse-crushing," which further exposes the wound to bacteria intrusion (Antinori et al. 2016).

Clinically, multiple febrile stages may occur with all three kinds of fevers. The severity may differ with trench fever causing milder symptoms to epidemic typhus being highly life-threatening. The condition known as trench fever is caused by *Bartonella quintana*, a bacterium specifically living in human. Lice infected with human blood that carry the bacterium have been identified as the only vector. Symptoms include relapsing fevers, bone pain in the legs, neck and back, and skin lesions. Untreated, the infection could sometimes infect the heart valves. Presence of the bacterium collected from homeless people and refugees reportedly ranges between 2.3 percent and 93 percent in samples collected from Algeria, Burundi, Congo, Democratic Republic of Congo, Ethiopia, Kenya, Madagascar, Rwanda, and Zimbabwe (CDC; Ouarti et al. 2023).

LBRF is caused by *Borrelia recurrentis* through louse infestation. Symptoms include chronic febrile episodes with intervals of 5–10 days, with beginning relapses being more severe or fatal than subsequent relapses. Historically, the epidemics occurred frequently in Europe and Russia in the early 1900s, infecting 13 million people and resulting in 5 million deaths. Today, LBRF remains endemic in Ethiopia, Sudan, Eritrea, and Somalia, with fatality reaching 40 percent in outbreaks, ranking the fifth cause of death in the region (ECDC; Grecchi et al. 2016).

The epidemic typhus, also known as louse-borne typhus, is caused by the bacterium *Rickettsia prowazaki*. The bacterium was named in honor of H.T. Ricketts and L. von Prowazek who contracted typhus while investigating the disease (Conlon 2007). The infectious agent is transmitted by body lice after feeding on infected humans. Symptoms include initial sudden fever of 105° F, severe headaches, chills, photophobia, blood clotting, skin infection leaving spotted rashes, infection of the central nervous system causing confusion, the liver, the lungs, and the heart. Left untreated, mortality could reach 50–70 percent in severe epidemics. One study estimates that the epidemic typhus may have been responsible for more deaths than all of the wars in history. Since the Second World War, epidemic typhus has been reduced to rare outbreaks, with a number of reemergence instances in the 1990s in Burundi, Ethiopia, Russia, Tibet, Nepal, and Peru (CDC; Raoult et al. 1999).

Louse-borne diseases, once a leading cause of death, had retreated to a few regions in East Africa. However, they are now reemerging as a global health concern. This resurgence is closely tied to worsening economic decline, social instability, and the resulting mass migration. By 2015, African refugees arriving in Europe reportedly reached 1 million, with nearly 11 million residing there by 2020 (Maunganidze 2021). Poor hygiene and overcrowded living conditions during their journeys from Africa are thought to have facilitated the spread of these diseases.

Cases of LBRF have been reported in Germany, Switzerland, Italy, the Netherlands, and Finland. These diagnoses likely represent only a fraction of the actual infections (Raoult et al. 1999; Grecchi 2016; Antinoli et al. 2016). Compounding the issue is the spread of louse-borne infections among homeless populations in developed countries, often due to systemic mismanagement. This complex context serves as a stark reminder that louse-borne diseases continue to be a global health issue today and need to be monitored.

Further Reading

Antinori, Spinello, Oleg Mediannikov, Mario Corbellino, and Didier Raoult. 2016. "Louse-Borne Relapsing Fever among East African Refugees in Europe." *ScienceDirect*, *14*(2): 110–14. http://dx.doi.org/10.1016/j.tmaid.2016.01.004.

Brouqui, Philippe, et al. 2005. "Ectoparasitism and Vector-Borne Diseases in 930 Homeless People from Marseilles." *Medicine*, *84*(1): 61–8. doi: 10.1097/01.md.0000152373.07500.6c.

Centers for Disease Control and Prevention. "Louse-Borne Relapsing Fever (LBRF)." https://www.CDC.gov.

Conlon, Joseph M. 2007. "The Historical Impact of Epidemic Typhus." https://www.montana.edu/historybug/documents/TYPHUS-Conlon.pdf.

ECDC. "Facts about Louse-Borne Relapsing Fever." https://www.ecdc.europa.eu/en/louse-borne-relapsing-fever/facts.

Grecchi, Cecilia, Paola Zanotti, Agostina Pontarelli, et al. 2016. "Louse-Borne Relapsing Fever in a Refugee from Mali." *Case Report*. doi https://10.1007/s15010-017-0987-2.

Jackons, Lisa A., and David H. Spach. 1996. "Emergence of Bartonella Quitana Infection among Homeless Persons." *Immerging Infectious Diseases*, *2*(2), April–June: 141–4.

KJCT News. 2020. "Trench Fever Identified among Homeless in Denver Area." July 20. https://www.kjct8.com/2020/07/20/trench-fever-identified-among-homeless-in-denver-area/.

Maunganidze, Ottilia Anna. 2021. "Policy Brief." *Institute for Security Studies*. http://issafrica.s3.amazonaws.com/site/uploads/PB-166.pdf.

Ouarti, Basma, Descartes Maxime Mbogning Fonkou, Linda Houhamdi, Oleg Mediannikov, and Philippe Parola. 2023. "Lice and Lice-Borne Diseases in Humans in Africa: A Narrative Review." *Acta Tropica*, *232*(2022): 106709. https://doi.org/10.1016/j.actatropica.2022.106709.

Raoult, Didier and Veronique Roux. 1999. "The Body Louse as a Vector of Reemerging Human Diseases Clinical Infectious Diseases." https://www.jstor.org/stable/4461025.

Toups, Melissa A., Andrew Kitchen, Jessica E. Light, and David L. Reed. 2010. "Origin of Clothing Lice Indicates Early Clothing Use by Anatomically Modern Humans in Africa." *Mol Biol Evol*. doi: 10.1093/molbev/msq234.

The 1918 Flu—How War Promotes Pandemics

The 1918 flu, smallpox, and measles had one thing in common—these pandemics once rode the wings of wars and devastated all continents. The devastation of the 1918 flu, however, dwarfed all pandemics in human history, infected more than 500 million people or one third of the world's population, and killed more than 50 million worldwide, including 675,000 deaths in the United States, according to the Centers for Disease Control and Prevention (CDC).

The 1918 flu has another popular nickname—the "Spanish Flu" not because the virus was originated in Spain, but rather due to Spanish media's candid reporting on the rampant infections. During the First World War, Spain's neutrality allowed its uncensored press to report openly on the flu, unlike the censored media in Allied and Central Powers nations. Neither the Germans nor the Americans were willing to talk about it, the war being the top priority for both sides. When King Alfonso XIII fell ill in 1918, Spanish coverage intensified, leading other countries to mistakenly assume Spain was the pandemic's origin. Meanwhile, the Spanish believed the virus came from France, dubbing it the "French Flu" (Andrews 2023).

Genetics research indicates that the H1N1 influenza virus that caused the 1918 flu was of avian origin. The virus may have jumped from birds to humans, possibly through an intermediate host, but the exact origin is still debated. The 1918 strain is considered a "founder virus," evolving into all subsequent influenza A viruses including 1957 (H2N2), 1968 (H3N2), and 2009 (H1N1pdm). In a sense, the impact of the 1918 flu far surpassed the 1918–19 pandemic era (Taubenberger et al. 2020; Jordan et al. 2023).

The 1918 flu spread rapidly through respiratory droplets in crowded settings, such as military camps and urban areas. High death rates were caused by severe viral pneumonia, overactive immune responses (cytokine storms) that damaged lung tissue, and secondary bacterial infections, which were untreatable at the time due to the lack of antibiotics, according to Cleveland Clinic. The wartime conditions provided a hotbed for the virus to spread fast. A report describes the living conditions in some of the camps as follows:

> All of these camp arrangements were implicated in late 1918 by Vaughan and Palmer who highlighted the assembly rooms as key to the transmission of airborne organisms in camp life. "The acute respiratory diseases are transmitted by the transference of organism from the respiratory tract of one man to those of another." To put it bluntly, "by spitting into one another's face." For example, "In an assembly hall in one of our camps where several thousand men are seated night after night, if every man sits upright and moves his head neither backward nor forward, the greatest distance between his nose and that of the man in front or behind is 26 inches, and to the right or left, 16 inches." Since, they added, "in such an assembly with one-half of the men coughing, one can have some idea of the extent to which respiratory bacteria are being transmitted." The men did a lot of regular spitting as well, coating the sidewalks and floors with bubbly sputum. (Humphreys 2018)

Researchers typically divide the 1918 pandemic into three waves; though some argue that more infectious outbreaks followed. According to the CDC's timeline, the three waves of infection occurred in spring and fall of 1918 for the first two waves, and the third wave occurred in spring and summer of 1919. Each wave created ideal conditions for the flu to rapidly expand. The second wave proved especially deadly, due to military personnel being actively transported within the United States and to European countries.

In April 1917, the United States joined allies France, Britain, and Russia in their battle against Germany. The U.S. military rapidly expanded from 378,000 to more than 4.7 million personnel by the end of the war, with most new soldiers coming through a massive draft system. Mobilization drew millions of civilians into military institutions, leading to the construction of large training camps and facilities across the country. These camps, often overcrowded and highly mobile, became ideal environments for the spread of influenza. Early cases in the United States were reported at sites such as Camp Funston in Kansas, where acute respiratory illnesses were observed before the global peak of the pandemic. These cases likely belonged to the first wave of the virus, which was milder and less deadly than the second wave that followed in the fall—when some infected soldiers carried the virus with them aboard ships to France (Byerly 2010; Tautenberger et al. 2020).

Flu symptoms were more severe in Europe, and, as the infections became more virulent in summer and fall 1918, military operations in battlefields had to be put on hold, as millions of soldiers on both sides were sickened.

The First World War was primarily a ground war dominated by trench warfare, where overcrowded conditions were common. The flu virus struck both Allied and German armies, overwhelming field hospitals and transport trains with sick, feverish soldiers along the Western Front. More American soldiers were hospitalized than injured in the battles. The epidemic peaked during the height of the American Expeditionary Force's (AEF) deployment, severely impacting the troops' performance in the Meuse-Argonne Offensive, their largest campaign of the war, according to one study. The flu disrupted transportation along the battlefront, overwhelmed hospitals, claimed thousands of lives, and rendered many soldiers unfit for duty. It drained troop's morale and resources, diverting attention from the war effort to fighting the disease. Ultimately, the flu killed more American military personnel than enemy weapons (Byerly 2010).

The flu virus did not only follow American military to the war, it also returned with the military personnel when the war drew to a close. Some of the most devastating symptoms were observed among soldiers coming home. Portal cities such as New York, Philadelphia, Boston, as well as many inland cities became epicenters in June and August 1918 as ships arrived. Vessels departing from Boston also went to New Orleans, Chicago, and out to the West Coast. As infected soldiers and civilians traveled by boats and trains, they spread the disease throughout the United States. Along the way, the flu quickly infected the port cities with extreme virulence and high mortality rate (Roos 2023).

An outbreak struck Philadelphia in September 1918 after a navy ship arrived from Boston, introducing the virus to the city. Despite the growing number of infections, public health officials downplayed the severity of the influenza threat. The city, home to 1.7 million people, went ahead with a planned Liberty Loan Parade to promote government-issued war bonds for funding the First World War. The event drew 200,000. Within six months, the city reported 500,000 cases and 16,000 deaths (Asmelash 2020).

The 1918 pandemic concluded with a third wave, which lasted from the fall through the winter of 1919. Symptoms during this phase were generally milder and shorter in duration than those of the devastating second wave. By the end of 1920, after a few more smaller outbreaks, the pandemic had largely subsided, likely due to population immunity and mutations that may have reduced the severity of the illness, according to scientists (Waxman 2020).

Several key lessons can be drawn from the 1918 pandemic, with the most significant being the link between war and pandemics. Overcrowded camps and trenches, poor sanitation, and weakened immune systems due to malnutrition made soldiers highly susceptible to infections, while overwhelmed medical facilities made the crisis even worse. War created ideal conditions for influenza to flourish and spread globally.

Another critical lesson is the importance of information transparency in disease control. Wartime censorship in many countries suppressed flu-related information to preserve morale, delaying public awareness and hindering response efforts. This emphasizes the need of open and transparent communication during health crises.

Further Reading

Andrews, Evan. 2023. "Why Was It Called the 'Spanish Flu?'" *History.com*. Updated 2023. https://www.history.com/news/why-was-it-called-the-spanish-flu.

Asmelash, Leah. 2020. "Philadelphia Didn't Cancel a Parade during a 1918 Pandemic. The Results Were Devastating." https://www.cnn.com/2020/03/15/us/philadelphia-1918-spanish-flu-trnd/index.html.

Barry, John M. 2005. *The Great Influenza: The Story of the Deadliest Pandemic in History*. New York: Penguin Books.

Byerly, Carol R. 2010. "The U.S. Military and the Influenza Pandemic of 1918–1919." *Public Health Rep*. https://pmc.ncbi.nlm.nih.gov/articles/PMC2862337/.

Centers for Disease Control (CDC). 2018. "History of 1918 Flu Pandemic." *CDC Archive*. https://archive.cdc.gov/www_cdc_gov/flu/pandemic-resources/1918-commemoration/1918-pandemic-history.htm.

Cleveland Clinic. "1918 Influenza Pandemic (Spanish Flu)." *Clevelandclinic.org*. https://my.clevelandclinic.org/health/diseases/21777-spanish-flu.

Jordan, Douglas, Terrence Tumpey, and Barbara Jester. 2023. "The Deadliest Flu: The Complete Story of the Discovery and Reconstruction of the 1918 Pandemic Virus." https://archive.cdc.gov/www_cdc_gov/flu/pandemic-resources/reconstruction-1918-virus.html.

Jordan, Edwin O. 1927. *Epidemic Influenza—A Survey*. Chicago: American Medical Association.

Humphrey, Margaret. 2018. "The Influenza of 1918." *Evolution, Medicine, and Public Health*, *2018*(1): 219–29. doi: 10.1093/emph/eoy024.

Roos, David. 2023. "How U.S. Cities Tried to Halt the Spread of the 1918 Spanish Flu." *History.org*. https://www.history.com/news/spanish-flu-pandemic-response-cities.

Taubenberger, Jeffery K. 2006. "The Origin and Virulence of the 1918 'Spanish' Influenza Virus." *Proceedings of American Philosophical Association*. 2006 March, 150(1): 86–112. https://pmc.ncbi.nlm.nih.gov/articles/PMC2720273/.

Taubenberger, Jeffery K., and David M. Morens. 2020. "The 1918 Influenza Pandemic and Its Legacy." *Cold Spring Harbor Laboratory Press*. doi: 10.1101/cshperspect.a038695.

Waxman, Olivia. 2020. "How Does a Pandemic End? Here's What We Can Learn from the 1918 Flu." *Time*. https://time.com/5894403/how-the-1918-flu-pandemic-ended/.

Forced to Flee, Left Behind: Health Consequences of the Syrian Refugee Crisis

In December 2010, the Arab Spring movement, a wave of anti-government protests, swept across the Arab world. In 2011, peaceful demonstrations erupted in Syria, driven by high unemployment, government corruption, and demands for greater freedom. The Assad regime responded with lethal force to suppress the protests, which escalated into a full-scale civil war. The conflict became increasingly complex, with armed clashes involving rebel groups both supporting and opposing the government. The situation worsened as extremist organizations, including the Islamic State and al-Qaeda, entered the conflict. This prolonged war triggered a massive humanitarian crisis, forcing around 5 million Syrians, or one-quarter of the population, to flee to neighboring countries including Lebanon, Jordan, Turkey, and Egypt, while millions more were displaced within Syria (BBC 2023).

The hardships endured by Syrian refugees testify to the profound devastation that war and forced migration can inflict on humanity. The impact on public health was particularly severe in three critical aspects. First, the destruction of medical infrastructure posed a major health challenge. The conflict led to a widespread decimation of hospitals, clinics, and medical facilities, drastically reducing access to health care and disrupting the supply of essential medications. Second, there was a significant shortage of health care professionals, as many of them were displaced or unable to continue practicing due to the ongoing conflict. This shortage contributed to dangerous gaps in vaccination coverage, increasing risks of deadly disease outbreaks. Finally, displacement resulted in malnutrition and overcrowding, creating conditions that facilitated the rapid spread of infectious diseases (WHO: "Syria Crisis").

A review study by Saleh and colleagues (2018) emphasized the widespread prevalence of diseases such as tuberculosis (TB) and leishmaniasis in overcrowded environments. Leishmaniasis, a parasitic infection endemic to Mediterranean regions and transmitted by sandflies, occurs in two forms: visceral (affecting internal organs) and cutaneous (affecting the skin). Both forms can be life-threatening or result in severe damage to bodily functions. In the region, leishmaniasis and TB disproportionately impact impoverished communities, where overcrowding and malnutrition are common. These conditions heightened the vulnerability of the refugee populations during the conflict (WHO: "Leishmaniasis").

Studies show that Syrian refugees faced significant challenges related to chronic conditions in accessing essential care and medications during the war. Among Syrian refugees, the most commonly reported non-communicable diseases (NCDs) were anemia, cancer, hypertension, diabetes, malnutrition, renal diseases, and blood disorders. War-related injuries were widespread, including gunshot wounds, burns, injuries from falls, and trauma caused by bombings, affecting approximately 5.7 percent of the refugee population. Moreover, data from refugee camps in Turkey, Lebanon, and Jordan revealed that an alarming 54 percent of Syrian refugees suffered from severe emotional disorders, a profound psychological toll of war and forced displacement (Saleh et al. 2018).

The war had a disproportionately greater impact on women, the study reveals. Nearly half of refugee women lacked access to contraceptives, resulting in a high rate of teenage pregnancies. Many pregnant women were unable to receive essential antenatal care, contributing to an elevated maternal mortality rate. The study also reported the prevalence of forced marriages, with some families resorting to this practice as a means of protecting girls from widespread sexual violence and as a strategy to alleviate poverty (Saleh et al. 2018).

The forced migration also profoundly affected communities in host countries. A common challenge was the overwhelming of local health care facilities and critical resources due to the sudden influx of refugees, which limited access to health care for local residents.

Helou and colleagues (2022) reported that Lebanon received over 1.2 million refugees between 2012 and 2015, equivalent to a 30 percent increase in the country's population. This sudden surge placed significant strain on both the Lebanese population and the refugees. The rapid population growth caught local governments unprepared. Unlike in other countries, most refugees in Lebanon were not accommodated in camps but were taken in by private households, many of whom were already suffering from economic difficulties and high unemployment. This situation created conditions that contributed to outbreaks of diseases such as measles, hepatitis A, and leishmaniasis.

These outbreaks were attributed to a critical shortage of resources for accommodation, including substandard housing for refugees, poor sanitation, water pollution, inadequate nutrition, and low immunization rates among both Syrian and Lebanese children. Additionally, the study indicates that poorly managed waste further contributed to the spread of diseases.

According to Helou and colleagues, between 2012 and 2015, as the refugee burden intensified, Lebanese unemployment rose to 20 percent. In Bekaa, where hepatitis A and leishmaniasis became endemic, Syrian refugees accounted for as much as 48 percent of the population.

The hardship further affected the supply of drinking water. The study reports that many refugees resorted to drawing drinking water from ground boreholes. This practice turned water pollution into a significant source of infectious diseases, exacerbated by poor management of wastewater and solid waste. In Syrian cities where landfill facilities were dysfunctional, trash often could accumulate for days before being removed and burned, a process that could easily lead to water sources being contaminated with toxins and pathogens (Helou et al. 2022).

Alarmingly low immunization rates caused concerns during the period. A 2015 study involving 135 households in Kobane, an area in the Aleppo governorate, revealed that only 20.3 percent of children under 59 months were fully vaccinated, just 36 percent of five-month-old children received their third polio vaccine on time, and only 34 percent of twelve-month-olds received their MMR vaccine as scheduled (Kampalath et al. 2023).

The Syrian refugee health crisis shows how war and displacement dismantle health systems and spread disease across borders. Without stronger surveillance, wider vaccination, and better care in conflict zones and host countries, these risks persist. As tensions builds up again in Syria today, global organizations must act to prevent these consequences from returning.

Further Reading

BBC. 2023. "Why Has the Syrian War Lasted 12 Years?" *BBC.com*. https://www.bbc.com/news/world-middle-east-35806229.

Centers for Disease Control and Prevention (CDC). "Syrian Refugee Health Profile." https://search.cdc.gov/search/?query=syria&dpage=1.

Helou, Mariana, Gerlant VanBerlaer, and Kaissar Yammine. 2022. "Factors Influence the Occurrence of Infectious Disease Outbreaks in Lebanon since the Syrian Crisis." *Pathogens and Global Health*, 116(1): 13–21. doi: https://doi.org/10.1080/20477724.2021.1957192.

Kampalath, Vinay, Ahmad Tarakji, Mohamed Hamze, Randa Loutfi, Keri Cohn, and Aula Abbara. 2023. "The Impacts of the Syrian Conflict on Child and Adolescent Health: A Scoping Review." *Journal of Public Health*, 45(3): 621–30. doi: https://doi.org/10.1093/pubmed/fdac132.

Saleh, Ayman, Serdar Aydin, and Orhan Kocak. 2018. "A Comparative Study of Syrian Refugees in Turkey, Lebanon, and Jordan: Healthcare Access and Delivery." *OPUS Journal*, 8(14): 448–64. doi: https://doi.org/10.26466/opus.376351.

World Health Organization (WHO). 2023. "Leishmaniasis." https://www.who.int/news-room/fact-sheets/detail/leishmaniasis.

World Health Organization (WHO). 2024. "Syria Crisis." https://www.who.int/emergencies/situations/syria-crisis.

The Surge of Covid, TB, and HIV in War-Torn Ukraine

Throughout history, wars have often led to outbreaks of diseases. Smallpox and the 1918 flu pandemic are striking examples, as these viruses followed wars and claimed more lives than the battles themselves. Similarly, since Russia's invasion of Ukraine in February 2022, the conflict has severely impacted health conditions in the country. Medical infrastructure has been bombarded, and the supply of medical resources and treatments has been severely disrupted.

The war has forced tens of thousands of civilians to take shelter in crowded and unsanitary conditions. Barrage of shelling left millions of homes in ruin; thousands of families were forced to flee, many spent weeks in confined to bunkers, basements, and subway stations, increasing their exposure to airborne pathogens. These conditions have disrupted immunization efforts and cut off supply lines for essential medicines needed to manage chronic diseases (Norwegian Refugee Council 2023).

The Covid-19 pandemic further exacerbated the crisis. Reports indicate that decreased testing and a low vaccination rate left only 36 percent of Ukrainians vaccinated as of February 2022. As of March 2023, the World Health Organization (WHO) reported 5.4 million confirmed Covid-19 cases and 111,457 related deaths. However, actual mortality and morbidity figures may be even higher, as the Russian invasion continued.

Reports indicate that crowded living conditions accelerated the spread of tuberculosis (TB) and related illnesses. Individuals living with HIV are particularly vulnerable to TB due to their weakened immune system. Even before the Russian invasion, Ukraine grappled with high rates of TB and HIV infections. Ukraine was ranked among the countries with the highest rates of multi-drug-resistant TB globally, reporting 32,000 new cases annually. One-third of TB patients were also living with HIV (Reuters 2022). Moreover, Ukraine had the second-highest HIV infection rate in Europe, with approximately 250,000 cases before the war (Roberts 2022). War-related displacement and overcrowding further intensified the spread of infections, while severe shortages of medical supplies undermined efforts to manage TB and HIV. Experts warned that prolonged drug shortages could fuel the rise of drug-resistant strains, posing a major public health threat.

The war also significantly disrupted polio immunization efforts for children in Ukraine, leading to an outbreak of circulating vaccine-derived poliovirus type 2 (cVDPV2). Polio is a highly contagious enterovirus that replicates in the intestinal tract and is shed in fecal matter. It can cause paralysis and death, primarily in children under the age of five. Vaccination is the only effective means of prevention. According to the World Health Organization, Ukraine had been experiencing an outbreak of cVDPV2 since October 2021, with cases confirmed in Rivne and Zakarpattia provinces. The ongoing conflict further disrupted immunization campaigns, exacerbating the situation (WHO 2022c).

Experts are also concerned that gaps in vaccinations among children, adolescents, and adults in Ukraine could lead to outbreaks of other infectious diseases, such as cholera and measles. The lack of access to clean water, sanitation, and hygiene (WASH), combined with crowded conditions in shelters and suboptimal vaccination coverage, increases the risk of such outbreaks (WHO 2022c).

War conditions have not only increased vulnerability to infectious diseases but have also severely disrupted the management of chronic diseases, likely contributing to a significant number of deaths. Reports indicate that noncommunicable diseases (NCDs) became a leading cause of morbidity and mortality in Ukraine. The five major NCDs—cardiovascular disease, diabetes, cancer, chronic respiratory diseases, and mental health conditions—accounted for 84 percent of all deaths. Patients with diabetes, in particular, faced life-threatening challenges due to continuous disruptions in the supply of essential, lifesaving medications (WHO 2022a).

Ukrainians have met the public health crisis with determination, aided by strong international support. Civil society secured global funding for HIV and TB programs, while NGOs delivered millions of antiretroviral doses. Groups such as the Red Cross and Médecins Sans Frontières provided essential training and supplies (Simoneau et al. 2022). Still, recovery depends on sustained local resilience, continued global support, and ultimately, the region's return to peace.

When the Russia-Ukraine war began, many expected the health disruptions and human suffering to be short-lived. Now, with the war nearing its third year, the global community faces an urgent responsibility to coordinate efforts to prevent further deterioration of public health in Ukraine – a crisis that could have far-reaching consequences beyond its borders.

Further Reading

Mann, Brian. 2022. "What It's Like Living in Ukraine's Warzone." *NPR*. May 2. Https://www.npr.org/2022/05/01/1095809104/what-its-like-living-in-ukraines-warzone.

Norwegian Refugee Council. 2023. "Ukraine: Millions Face Winter in Damaged Homes, under Threat of Air Raids, beyond the Reach of Aid." https://www.nrc.no/news/2023/november/ukraine-millions-face-winter-in-damaged-homes-under-threat-of-air-raids-beyond-the-reach-of-aid/.

Reuters (a). 2022. "Covid-19 Tracker—Ukraine." Ukraine: the latest coronavirus counts, charts and maps (reuters.com). Last update July 15, 2022.

Reuters (b). 2022. "Fears of Medicine Shortages and Disease Outbreak in Ukraine after Russian Invasion." *Alarabiya News*. Fears of medicine shortages and disease outbreak in Ukraine after Russian invasion | Al Arabiya English.

Roberts, Leslie. 2022. "Surge of HIV, Tuberculosis and Covid Feared amid War in Ukraine." *Nature*. doi: https://doi.org/10.1038/d41586-022-00748-6.

Science Daily. 2022. "Polio Outbreak Risk Increases in Western Ukraine as War Ensues." https://www.sciencedaily.com/releases/2022/06/220615211330.htm.

Simoneau, Michaela, and Humzah Khan. 2022. "War amid a Pandemic: The Public Health Consequences of Russia's Invasion of Ukraine." *Center for Strategic & international Studies*. Https://www.csis.org/analysis/war-amid-pandemic-public-health-consequences-russias-invasion-ukraine.

World Health Organization (WHO). 2022c. "Guidance on Vaccination and Prevention of Vaccine-Preventable Disease Outbreaks for Countries Hosting Refugees from Ukraine." https://iris.who.int/bitstream/handle/10665/353408/WHO-EURO-2022-5321-45085-64306-eng.pdf.

World Health Organization (WHO). 2022a. "Ukraine Crisis Strategic Response Plan for June-December 2022." https://reliefweb.int/node/3863941.

World Health Organization (WHO). 2022b. "Ukraine: Immediate Steps Needed to Prevent a Measles Outbreak due to the Ongoing War and Low Vaccination Rates, Warns WHO." https://www.who.int/europe/news/item/27-04-2022-ukraine-immediate-steps-needed-to-prevent-a-measles-outbreak-due-to-the-ongoing-war-and-low-vaccination-rates–warns-who.

World Health Organization (WHO). 2023. "Ukraine: WHO Coronavirus Disease (COVID-19) Dashboard with Vaccination Data." https://covid19.who.int/region/euro/country/ua.

Addressing the Health Needs of Migrant Populations

Migration is driven by a variety of political, economic, and social pressures, ranging from the search for better livelihoods to the urgent need to escape violence, persecution, or climate-related disasters. For many, especially those forced to flee, the journey comes with immense risks: unsafe travel routes, exploitation, inadequate shelter, and limited access to health care. These vulnerabilities can have lasting effects on physical and mental well-being. Protecting the health and dignity of migrant populations is not only a humanitarian imperative but also essential for building stable, inclusive societies (European Parliament 2024).

The dangers migrants face are reflected in alarming mortality rates. A systematic review published in *The Lancet* reported that, of the 250 million people living outside their birth countries, age-standardized all-cause mortality rates ranged from 420 to 874 per 100,000 population in high-income countries. The study suggests that while migrants often arrive healthier—a phenomenon known as the "healthy migrant effect"—certain subgroups may face increased risks due to factors like limited access to healthcare, higher exposure to infectious disease, socioeconomic challenges, and exposure to hazardous conditions. (Aldridge et al. 2018). The Migrant Data Portal further notes that over 4,000 migrant fatalities have been recorded annually on global migratory routes since 2014, with more than 75,000 deaths documented globally since 1996. These figures are likely underestimates, as many migrant deaths go unrecorded (Migrant Data Portal 2024).

Beyond the risks during transit, migrants often encounter significant challenges in destination countries. According to the World Health Organization (WHO), refugees and migrants are among society's most vulnerable, frequently facing xenophobia, discrimination, poor living and working conditions, and inadequate access to health care. These challenges exacerbate the risk of communicable diseases, injuries, pregnancy complications, and mental health disorders, including depression, anxiety, and posttraumatic stress disorder (WHO 2024). Migrant workers, in particular, are vulnerable to hazardous working conditions, poverty, insufficient support systems, and unsafe housing. Undocumented workers face additional risks, such as deportation and exploitation, often taking dangerous jobs with little recourse (Underwood 2018).

Migrant populations also face heightened risks of infectious diseases like tuberculosis, malaria, and HIV/AIDS due to poor living conditions and limited access to health care. Chronic illnesses, including diabetes,

Why People Migrate

The twentieth and the twenty-first centuries are marked by rising global migration. In a 2021 publication "The Future of Migration," the U.S. Office of the Director of National Intelligence offered a comprehensive analysis of the underlying driving factors.

According to this research, the forces driving migration are a mix of economic, demographic, and environmental factors, with economic migrants comprising about two-thirds of global migrants, while refugees fleeing conflict making up 11 percent. Economic opportunities are a strong pull factor, particularly in high-income countries where per-capita income averages fifty-four times that of low-income countries. This significant income gap, combined with better health care, social services, and civil liberties, makes destinations like the United States and other OECD countries highly attractive for migrants. Rapid internet expansion further fuels migration by exposing individuals in low-income countries to the lifestyles and prospects abroad.

Migration is also driven by demand. The developed world's aging populations drive demand for migrants, particularly in countries like Japan and South Korea, where low birth rates have shrunk working-age populations. By 2040, people aged sixty-five and over will make up about a quarter of the population in developed regions, prompting countries to relax visa restrictions to attract foreign workers. For example, OECD anticipates a shortage of 2.5 million nurses and 400,000 doctors over the next decade, shortages that could be partially alleviated by a surplus of health care professionals from sub-Saharan Africa.

On the push side, rapid population growth in developing countries, which will add 1.4 billion people by 2040, outpaces economic opportunities, especially in sub-Saharan Africa where urbanization has led to large slum populations. Overburdened urban centers and limited job creation encourage migration, as illustrated by the Northern Triangle region (El Salvador, Guatemala, and Honduras) where only 10 percent of new workforce entrants could find formal employment. Environmental and security stresses further drives up migration pressures, displacing millions annually.

Recipient countries see benefits from immigration through economic contributions, especially after integration. For instance, migrants in New Zealand start contributing to the economy within five years. Migrants to Canada, Germany, and the UK contribute more in taxes than they consume in social services, helping sustain social security systems and filling labor-intensive roles that might otherwise go unfilled. Long-term migrants have been shown to boost GDP growth by enhancing labor force participation and introducing entrepreneurship, contributing approximately 9.4 percent of global GDP in 2015 alone.

Further Reading

Office of the Director of National Intelligence. 2021. "The Future of Migration." *Dni.gov.* https://www.dni.gov/index.php/gt2040-home/gt2040-deeper-looks/future-of-migration.

hypertension, cardiovascular diseases, and cervical cancer, are more prevalent in migrant populations and the conditions are often diagnosed at advanced stages (WHO 2019).

Addressing the Health Needs of Vulnerable Communities

Studies show that mitigating the health challenges associated with migration requires a holistic approach that integrates migration into broader frameworks of globalization, trade, economics, security, and environmental change. Providing legal avenues for migration can help reduce the unpredictability of human movement, addressing labor and economic needs while alleviating demographic challenges in developed nations. Contemporary migration trends, characterized by larger scale and more diverse health demographics, necessitate targeted and coordinated efforts to enhance migrant health (Gushulak et al. 2010).

The European Union (EU) has implemented initiatives such as the EU Blue Card and the Single Permit program to encourage legal migration, fill labor shortages, and boost economic growth. These programs provide work and residency permits to non-EU citizens, facilitating access to employment and stability within the EU (European Parliament 2024).

In parallel, global institutions like WHO and the Pan American Health Organization (PAHO) advocate for a comprehensive strategy to address migrant health. This includes training health care providers in cultural competency, ensuring language access through interpreters and translated materials, and conducting community outreach via health workers, mobile clinics, and awareness campaigns. According to PAHO, efforts should focus on addressing infectious diseases, mental health, and chronic conditions while promoting policies that ensure health care access for migrants, regardless of immigration status. Robust data collection systems are crucial for identifying health disparities and shaping effective policies. Collaboration with community organizations can help deliver integrated support services, including housing and employment assistance. The WHO and PAHO also stress the importance of addressing key barriers—such as fear of deportation, lack of insurance, language obstacles, and social determinants like poverty and housing instability—to improve the overall care of migrant populations (PAHO 2024).

Further Reading

Aldridge, Robert W., Laura B. Nellums, Sean Bartlett, Anna Louise Barr, Parth Patel, Rachel Burns, Sally Hargreaves, and J. Jaime Miranda. 2018. "Global Patterns of Mortality in International Migrants: A Systematic Review and Meta-Analysis." *The Lancet*, 392(10164): 2553–6. doi: http://dx.doi.org/10.1016/S0140-6736(18)32781-8.

European Parliament. 2024. "Exploring Migration Causes: Why People Migrate." https://www.europarl.europa.eu/pdfs/news/expert/2020/7/story/20200624STO81906/20200624STO81906_en.pdf.

Gushulak, B., J. Weekers, and D. Macpherson. 2010. "Migrants and Emerging Public Health Issues in a Globalized World: Threats, Risks and Challenges, An Evidence-based Framework." *Emerging Health Threats, 2*: e10. doi: 10.3134/ehtj.09.010.

Migrant Data Portal. 2024. "Migrant Deaths and Disappearances." Updated 2024. https://www.migrationdataportal.org/themes/migrant-deaths-and-disappearances.

Pan American Health Organization (PAHO). 2024. "PAHO Report Highlights Urgent Need to Improve Access to Health for Migrant Populations in the Darien Region." https://www.paho.org/en/news/15-10-2024-paho-report-highlights-urgent-need-improve-access-health-migrant-populations-darien#:~:text=Strengthen%20inter%2Dcountry%20coordination%20and,and%20Health%20in%20the%20Americas.

The World Health Organization (WHO). 2019. "10 Things to Know about the Health of Refugees and Migrants." https://www.who.int/news-room/feature-stories/detail/10-things-to-know-about-the-health-of-refugees-and-migrants.

The World Health Organization (WHO). 2024. "Refugee and Migrant Health." Updated 2024. https://www.who.int/health-topics/refugee-and-migrant-health#tab=tab_1.

Underwood, Emily. 2018. "Unhealthy Work: Why Migrants Are Especially Vulnerable to Injury and Death on the Job." *Knowable Magazine*. https://knowablemagazine.org/article/society/2018/unhealthy-work-why-migrants-are-especially-vulnerable-injury-and-death-job.

4

Globalization and Public Health

Our era, characterized by globalization, symbolizes a shift away from Cold War divides and isolationism. This interconnected world, defined by global trade and travel, has broadly elevated living standards while also introducing significant health challenges. The combined effects of globalization, migration, conflict, climate change, and zoonotic diseases have intensified the risk of infectious disease outbreaks, necessitating coordinated global responses.

The 2013–16 Ebola outbreak in West Africa demonstrates how weak health care systems and local cultural practices can magnify the impact of infectious diseases. Originating from zoonotic transmission in Guinea, the virus spread rapidly across borders to Liberia and Sierra Leone. Traditional burial customs, distrust of modern health care, and insufficient resources exacerbated the crisis, resulting in over 28,000 cases and 11,000 deaths. Despite its devastating toll, global intervention efforts, including vaccine development, highlighted the necessity of international cooperation to manage such epidemics effectively.

Prion diseases reveal the grave risks associated with global food systems and industrial farming practices. These fatal neurodegenerative disorders, including bovine spongiform encephalopathy (BSE), illustrate how zoonotic transmission can affect humans through contaminated food. The emergence of variant Creutzfeldt-Jakob Disease (vCJD) during the BSE epidemic exemplifies these risks. Global trade and lax biosecurity measures facilitated the spread of prion diseases, necessitating stricter regulations and increased public awareness to mitigate future outbreaks.

Influenza pandemics, such as those caused by swine flu (H1N1) and bird flu (H5N1), demonstrate the rapidity with which zoonotic viruses can spread in a globalized world. The 2009 H1N1 pandemic affected millions globally, fueled by urbanization and international travel. Meanwhile, H5N1 poses a localized but severe threat, with limited human-to-human transmission but alarmingly high fatality rates. These outbreaks emphasize the critical need for a

One Health approach, addressing the interconnectedness of human, animal, and environmental health, alongside improving access to vaccines and biosecurity.

Tuberculosis remains a potent health threat, compounded by the forces of globalization and forced migration. Overcrowded refugee camps, malnutrition, and inadequate health care have created fertile conditions for TB to persist and spread, particularly in developing regions. Recent years have seen a resurgence of TB due to health care disruptions, including those caused by the Covid-19 pandemic. Addressing this challenge requires global efforts to tackle multidrug-resistant TB strains and improve health care equity for at-risk populations.

As these examples demonstrate, infectious diseases like Ebola, mpox, prion diseases, influenza, and tuberculosis transcend borders and demand a global response. International collaboration in disease prevention, early detection, and equitable access to health care resources is essential to combat the growing health threats amplified by globalization. Through collective action, countries can strengthen global health systems and mitigate the risks of future pandemics.

Mpox: Understanding Its Origins, Global Spread, and Strategies for Control

Mpox, formerly known as monkeypox, is a viral zoonotic disease that has drawn growing global attention due to its similarities to smallpox and its potential for widespread transmission. The mpox virus is part of the *Orthopoxvirus* genus of the *Poxviridae* family, which also includes the variola virus that causes smallpox. Although mpox is endemic to Africa, numerous outbreaks have been reported worldwide, driven in part by global travel and trade (WHO 2024).

Since January 1, 2024, the Democratic Republic of the Congo (DRC) and neighboring countries in Central and Eastern Africa have reported over 50,000 suspected mpox cases, including 1,000 deaths. Of these, approximately 13,000 cases and more than forty deaths have been confirmed through laboratory testing. Additionally, travel-related cases have been detected in other regions, including parts of Africa, Europe, Asia, and North America, according to the Centers for Disease Control and Prevention (CDC).

Mpox was first identified in 1958 in research monkeys, which led to its name. However, it is now known that the primary reservoirs of the virus are small mammals, particularly rodents, rather than monkeys. Various species of rodents, including Gambian pouched rats and dormice, are believed to be the main animal hosts. Transmission to humans can occur through bites, scratches, or direct contact with the blood, bodily fluids, or lesions of an infected animal. Consuming undercooked meat from infected animals also poses a significant risk (CDC).

However, the main venue of transmission is through person-to-person contact, according to the CDC. Mpox can be transmitted through direct skin-to-skin contact with the bodily fluid, rash, scabs of an infected person. Pregnant individuals with mpox can pass the virus to their fetus during pregnancy or to their newborn during and after birth. Touch of infected objects can also lead to infection, according to the CDC.

Symptomatically, mpox manifests with fever, headache, muscle aches, and a characteristic rash that progresses from macules to pustules and eventually forms crusts. However, mpox is generally less severe than smallpox, with lower mortality rates. Smallpox was declared eradicated globally in 1980 through an extensive vaccination campaign led by the World Health Organization (WHO). However, the cessation of smallpox vaccination has made populations increasingly susceptible to mpox, as the smallpox vaccine also provides cross-protection against mpox due to the genetic similarities between the two viruses (Ladnyj et al. 1972).

Mpox emerged as an increasing public health concern following several notable outbreaks that demonstrated how zoonotic spillovers can be amplified in a globalized world. The first human case was reported in 1970 in the DRC, where a nine-month-old boy in a region that had eradicated smallpox presented with a smallpox-like illness, later confirmed to be mpox. This case marked the recognition of mpox as a disease capable of affecting humans. During the 1970s and 1980s, additional cases were reported in Central and West Africa, though these were relatively sporadic and localized (Ladnyj et al. 1972).

In 2003, the first cases of mpox outside Africa were reported in the United States. This outbreak was traced to the importation of infected exotic pets, specifically Gambian pouched rats and dormice from Ghana, which were housed with prairie dogs. These prairie dogs were sold as pets, leading to human infections. A total of forty-seven confirmed and probable cases were reported across six states, with no fatalities (Reed et al. 2004).

After a prolonged period with few reported cases, mpox reemerged in Nigeria in 2017, leading to the largest outbreak in the country's history at the time. Over 200 confirmed cases, more than 500 suspected cases, and several deaths were reported. Scientists have observed that the global population has become increasingly vulnerable to mpox due to the discontinuation of widespread smallpox vaccination, particularly in regions where the virus is endemic (Rimoin et al. 2010).

In 2022, mpox gained unprecedented global attention as cases began to appear in countries outside Africa, including Europe, North America, and Australia. Unlike previous outbreaks, the 2022 spread was marked by human-to-human transmission in non-endemic regions, raising concerns about the virus's potential to establish a broader foothold. In response, the World Health Organization (WHO) declared the outbreak a Public Health Emergency of International Concern, triggering enhanced surveillance, contact tracing, and vaccination efforts worldwide (WHO 2022).

The prevalence of mpox varies worldwide, with most cases historically concentrated in Central and West Africa. In the DRC, mpox is endemic, with thousands of suspected cases reported annually. According to data from the CDC and the World Health Organization (WHO), mpox has been relatively rare in the United States, with the 2003 outbreak being the most notable until recently. However, the 2022 outbreak marked a turning point, with thousands of cases reported across multiple states, prompting a swift public health response. Globally, the severity of mpox ranges from mild to severe, with potential complications including secondary bacterial infections, respiratory distress, and, in some cases, death. Children, pregnant women, and immunocompromised individuals are particularly vulnerable to severe outcomes.

From January to August 2024, a significant mpox outbreak prompted the WHO to declare it a Public Health Emergency of International Concern. This outbreak was particularly severe in several African countries, with the DRC being the most affected. By July, the DRC had reported over 13,791 cases and 450 deaths. The fatality rate for this outbreak was notably higher than in previous outbreaks, estimated at 3-4 percent, compared to less than 1 percent during the 2022-3 outbreak. According to WHO's key epidemiological findings, sexual contact was identified as a primary mode of transmission in this outbreak. It accounted for 83.8 percent of reported cases (19,102 of 22,801), followed by person-to-person non-sexual contact. This trend continued during the first six months of the year, with 95.6 percent of new cases (483 of 505) linked to sexual contact (WHO 2024).

Mpox's connection to global travel and trade has become increasingly apparent, particularly during the 2003 and 2022 outbreaks in the United States. These outbreaks were linked to the international trade of exotic animals and person-to-person transmission. Another example occurred in 2018 when a traveler returning to the UK from Nigeria contracted the virus through contact with an infected animal. Upon their return, the traveler developed symptoms and subsequently transmitted the virus to a health care worker. Such incidents demonstrate how zoonotic diseases like mpox can spread through travel, leading to secondary infections in non-endemic regions (Yinka-Ogunleye et al. 2018).

Certain groups are more vulnerable to mpox, as indicated by the distribution of cases. Individuals living in endemic regions, such as Central and West Africa, face the highest risk. Health care workers are also at elevated risk due to their exposure to infected individuals. Young children are more likely to develop severe disease, likely due to their developing immune systems. Immunocompromised individuals, including those living with HIV, are particularly susceptible to severe outcomes, according to the CDC and the WHO.

Prevention of mpox can be achieved through vaccines originally developed for smallpox, such as JYNNEOS. Vaccination campaigns targeting high-risk groups, including health care workers and close contacts of confirmed cases, have been implemented during outbreaks. However, treatment remains primarily supportive, focusing on symptom relief (CDC 2022).

Global health organizations emphasize a multifaceted approach to controlling mpox, focusing on surveillance, vaccination, public education, and international collaboration. Efforts include regulating animal trade and educating travelers from endemic regions to reduce exposure. The WHO also warns against the harmful effects of stigma, which can lead to discrimination, delay in seeking care, and unsafe behaviors. To combat this, WHO advocates for trust in health services, empathy for those affected, and practical measures to ensure safety (Farge 2024).

Further Reading

Centers for Disease Control and Prevention (CDC). "Monkeypox." https://www.cdc.gov/mpox/index.html.

Farge, Emma. 2024. "Fighting Mpox Stigma Key to Ending Burundi Outbreak Quickly, UNICEF Says." *Reuters*. https://www.reuters.com/world/africa/fighting-mpox-stigma-key-ending-burundi-outbreak-quickly-unicef-says-2024-09-20/.

Ladnyj, I. D., P. Ziegler, and E. Kima. 1972. "A Human Infection Caused by Monkeypox Virus in Basankusu Territory, Democratic Republic of the Congo." *The Lancet*, 299(7750): 76–8. doi: 10.1016/S0140-6736(72)92360-2.

Reed, Kurt D., John W Melski, Mary Beth Graham, et al. 2004. "The Detection of Monkeypox in Humans in the Western Hemisphere." *New England Journal of Medicine*, 350(4): 342–50. doi: 10.1056/NEJMoa032299.

Rimoin, Anne W., Prime M. Mulembakani, Sara C. Johnston, and Jean-Jacques Muyembe. 2010. "Major Increase in Human Monkeypox Incidence 30 Years after Smallpox Vaccination Campaigns Cease in the Democratic Republic of Congo." *PLoS One*, 5(10): e13522. doi:10.1371/journal.pone.0013522.

World Health Organization (WHO). 2022. Monkeypox Outbreaks 2022. Retrieved from https://www.who.int/emergencies/situations/monkeypox-2022.

World Health Organization (WHO). 2024. "Mpox." https://www.who.int/news-room/fact-sheets/detail/mpox.

World Health Organization (WHO). 2024. "Multi-country Outbreak of Mpox, External Situation Report #35—August 12, 2024." August 12. https://www.who.int/publications/m/item/multi-country-outbreak-of-mpox–external-situation-report-35–12-august-2024.

Yinka-Ogunleye, Adesola, Olusola Aruna, Mahmood Dalhat, Dimie Ogoina, et al. 2018. "Outbreak of Human Monkeypox in Nigeria in 2017–18: A Clinical and Epidemiological Report." *The Lancet Infectious Diseases*, 19(8): 872–9. doi: 10.1016/S1473-3099(19)30294-4.

Prion Diseases—Navigating Global Health Risks in an Era of Zoonotic Threats and Globalization

Prion diseases, also known as transmissible spongiform encephalopathies (TSEs), are a group of fatal neurodegenerative disorders affecting both animals and humans. They are caused by prions—infectious proteins that propagate by inducing the misfolding of normal cellular prion proteins into their disease-causing form. Unlike other pathogens, prions lack nucleic acids, relying solely on their protein structure to cause infection and spread. Consequently, these diseases cannot be prevented with vaccines or treated with medication, as noted by the Centers for Disease Control and Prevention (CDC). The zoonotic transmission of prion diseases between animals and humans raises substantial public health concerns, particularly in our increasingly globalized world.

In animals, prion diseases such as Bovine Spongiform Encephalopathy (BSE), Scrapie in sheep, and Chronic Wasting Disease (CWD) in deer and elk are well-documented. These diseases share a common pathological hallmark: spongiform changes in brain tissue caused by the accumulation of misfolded prion proteins. In humans, prion diseases include Creutzfeldt-Jakob Disease (CJD), Gerstmann-Sträussler-Scheinker Syndrome (GSS), Fatal Familial Insomnia (FFI), and Kuru.

The emergence of variant Creutzfeldt-Jakob Disease (vCJD) in the 1990s, linked to the consumption of beef contaminated with the BSE agent, illustrates the zoonotic potential of these diseases (Belay et al. 2005).

Symptoms of prion diseases typically manifest as a spectrum of neurological disorders, reflecting the progressive neurodegeneration caused by the buildup of misfolded prions in the brain. Common symptoms include rapidly progressing dementia, memory loss, personality changes, and hallucinations. Motor symptoms are also prevalent, such as myoclonus (involuntary muscle jerks), ataxia (loss of coordination and balance), and akinetic mutism (loss of voluntary movement and speech). As the disease advances, patients often become bedridden and unable to perform basic self-care, ultimately resulting in death (Belay et al. 2005).

In animals, prion diseases are transmitted through direct contact with infected animals, consumption of contaminated feed, or exposure to contaminated environments. For example, BSE, commonly known as "mad cow disease," was primarily spread through the consumption of meat-and-bone meal made from infected cattle. This route of transmission amplified the disease within cattle herds and introduced it to humans through the food chain. In wild animals, CWD affects deer and elk, with transmission occurring through direct contact with contaminated bodily fluids such as saliva, urine, or feces, as well as through environmental contamination. The spread of CWD to new regions, often facilitated by animal translocation or trade in animal products, highlights the role human activities can play in disseminating prion diseases among animal populations (Belay et al. 2004).

In humans, prion diseases can be acquired through various pathways. Sporadic Creutzfeldt-Jakob Disease (sCJD) arises without a known cause and is believed to result from spontaneous misfolding of prion proteins. Familial forms of prion diseases, such as CJD, GSS, and FFI, are inherited and associated with specific mutations in the *PRNP* gene, which predispose individuals to prion misfolding, as noted by the CDC.

Acquired forms of prion diseases, such as vCJD, have been linked to the consumption of beef products contaminated with the BSE agent, as seen during the BSE epidemic in the United Kingdom. Another transmission route is iatrogenic CJD, which occurs through exposure to contaminated medical instruments, dura mater grafts, or human growth hormone derived from cadaveric pituitary glands (Belay et al. 2005). Additionally, concerns about the zoonotic potential of prion diseases extend to CWD in deer and elk. This disease is closely monitored for possible transmission, particularly among hunters and others who handle or consume meat from infected animals (Belay et al. 2004; Belay et al. 2003).

Prion diseases, although rare, remain incurable. The global incidence of sCJD is approximately 1 to 2 cases per million people annually. vCJD, linked to BSE, has accounted for fewer than 250 cases worldwide, the majority of which occurred in the United Kingdom. Despite their rarity, prion diseases are almost universally fatal, with most patients succumbing within months to a few years of symptom onset (Belay et al. 2005).

In animals, the prevalence of prion diseases varies significantly. The BSE epidemic in the UK during the 1980s and 1990s led to the culling of millions of cattle to contain the outbreak. CWD, which continues to spread among deer and elk in North America, has raised concerns about its potential transmission to humans and other species. In the context of animal prion diseases, farmers, hunters, and others who could be potentially exposed to infected animals are at greater risks. This includes hunters who handle or consume deer or elk in areas where CWD is endemic, although no human cases have been confirmed(Belay et al. 2005; Belay et al. 2004).

Certain populations are more vulnerable to prion diseases than others. Individuals with specific genetic mutations affecting the PRNP gene are at higher risk for developing familial forms of prion diseases. Populations exposed to contaminated food products, such as those affected by the BSE outbreak, are also at increased risk for vCJD. Health care workers and patients undergoing certain medical procedures may be at risk of iatrogenic transmission if proper sterilization procedures are not followed (Belay 1999).

Prion diseases are closely linked to globalization in multiple ways. The global trade of livestock, animal products, and foodstuffs has facilitated the cross-border spread of prion diseases, exemplified by the BSE epidemic in Europe and the ongoing spread of CWD in North America. International travel and migration further contribute to the potential dissemination of prion diseases, as individuals exposed to prions in one country can introduce the disease to new regions (CDC; Belay et al. 2005). The interconnected nature of global food markets amplifies the impact of prion disease outbreaks, as seen during the BSE crisis in the UK, which led to a ban on British beef exports, significant economic losses, and widespread fear about the safety of the global food supply (Belay 1999).

The CDC and WHO have developed infection control guidelines (CDC; WHO 1999), recommending a combination of infection control, food safety, and global cooperation to prevent prion diseases, particularly in an era of globalization. In health care, strict decontamination of medical instruments with sodium hydroxide or sodium hypochlorite combined with autoclaving is essential. Rules for proper disposal of contaminated materials through incineration and safe handling of infectious must be strictly followed. For the public, food safety measures include avoiding high-risk animal tissues, such as brain and spinal cord, sourcing meat from trusted suppliers, and adhering to regulations banning animal-derived proteins in livestock feed to prevent diseases like BSE.

The WHO encourages countries to work together to monitor and regulate the trade of food and medicines, improve prion disease surveillance, and share information about outbreaks openly. Raising public awareness and maintaining strong biosecurity in farming and health care are also important steps to help prevent the spread of prion diseases in today's connected world.

Further Reading

Belay, Ermias D. 1999. "Transmissible Spongiform Encephalopathies in Humans." *Annual Review of Microbiology*, 60(2): 176–81. https://www.cdc.gov/prions/pdfs/tse-in-humans.pdf.

Belay, Ermias D., and Lawrence B. Schonberger. 2005. "The Public Health Impact of Prion Diseases." *Annual Review of Public Health*, 26(1): 191–212. doi: 10.1146/annurev.publhealth.26.021304.144536.

Belay, Ermias D., Ryan A. Maddox, Pierluigi Gambetti, and Lawrence B. Schonberger. 2003. "Monitoring the Occurrence of Emerging Forms of Creutzfeldt-Jakob Disease in the United States." *Neurology*, 60(2): 176–81. doi: 10.1212/01.wnl.0000039953.15052.3b.

Belay, Ermias D., Ryan A Maddox, Elizabeth S Williams, Michael W Miller, Pierluigi Gambetti, and Lawrence B. Schonberger. 2004. "Chronic Wasting Disease and Potential Transmission to Humans." *Emerging Infectious Diseases*, 10(6): 977–84. doi: 10.3201/eid1006.030707.

Centers for Disease Control and Prevention (CDC). 2024. "Prion Diseases." https://www.cdc.gov/prions/about/index.html.

The World Health Organization (WHO). 1999. "WHO Infection Control Guidelines for Transmissible Spongiform Encephalopathies." https://iris.who.int/handle/10665/66707.

Watson, Neil, Jean-Philippe Brandel, Alison Green, Peter Hermann, Anna Ladogana, Terri Lindsay, Janet Mackenzie, Maurizio Pocchiari, Colin Smith, Inga Zerr, and Suvankar Pal. 2021. "The Importance of Ongoing International Surveillance for Creutzfeldt–Jakob Disease." *Nature Reviews Neurology*, 17(6): 362–79. doi: https://doi.org/10.1038/s41582-021-00488-7.

Influenza in a Globalized World—Swine Flu and Bird Flu

Swine flu and bird flu are caused by the avian influenza viruses H1N1 and H5N1, respectively. These viruses have demonstrated the ability to transmit from birds or domestic animals, such as pigs and cattle, to humans. The H1N1 virus responsible for the 2009 swine flu pandemic originated in pigs and crossed over to humans, resulting in a global outbreak (CDC 2023). Similarly, the H5N1 bird flu has shown the potential to infect humans, as evidenced by a growing number of cases as of early 2025.

The United States reported its first death linked to H5N1 avian influenza on January 6, 2025. An elderly individual in Louisiana, who had underlying health conditions, died from the infection, likely due to exposure to infected backyard poultry and wild birds. Of the sixty-six human infections reported in the United States, most occurred among farm workers who had contact with sick poultry or cattle. However, human-to-human transmission, a critical factor for a potential pandemic, had not been identified, according to the Centers for Disease Control and Prevention (CDC 2025).

The pathogenesis of H1N1 and H5N1 influenza viruses demonstrates how global travel and trade can accelerate the emergence, spread, and impact of zoonotic diseases. These viruses can be transmitted through respiratory pathways or direct contact with sources of infection. During the 2009 H1N1 pandemic, global travel and trade facilitated the rapid spread of the virus to over 200 countries within a few months, resulting in approximately one billion infections and half a million deaths, according to the WHO.

H5N1, first detected in birds in 1996, is believed to have spread globally through migratory birds and the poultry trade, leading to sporadic human infections with high case fatality rates and significant economic losses in the poultry industry. The interconnected nature of the modern world through travel, trade, urbanization, and industrial farming has amplified the risks and impacts of these viruses (WHO 2009; CDC 2024).

Flu pandemics have occurred frequently throughout history. The 1918 Spanish Flu caused an estimated 50 to 100 million deaths worldwide, making it one of the deadliest pandemics in human history. Descendants of this virus, including the current H1N1 swine flu virus and the H3N2 virus, continue to circulate today. H3N2 was responsible for the 1968 global pandemic, popularly known as "Hong Kong Flu." These descendant strains have not resulted in the same level of mortality, largely due to widespread immunity, advancements in

How Flu Strains Are Named

Flu strains are identified using a standardized system that includes the virus type, origin, isolate number, and protein subtype. Influenza A viruses, responsible for pandemics, are classified by two surface proteins: hemagglutinin (H) and neuraminidase (N), with 18 H and 11 N subtypes forming combinations like H1N1 and H3N2. Isolate numbers specify unique strains, though "isolate" and "strain" are often used interchangeably.

Example: A/California/07/2009 (H1N1)
"A": Virus type (Influenza A).
"California": Geographic origin of the first identified sample.
"07": The 7th isolate from this location and year.
"2009": Year the virus was isolated.
"H1N1": Specific protein combination.

Notable Flu Strains:
H1N1: Linked to the 1918 "Spanish Flu" and 2009 "swine flu" pandemics.
H2N2: Caused the 1957 "Asian FLu" pandemic.
H3N2: Associated with the 1968 "Hong Kong Flu" pandemic.
H5N1: Known as "avian flu," originating from birds.
H7N9: Another avian flu strain with human cases.

The names of locations mentioned in these examples are provided for explanatory purposes. It should be noted that the WHO and CDC discourage using names based on geographical locations or animals to prevent stigmatization. Instead, they advocate for neutral scientific terms to promote clear and unbiased communication about flu risks. For more information, refer to CDC and WHO resources.

Further Reading

The World Health Organization (WHO). 2024. "A Revised System of Nomenclature for Influenza Viruses." *Bulletin of the World Health Organization.* https://iris.who.int/handle/10665/262638.

---

medical care, and evolutionary changes in the virus over time (Taubenberger and Morens 2006; CDC 2023).

H5N1 and H1N1 are influenza A viruses with distinct evolutionary origins and behaviors, according to the CDC. H5N1 primarily originated from avian reservoirs and is adapted to birds, whereas H1N1 evolved through reassortment involving swine, avian, and human influenza viruses, making it more suited to mammals. These differences appear to influence their transmission and fatality rates.

H5N1 exhibits limited zoonotic transmission, typically requiring direct contact with infected birds or contaminated environments. It rarely spreads between humans but has a high fatality rate, exceeding 50 percent in confirmed cases. In contrast, H1N1 spreads efficiently among humans via airborne droplets and surface contact, facilitating pandemics like the 2009 outbreak. However, its fatality rate is much lower, comparable to that of seasonal flu. H5N1, while posing a localized and deadly threat, would need significant mutation to become a pandemic risk, according to the CDC. In comparison, H1N1's adaptation to mammals enables widespread transmission, albeit with relatively low lethality.

In our interconnected world, the evolution and spread of influenza viruses such as H1N1 and H5N1 are influenced by a number of factors including climate change, urbanization, and health inequalities, scientists believe.

Climate change is altering ecosystems and influencing the migratory patterns of wild birds, which serve as natural reservoirs for avian influenza viruses such as H5N1. As global temperatures rise, these birds may adjust their migration routes, potentially introducing the virus to new regions and heightening the risk of transmission to domestic poultry and humans (Boodhoo et al. 2024).

Urbanization creates densely populated areas that facilitate the rapid transmission of viruses, as demonstrated during the 2009 H1N1 pandemic, where close human contact and global travel networks accelerated the virus's spread. Additionally, health inequalities in urban settings can significantly worsen the impact of such outbreaks. Populations with limited access to health care, inadequate sanitation, and poor living conditions are more vulnerable to infection and less likely to receive timely treatment. During the H1N1 pandemic, marginalized communities experienced higher infection rates and faced greater difficulties accessing vaccines and antiviral medications (Anguelov 2012).

To prevent and control H1N1 and H5N1, the CDC and the WHO emphasize several critical actions. These include strengthening surveillance systems to enable early detection of outbreaks in both humans and animals, enhancing biosecurity measures in agriculture—particularly in poultry and livestock farming—and ensuring equitable access to health care, vaccines, and antiviral treatments, with a focus on marginalized communities. Additionally, addressing climate change through policies to reduce greenhouse gas emissions and promote sustainability is essential. A One Health approach, which acknowledges the interconnectedness of human, animal, and environmental health, is vital for developing comprehensive prevention and response strategies. The scientific community stresses the need to implement these measures proactively—before the threat escalates beyond control (Williams et al. 2024).

Further Reading

Boodhoo, Nitish, and Shayan Sharif. 2024. "Climate Change Is Helping the H5N1 Bird Flu Virus Spread and Evolve." *Phys.org*. https://phys.org/news/2024-06-climate-h5n1-bird-flu-virus.html.

Centers for Disease Control and Prevention (CDC). 2022. "1918 Pandemic (H1N1 Virus)." CDC. https://www.cdc.gov/flu/pandemic-resources/1918-pandemic-h1n1.html.

Centers for Disease Control and Prevention (CDC). 2023. "Avian Influenza (Bird Flu): Current Situation." CDC. https://www.cdc.gov/flu/avianflu/h5n1-virus.htm.

Centers for Disease Control and Prevention (CDC). 2025. "First H5 Bird Flu Death Reported in United States." *CDC Newsroom*. https://www.cdc.gov/media/releases/2025/m0106-h5-birdflu-death.html.

Centers for Disease Control and Prevention (CDC). "Influenza (Flu): Types of Influenza Viruses." CDC. https://www.cdc.gov/flu/about/viruses/types.htm.

Centers for Disease Control and Prevention (CDC). 2023. "Key Facts about Swine Influenza (Swine Flu) in Humans." CDC. https://www.cdc.gov/flu/swineflu/keyfacts_pigs.htm.

Centers for Disease Control and Prevention (CDC). 2024. "Past Reported Global Human Cases with Highly Pathogenic Avian Influenza A(H5N1) (HPAI H5N1) by Country, 1997–2024." *CDC*. https://www.cdc.gov/flu/avianflu/h5n1-virus.htm.

Sparke, Matthew, and Dimitar Anguelov. 2012. "H1N1, Globalization and the Epidemiology of Inequality." *Health and Place,* 18(4): 726–36. doi: https://doi.org/10.1016/j.healthplace.2011.09.001.

Taubenberger, Jeffrey K., and David M. Morens. 2006. "1918 Influenza: The Mother of All Pandemics." *Emerging Infectious Diseases* 12(1) (January 2006): 15–22. doi: https://doi.org/10.3201/eid1201.050979.

Williams, Adeline, Allison Berke, Casey Aveggio, Saskia Popescu, and Aurelia Attal-Juncqua. 2024. "Getting Ahead of H5N1: Declare a Public Health Emergency, Expand Wastewater Testing, and Increase Vaccine Research and Availability—Sooner Rather Than Later." *Rand.org*. https://www.rand.org/pubs/commentary/2024/12/getting-ahead-of-h5n1-declare-a-public-health-emergency.htm.

World Health Organization (WHO). 2023. "Avian Influenza (Bird Flu)." WHO. https://www.who.int/news-room/fact-sheets/detail/avian-influenza.

World Health Organization (WHO). 2024. "Cumulative Number of Confirmed Human Cases for Avian Influenza A(H5N1) Reported To WHO, 2003–2024, December 12, 2024." https://www.who.int/publications/m/item/cumulative-number-of-confirmed-human-cases-for-avian-influenza-a(h5n1)-reported-to-who–2003-2024–December20, 2024.

World Health Organization (WHO). 2022. "Influenza (Seasonal)." WHO. https://www.who.int/news-room/fact-sheets/detail/influenza-(seasonal).

World Health Organization (WHO). "Influenza A (H1N1)." https://www.who.int/emergencies/situations/influenza-a-%28h1n1%29-outbreak.

World Health Organization (WHO). 2010. "Pandemic (H1N1) 2009—Update 112." WHO. https://www.who.int/csr/don/2010_08_06/en/.

World Organization for Animal Health (OIE). 2006. "Economic Impact of Highly Pathogenic Avian Influenza." *OIE*. https://www.oie.int/en/document/economic-impact-hpai/.

Globalization, Forced Migration, and the Growing Threat of Tuberculosis Outbreaks

Tuberculosis (TB) remains one of the world's most enduring and deadly infectious diseases. Despite advancements in medicine, TB continues to be a major cause of illness and death, particularly in regions with limited health care resources. Over the past two decades, globalization, coupled with forced migration driven by conflicts and natural disasters, has resulted in overcrowded living conditions and poor hygiene in many areas. These circumstances create an environment highly favorable for the transmission of airborne diseases like TB, significantly raising the risk of outbreaks.

TB is an ancient disease, with evidence of its existence found in human remains dating back thousands of years. Although the term "tuberculosis" was coined in the nineteenth century, the disease was previously known by various names, including "consumption" and "phthisis." During the Industrial Revolution of the eighteenth and nineteenth centuries, rapid urbanization and poor living conditions caused a surge in TB cases, making it one of the most devastating diseases in Europe and North America. A major breakthrough came in 1882 when Robert Koch discovered the bacterium *Mycobacterium tuberculosis*, revolutionizing the understanding and treatment of the disease. The development of antibiotics, particularly streptomycin in the 1940s, led to a significant decline in TB cases in developed countries (Barberis et al. 2017).

TB primarily affects the lungs, with pulmonary TB being the most common and contagious form of the disease. Key symptoms of pulmonary TB include a persistent cough lasting over three weeks, chest pain, and sputum production, which may sometimes contain blood. General symptoms include unexplained weight loss, fever, night sweats, and fatigue. In some cases, TB can spread to other parts of the body, such as the kidneys, spine, or brain, resulting in extrapulmonary TB, according to the CDC.

The bacterium that causes TB spreads through airborne particles released when an infected person coughs, sneezes, or speaks. These tiny droplets, known as droplet nuclei, can remain suspended in the air for several hours, especially in enclosed, poorly ventilated spaces. People nearby may inhale these droplets, potentially leading to infection. TB is particularly contagious in settings where individuals live or work in close quarters, such as prisons, shelters, and densely populated urban areas.

Globally, tuberculosis (TB) continues to impose a significant burden on public health. According to the World Health Organization (WHO), an estimated 10.6 million people contracted TB in 2022, marking a troubling increase compared to previous years. This surge is partly attributed to disruptions in health care services caused by the Covid-19 pandemic, which delayed diagnosis and treatment in many regions. The WHO reported that TB was the second leading cause of death from a single infectious agent, responsible for approximately 1.3 million deaths in 2022. It ranks the second deadliest infectious disease after Covid-19, surpassing HIV/AIDS. The disease disproportionately affects low- and middle-income countries, with India, China, Indonesia, the Philippines, and Nigeria collectively accounting for nearly 50 percent of global TB cases (WHO 2023).

CDC data shows tuberculosis is less common in the United States but continues to pose public health challenges, particularly among high-risk populations such as immigrants, individuals living with HIV, and those with weakened immune systems. In 2022, CDC reported approximately 8,300 new TB cases nationwide, with a case rate of about 2.5 per 100,000 people. While mortality rates in the United States are relatively low due to the country's advanced health care infrastructure, TB still causes deaths each year, particularly among vulnerable groups.

Globalization contributes to the spread of tuberculosis by enabling the rapid movement of people, goods, and services across borders. Increased mobility heightens the risk of TB spreading to new regions, as individuals travel from high-burden to low-burden areas. Forced migration worsens this trend by displacing large populations into conditions that foster TB transmission. Migrants from countries with high TB prevalence could carry latent TB infections, which can become active under stress or weakened immunity. Countries receiving substantial numbers of migrants, such as the United States and European countries, have experienced a notable rise in TB cases among foreign-born individuals. In the United States, foreign-born individuals accounted for over 70 percent of reported TB cases in 2022, according to the CDC.

Forced migration caused by wars, persecution, and natural disasters often results in overcrowded refugee camps and informal settlements with poor sanitation and limited access to health care, creating ideal conditions for TB transmission. Refugees and displaced populations are especially vulnerable due to the stress of displacement, malnutrition, and exposure to environments where TB prevalence may be higher. Globalization has also driven rapid urbanization, particularly in developing countries where population growth frequently outpaces infrastructure development, making overcrowded urban areas with insufficient health care services become hotspots for TB transmission. Additionally, global trade has contributed to the spread of drug-resistant TB strains. In recent years, supply chain disruptions during the Covid-19 pandemic revealed vulnerabilities in TB drug distribution systems, increasing the risk of outbreaks of multidrug-resistant TB (MDR-TB), according to the World Trade Organization.

The historical trend of TB infections in the UK provides a compelling example of how domestic economic stress and globalization have influenced the pathogenesis of the disease.

TB prevalence in the UK peaked during the eighteenth century, as the Industrial Revolution brought unprecedented migration and urbanization. In major cities like London, migrant workers often lived in overcrowded, unsanitary conditions where malnutrition and close contact fueled the spread. Historical records from 1913 indicate the TB prevalence rate exceeding 300 cases per 100,000 people, with one in four deaths attributed to the disease. However, prevalence rates began to decline rapidly due to advancements in medical technology, such as the introduction of chemotherapy and the use of X-rays for diagnosis. By the 1980s, TB prevalence in the UK had fallen to approximately 10 cases per 100,000 people (Glaziou et al. 2018).

In the early 2000s, the UK saw a resurgence of tuberculosis, with incidence rates exceeding 20 cases per 100,000 people by 2011–12, and even higher in metropolitan areas. Contributing factors included international migration, the spread of HIV, and the rise in Type II diabetes – conditions that increase susceptibility to TB. In response, the UK implemented pre-entry screening for immigrants and reduced the number of new arrivals from high TB burden countries. These measures successfully brought the prevalence rate back to pre-surge levels (Glaziou et al. 2018).

A study by Anderson and colleagues, analyzing data from 1999 to 2003 in London, highlighted the significant role of infections acquired abroad in the spread of TB. Their research revealed that in 2003, London recorded 3,048 TB cases, representing 45 percent of the UK's national total and nine times the average level. Notably, 75 percent of those with TB in London were born abroad, with nearly half having lived in the UK for less than five years and a third for more than ten years.

The study also found that 86 percent of cases occurred among ethnic minority groups, with the highest incidence rate of 283 per 100,000 among Black Africans, followed by 141 per 100,000 among both Pakistanis and Indians, and just 8 per 100,000 among Whites. Other vulnerable groups identified in the research included the homeless, prisoners, hard drug and alcohol users, and individuals with suppressed immune systems (Anderson et al. 2007).

Researchers warn that in today's globalized world, where travel is easily accessible, infectious diseases like TB can be quickly acquired or spread across borders. This underscores the need for effective TB control measures that involve coordinated global efforts and focus on addressing the needs of at-risk populations (Glaziou et al. 2018; Anderson et al. 2007). Furthermore, while TB is more commonly detected among foreign-born populations, the disease is not linked to race or gender but is instead associated with challenging socioeconomic conditions.

Further Reading

Anderson, Sarah R, Helen Maguire, and Jacqui Carless. 2007. "Tuberculosis in London: A Decade and a Half of No Decline." *Thorax*. https://www.ncbi.nlm.nih.gov/pmc/articles/PMC2111261/.

Barberis, I., N. L. Bragazzi, L. Galluzzo, and M. Martini. 2017. "The History of Tuberculosis: From the First Historical Records to the Isolation of Koch's Bacillus." *Journal of Preventive Medicine and Hygiene*. https://www.ncbi.nlm.nih.gov/pmc/articles/PMC5432783/.

Boyd, Andrew T., Susan T. Cookson, Ibrahim Almashayek, Hiam Yaacoub, M. Saiful Qayyum, and Aleksandar Galev. 2019. "An Evaluation of a Tuberculosis Case-Finding and Treatment Program among Syrian Refugees—Jordan and Lebanon, 2013–2015." *Conflict and Health*. https://doi.org/10.1186/s13031-019-0213-1.

Centers for Disease Control and Prevention (CDC). "Tuberculosis (TB)." https://www.cdc.gov/tb/index.html.

Glaziou, Philippe, Katherine Floyd, and Mario Raviglione. 2018. "Trends in Tuberculosis in the UK." *Thorax*. https://doi.org/10.1136/thoraxjnl-2018-211537.

World Health Organization (WHO). 2023. "Tuberculosis—Key Facts." November 7. https://www.who.int/news-room/fact-sheets/detail/tuberculosis.

Ebola in West Africa—
The Clash of Globalization and Tradition

Globalization has driven remarkable economic progress, enhancing the quality of life for many, particularly in middle- and low-income countries. However, it has also introduced new public health challenges, particularly in the context of climate change and the increasing spread of zoonotic diseases. Addressing these challenges requires proactive and comprehensive strategies. The recurring Ebola outbreaks during 2013–16 in Africa stand as a striking example of the urgent need for such efforts.

Ebola virus is a highly infectious pathogen that causes Ebola Virus Disease (EVD), a severe and often fatal illness that affects both humans and nonhuman primates. It is part of the *Filoviridae* family and includes several lethal strains, such as Zaire ebolavirus, Sudan ebolavirus, Taï Forest ebolavirus, Bundibugyo ebolavirus, and Reston ebolavirus. Ebola outbreaks are infamous for their high mortality rates, with case fatality rates (CFR) in some African countries ranging from 25 percent to 90 percent, depending on the strain and specific outbreak. Symptoms of EVD may begin with the sudden onset of fever, severe weakness, muscle pain, and headache, followed by vomiting, diarrhea, rash; and, in advanced cases, internal and external bleeding (Jacob et al. 2020).

The Ebola virus is closely linked to its zoonotic origins, with fruit bats believed to be the most likely natural reservoir. Transmission to humans occurs through direct contact with the blood, secretions, or other bodily fluids of infected animals, such as bats, or other nonhuman primates. Once the virus enters the human population, it spreads primarily through human-to-human transmission, involving direct contact with the blood, bodily fluids, or tissues of infected individuals, or contact with surfaces and materials contaminated with these fluids. The virus infects multiple cell types, causing immune system dysregulation, widespread inflammation, and damage to the vascular system, leading to severe symptoms and high fatality rates (Jacob et al. 2020; WHO 2023). Vaccines are now available for the Zaire strain, and others are currently under development (CDC 2023).

A major Ebola outbreak began in 2013 in West Africa and lasted for three years. This outbreak was the most severe in history in terms of both the number of cases and fatalities. The epicenter was located in southeastern Guinea, specifically in the small village of Meliandou, within the Guéckédou district. The outbreak is believed to have started in December 2013, with the first known case involving a two-year-old child who likely contracted the virus from a bat

(Baize et al. 2014). This initial infection rapidly spread within the community and across borders into neighboring countries.

The Ebola virus spread from Guinea to neighboring Liberia and Sierra Leone, escalating into a full-blown epidemic in these countries. The outbreak was intensified by traditional burial practices, which involved direct contact with the bodies of the deceased, as well as the lack of early detection and proper containment measures. Guinea reported a total of 3,814 cases and 2,544 deaths. In Liberia, the capital city Monrovia was one of the hardest-hit areas due to its high population density and inadequate health care infrastructure, resulting in 10,678 cases and 4,810 deaths. Sierra Leone experienced rapid transmission of the virus, particularly in its capital, Freetown, and reported the highest number of cases, with 14,124 infections and 3,956 deaths (Jacob et al. 2020).

The Ebola outbreak also reached Europe and the United States in 2014, though its impact was far less severe than in West Africa. In the United States, four cases were confirmed, including two health care workers who contracted the virus while treating an Ebola patient in Dallas, Texas, according to the CDC. Europe also recorded a few cases, notably in Spain, where a health care worker became infected while caring for a repatriated Ebola patient (IDSA).

The 2013–16 Ebola outbreak in Africa drew global attention to contemporary health challenges. The virus's rapid and widespread transmission was a demonstration of how highly infectious diseases can easily cross geographical and administrative boundaries. Notably, Ebola's spread far exceeded the anticipated scale, given its relatively low basic reproduction number (R_0) of approximately 2 (Doucleff 2014). This R_0 is significantly lower than those of other diseases such as HIV and SARS (5), mumps (10), or measles (18). The outbreak's swift cross-border transmission and high mortality rate suggest that additional factors—such as inadequate health care infrastructure, delayed containment efforts, and cultural practices—contributed significantly to its devastating impact.

The WHO's report, "Factors That Contributed to Undetected Spread of the Ebola Virus and Impeded Rapid Containment" (2015), identified five key factors that facilitated the rapid spread of the infection.

Poverty and Dysfunctional Infrastructure

Guinea, Liberia, and Sierra Leone—the three countries most affected by the outbreak—had been devastated by years of civil war and unrest, leaving their basic health care systems in disarray. Weak transportation and telecommunication networks, particularly in rural areas, severely delayed patients' access to treatment centers and laboratories. These challenges also hindered the effective dissemination of alerts, reports, calls for assistance, and public information campaigns.

Migration Pressure

West Africa faced intense migration across porous borders, with mobility levels estimated to be seven times higher than the global average. Driven largely by poverty, individuals frequently traveled in search of work or food, while extended families often spanned multiple countries. This high mobility complicated efforts to control the outbreak, rendering cross-border contact tracing nearly impossible. As conditions improved in one country, patients from neighboring countries often sought treatment there, inadvertently reigniting transmission chains.

Inadequate Preparation

The affected societies were unprepared for an Ebola outbreak on all fronts. The general population had little to no knowledge of the disease or the available treatments. Fear led many to flee and abandon their villages, inadvertently worsening the situation as their movements facilitated the wider transmission of the virus.

Prevalence of Traditional Practices

Traditional customs, such as returning to one's native village to die and be buried near ancestors, significantly increased the risk of Ebola transmission. In Guinea, funeral practices were linked to 60 percent of cases, while in Sierra Leone they accounted for 80 percent. These deeply rooted cultural traditions often disregarded medical advice. In Liberia and Sierra Leone, burial rites, particularly those associated with secret societies, involved highly hazardous practices. For example, some mourners bathed in or anointed others with water used to wash corpses. In addition, apprentices of influential society members might sleep near a highly infectious body for several nights, believing the ritual would transfer powers from the deceased.

Trust Deficit in Modern Health Care

Traditional medicine holds a deep cultural significance in Africa, and due to limited access to government-run health facilities, many people—particularly the poor—relied on traditional healers or self-medication. Numerous spikes in

Ebola cases were linked to contact with traditional healers. Once the outbreaks began, the high mortality rate fueled a false perception that hospitals were centers of contagion and death, discouraging early medical care. Furthermore, many treatment centers, surrounded by high fences and barbed wire, appeared more like prisons than places of healing in the eyes of local communities.

Critical Health Care Workforce Crisis

Before the Ebola outbreaks, Guinea, Liberia, and Sierra Leone had fewer than two doctors per 100,000 people. This already dire situation worsened as the epidemic unfolded, with many health care workers becoming infected, and some losing their lives. For example, Médecins Sans Frontières deployed 3,400 staff in the affected countries, of whom twenty-seven were infected and thirteen died. The crisis was further exacerbated by strikes among hospital workers protesting unpaid wages and unfulfilled promises of hazard pay. Adding to the challenges, local distrust of foreign medical teams, unfamiliar disinfection protocols, and fever checks hindered response efforts. Many community members viewed treatment centers with suspicion, especially as few patients survived after being admitted.

The Ebola outbreaks of 2013–16 illustrates the complex challenges the world faces in combating infectious diseases. These events demonstrate that providing medical resources alone is insufficient to contain diseases like Ebola in Africa without a thorough understanding of local cultures and practices. International organizations must engage communities through culturally sensitive communication to build trust. Collaborating with local political leaders and traditional healers is also crucial for effective disease control (DuBose et al. 2021).

Further Reading

Baize, Sylvain, Delphine Pannetier, Pharm. D., et al. 2014. "Emergence of Zaire Ebola Virus Disease in Guinea." *The New England Journal of Medicine, 371*: 1418–25. doi: 10.1056/NEJMoa1404505.
Centers for Disease Control and Prevention (CDC). 2022. "Ebola (Ebola Virus Disease)." *CDC.* May 27. https://www.cdc.gov/vhf/ebola/index.html.
Doucleff, Michaeleen. 2014. "No, Seriously, How Contagious Is Ebola?" National Public Radio. October 2. https://www.npr.org/sections/health-shots/2014/10/02/352983774/no-seriously-how-contagious-is-ebola.
DuBoise, Kennedy, Julia Duffy, Sania Farooq, Sucaad Mohamud, and Maggie Sanders. 2021. "Why Africa Still Has Ebola Outbreaks." *University of Michigan School of*

Public Health. https://sph.umich.edu/pursuit/2021posts/why-africa-still-has-ebola-outbreaks.html.

Infectious Diseases Society of America. "Ebola Facts." https://www.idsociety.org/public-health/ebola/ebola-resources/ebola-facts/#:~:text=Two%20died%20%E2%80%93%20a%20Liberian%20visiting,American%20soil%2C%20and%20neither%20died.

Jacob, Shevin T., Ian Crozier, William A. Fischer II, Angela Hewlett, Colleen S. Kraft, Marc-Antoine de La Vega, Moses J. Soka, Victoria Wahl, Anthony Griffiths, Laura Bollinger, and Jens H. Kuhn. 2020. "Ebola Virus Disease." *Nature Reviews Disease Primers*, 6(1): 1–31. doi: https://doi.org/10.1038/s41572-020-0147-3.

World Health Organization (WHO). 2023. "Ebola Virus Disease." *WHO.* https://www.who.int/news-room/fact-sheets/detail/ebola-virus-disease.

World Health Organization (WHO). 2015. "Factors That Contributed to the Undetected Spread of the Ebola Virus and Impeded Rapid Containment." https://www.who.int/news-room/spotlight/one-year-into-the-ebola-epidemic/factors-that-contributed-to-undetected-spread-of-the-ebola-virus-and-impeded-rapid-containment. Accessed August 23, 2024.

5

Spatial Technology and Public Health

Spatial technologies represent one of the most transformative advancements of our time. In an era marked by the confluence of conflict, migration, climate change, and zoonosis, humanity faces an unprecedented exposure to infectious diseases. Technologies such as Geographic Information Systems (GIS) and other spatial tools have emerged as effective methods for tracking and managing these threats. Among various global frameworks, the United Nations' One Health vision stands out as a comprehensive solution. One Health integrates human, animal, and environmental health under a unified approach, enabling early detection, prevention, and control of zoonotic diseases, which make up a significant portion of human infections. However, implementing this framework on a global scale would be impossible without the application of spatial technologies, which offer critical tools for mapping, monitoring, and responding to health crises.

The application of spatial technology in public health has evolved significantly since the pioneering work of John Snow, who used spatial analysis to trace the source of a cholera outbreak in 1854 in London. Snow's groundbreaking mapping of cholera cases marked the beginning of spatial epidemiology and demonstrated the power of geographical approach in identifying disease patterns and pinpointing causes. Today, GIS builds upon these foundations with advanced mapping, data integration, and visualization capabilities. Public health organizations like the CDC and the WHO rely on these technologies to track infectious diseases, identify risk factors, and implement data-driven interventions. For example, GIS has been instrumental in managing chronic diseases by mapping environmental and social determinants, such as access to healthy food, health care, and physical activity facilities.

The role of spatial technologies became particularly evident during the Covid-19 pandemic. Both China and Western countries deployed GIS and related tools to manage the health crisis. China integrated GIS into its Zero-Covid strategy, using health QR codes to monitor population movement, enforce testing, and manage quarantine measures. These technologies enabled the rapid identification of infection hotspots and guided resource allocation, such as hospital beds and testing kits. Meanwhile, Western countries like the United States used GIS to track infection rates, visualize health care disparities, and support public awareness through platforms such as the Johns Hopkins University Coronavirus Resource Center.

Beyond infectious diseases, spatial technologies have reshaped how chronic conditions are managed. GIS has facilitated the identification of geographical disparities in health outcomes, such as obesity and diabetes, by analyzing environmental factors and socioeconomic vulnerabilities. It has allowed researchers to analyze how community design, including walkability and access to recreational spaces, impacts public health. Initiatives like the CDC's diabetes atlas leverage GIS to map trends and disparities, enabling targeted interventions in underserved areas. These insights are crucial for addressing systemic health inequities and improving population health.

The utility of spatial technologies extends to global collaboration in managing health emergencies. Organizations such as the World Health Organization, the Food and Agriculture Organization of the United Nations (FAO), and the World Organization of Animal Health (WOAH) rely on these tools to address the interconnected challenges of human, animal, and environmental health. During the Covid-19 pandemic, GIS enabled the monitoring of food supply disruptions, zoonotic disease risks, and health care infrastructure capacity. The One Health framework, championed by these organizations, benefits greatly from the ability to integrate diverse data sources through GIS. For example, FAO's hunger maps and WOAH's animal health databases demonstrate how spatial data can inform global health strategies and enhance emergency preparedness.

However, the widespread use of spatial technologies is not without challenges. Concerns about effective data integration, interoperability, and privacy have emerged as critical issues. The Covid-19 pandemic highlighted disparities in how different countries and organizations adopted and utilized these tools. In some cases, privacy concerns reduced the effectiveness of contact tracing and surveillance efforts. Nevertheless, the overall success of spatial technologies in global health management suggests that these tools have become essential.

John Snow's Legacy in Modern Disease Control and Prevention

The defeat of cholera stands as a monumental triumph of nineteenth-century medical science, saving millions of lives and significantly expanding our understanding of infectious diseases and their spread. At the forefront of this progress was John Snow, who played a pivotal role in overturning the miasma theory, which attributed disease to "bad air," and establishing the germ theory. Thanks to Snow's contributions, public health became a cornerstone of urban development worldwide. Moreover, John Snow is also credited with pioneering the field of geographical epidemiology by applying rigorous scientific methods to the study of disease outbreaks.

Cholera, caused by the bacterium *Vibrio cholerae* (*V. cholerae*), is an acute diarrheal illness that can rapidly lead to severe dehydration and, if untreated, death within hours. The disease primarily spreads through the consumption of water or food contaminated with fecal matter. Cholera outbreaks can be especially devastating in regions characterized by poverty, poorly planned urban development, climate-related disasters, and complex humanitarian crises. Under all these circumstances, access to safe water and basic sanitation is limited. According to the World Health Organization (WHO), an estimated 2.3 to 4.0 million cases occur annually worldwide, resulting in 12,000 to 143,000 deaths, despite the availability of vaccines (WHO 2023).

John Snow made his landmark contribution in 1854 by pinpointing cholera's mode of transmission during an outbreak in London through a detailed geographical analysis of infection cases. At the time, London's rudimentary sewage system frequently discharged into the Thames River, which was also the city's main source of drinking water, thus contaminating wells and water pumps. The Broad Street pump, which Snow investigated, drew water tainted by nearby cesspools, which were themselves polluted by the Thames. By examining government death records, Snow mapped the cases of infection and traced them back to the Broad Street pump. He concluded that its contaminated water was the source of the outbreak. Acting on Snow's recommendation, local authorities removed the pump's handle, effectively ending the epidemic (Bynum 2013).

John Snow's contributions to epidemiology are notable for establishing evidence of both association and causation in disease transmission. This was one of the earliest uses of data and spatial analysis to demonstrate a causal link between an environmental source and a disease outbreak.

In disease investigations, identifying factors associated with an illness typically precedes determining its causes. Although symptoms may show a statistical correlation with a particular exposure, such an association does not necessarily confirm that the exposure causes the symptoms. The observed link could reflect direct causation, indirect causation (where the exposure leads to another factor that causes the symptoms), or a confounding effect (where both the exposure and symptoms are tied to a third factor).

Before John Snow's work, the dominant belief was the miasma theory, which posited that diseases like cholera were spread through "bad air" or miasmas. Snow challenged this established view by proposing that cholera was transmitted via contaminated water. His meticulous data collection and analysis established a strong association between the source of drinking water and cholera cases. Snow's scientific approach stood in sharp contrast to the miasma theory, marking the beginning of a new era in understanding disease transmission. (Tulchinsky 2018).

In his investigation of the cholera outbreak, John Snow made an indirect but critical contribution to the development of germ theory, which was later formalized by Louis Pasteur and Robert Koch in the 1860s through their research on microorganisms. Germ theory posits that many diseases are caused by specific pathogens. This breakthrough paved the way for the use of antibiotics and more effective public health measures. Snow hypothesized that cholera was caused by living organisms capable of reproducing—an insight that was remarkably ahead of its time (Bynum 2013).

Thanks to John Snow's research, municipal authorities in London were prompted to improve sanitary conditions by developing new sewage systems and water purification methods. Building on London's example, large cities worldwide, especially in industrialized countries, began establishing water supply systems that kept sewage separate from drinking water. Complementary efforts, including the implementation of waste water management programs to protect water source, the enforcement of sanitation-focused public health policies, and the design of urban infrastructure to maintain hygienic living conditions, have all contributed to healthier urban environments.

One key milestone in water sanitation came in 1897, when chlorine was first used to disinfect drinking water in England. In the United States, widespread chlorination during the first half of the twentieth century led to a sharp decline in typhoid cases. These measures significantly reduced the threats posed by cholera, typhoid, and other waterborne diseases, with their benefits eventually extending beyond industrialized nations. John Snow's groundbreaking investigation of the

1854 cholera outbreak laid the foundation for these advances and earned him recognition as "the father of modern epidemiology" (Tulchinsky 2018).

Despite ongoing efforts to control it, cholera remains a major public health concern in many parts of the world, particularly in areas lacking safe water and adequate sanitation. Outbreaks can escalate rapidly and become especially deadly during humanitarian crises, such as in refugee camps or in the aftermath of natural disasters like floods and earthquakes, that compromise water supplies and sanitation infrastructure. A notable example is the repeated outbreaks in Haiti. The 2010 earthquake resulted in around half a million cholera cases and thousands of deaths. In 2022, shortly after Haiti had been declared cholera-free, social unrest in Port-au-Prince coincided with a significant resurgence of the disease, leading to hundreds of fatalities (Denisse 2023).

Although the World Health Organization reports thousands of cholera cases each year, the true number is likely much higher due to underreporting and weak surveillance in many regions. This persistent gap underscores the urgent need for sustained investment in water and sanitation infrastructure, stronger health care systems, and coordinated global efforts to promote social stability. More than a century ago, John Snow's groundbreaking work on cholera established the critical link between water and disease—an insight that remains central to prevention today. Addressing these challenges remains essential to reducing the burden of cholera and averting future outbreaks.

Further Reading

Awofeso, Niyi and Kafeh Aldabk. 2018. "Cholera, Migration, and Global Health—A Critical Review." *International Journal of Travel Medicine and Global Health*, 6(3): 92–9. https://www.ijtmgh.com/article_69629_fd29fbe6a9c321c7b5d48a4428a76ec9.pdf.

Bynum, William. 2013. "In Retrospect: On the Mode of Communication of Cholera." *Nature*. https://www.nature.com/articles/495169a.

Harris, Jim. 2020. "Cholera and the Roots of Public Health." https://origins.osu.edu/connecting-history/cholera-covid-public-health-response?language_content_entity=en.

History.com. 2017. "Cholera." https://www.history.com/topics/inventions/history-of-cholera#section_4.

Newsom, SWB. 2005. "The History of Infection Control: Cholera—John Snow and the Beginnings of Epidemiology." *British Journal of Infection Control*, 6(6): 12–15. https://journals.sagepub.com/doi/pdf/10.1177/14690446050060060401.

Tulchinsky, Theodore H. 2018. "John Snow, Cholera, the Broad Street Pump; Waterborne Diseases Then and Now." *Case Studies in Public Health*, 30: 77–99. doi: 10.1016/B978-0-12-804571-8.00017-2.

Vega Oscasio, Denisse, et al. 2023. "Cholera Outbreak—Haiti, September 2022—January 2023." *Morbidity and Mortality Weekly Report*. https://www.cdc.gov/mmwr/volumes/72/wr/mm7202a1.htm.

Wilford, John Noble. 2008. "How Epidemics Helped Shape the Modern Metropolis." https://www.nytimes.com/2008/04/15/science/15chol.html.

World Health Organization (WHO). 2023. "Cholera." https://www.who.int/news-room/fact-sheets/detail/cholera.

Enhancing Public Health through Geographic Information Systems (GIS)

Geographic Information Systems (GIS) are widely used in modern public health care and medical research. GIS technology is employed for the collection, analysis, and visualization of spatial data. By integrating geographic information with other data types, such as demographics or healthcare resources, public health authorities can make more informed decisions regarding disease prevention, health promotion, and resource allocation.

The earliest application of what is now considered a form of GIS in public health is attributed to John Snow, a British physician in the nineteenth century. In 1854, during a cholera outbreak in London, Snow created a hand-drawn map to plot cholera cases and clusters of infection. This geographic approach enabled him to pinpoint the area with the highest concentration of cases centered around a specific water pump on Broad Street. His discovery led to the removal of the pump handle, after which cholera cases declined. Snow's spatial method gave rise to the field of spatial epidemiology and laid the foundation for the modern use of GIS in public health.

Modern GIS has transformed the manual methods once used by John Snow, replacing them with advanced digital tools. Technological advancements have made disease tracking more accurate, efficient, and comprehensive. GIS technologies can be classified into four main types based on their functions:

1. Mapping tools create electronic maps that integrate multiple layers of information, such as ZIP codes, census data, household details, health records, and socioeconomic status.
2. Story-mapping platforms enrich descriptions of specific locations by incorporating photographs, text, videos, and charts.

3. Crowdsourcing applications enable residents and stakeholders to contribute data and report issues in real time using mobile devices.
4. Data dashboards offer researchers flexible tools for analyzing information from various perspectives, combining maps, charts, gauges, and lists (Gibson 2020).

Organizations such as the U.S. Centers for Disease Control and Prevention (CDC) and the World Health Organization (WHO) use GIS to monitor and manage public health, track the spread of diseases, map risk factors, and plan interventions.

The CDC's Geospatial Research, Analysis, and Services Program (GRASP) employs GIS to monitor infectious diseases like influenza, Covid-19, and other pandemics. GRASP develops real-time maps that display infection rates, vaccination coverage, and the availability of medical resources. Additionally, the CDC's Division for Heart Disease and Stroke Prevention applies GIS to track and document risk factors in specific geographic areas.

The Division of Population Health develops applications to use statistical methods to analyze the epidemiology of chronic disease. It monitors factors such as geographic access to health care providers, variations in sleep duration across regions, the prevalence of chronic obstructive pulmonary disease (COPD), patterns of chronic conditions among Medicare beneficiaries, and the relationship between alcohol outlet density and violent crime. These are some of the applications. The CDC also employs GIS to investigate health impact of environmental factors, such as airport noise on sleep insufficiency.

Travelers may find the information provided on the CDC's "Traveler's Health" page particularly useful, such as recommended immunizations for various destinations. In a more comprehensive dimension, the CDC's Division of Global Migration and Quarantine publishes and updates a Yellow Book, which includes global continental disease maps, country-specific malaria maps, and fever maps. For nearly sixty years, this Yellow Book has been a trusted, must-consult resource for the public.

The World Health Organization (WHO) has a long history of using GIS to map and analyze the spatial distribution of diseases and risks. GIS enables the World Health Organization to monitor a wide range of factors, including air and water quality, sanitation, and neglected tropical diseases such as malaria, Guinea worm disease, and snakebites. It also plays a critical role in tracking polio outbreaks and managing health emergencies, offering a comprehensive tool for real-time decision-making and resource allocation (WHO GIS Centre).

In the realm of community health improvement, GIS is extensively used to analyze both community health and environmental context. For example, by mapping air quality, pollution levels, and health data, researchers can identify areas where environmental factors contribute to respiratory issues. Similarly, GIS has been applied in studies on effects of urban planning for better health outcomes. Public health authorities may use GIS to visualize the geographic distribution of health care resources and identify underserved areas.

The application of GIS in community health profiling yields valuable information of public health at the local level. This process typically involves compiling and mapping data on various health indicators within a specific community. The resulting information helps identify geographic strengths and gaps, supporting decisions about the allocation of health services and helping to justify funding for new facilities. For instance, in areas with limited green space, promoting exercise programs through local gyms may be an effective alternative when safe outdoor environments for activities such as walking are unavailable (Shaw et al. 2017).

A key strength of GIS technology lies in its ability to organize and visualize disease- and health-related data through powerful mapping and modeling tools. Researchers can use GIS to track and analyze cancer incidence across geographic regions by integrating data from cancer registries with environmental and demographic variables to identify cancer hotspots. This capability is invaluable for both research and public communication of findings.

A specific example is the use of Story Maps to visualize rural-urban disparities in cancer incidence across the United States. This web-based tool offers insights into differences in cancer rates between rural and urban populations, breaking down the data by patient demographics such as gender, race, socioeconomic status, tobacco use, and vaccination rates. It also presents the geographic distribution of various cancer types. This GIS-based approach goes beyond traditional epidemiological analysis by embedding a spatial dimension into the understanding of disease incidence and risk factors. Moreover, it makes complex data more accessible to broader audience (NCI—GIS Portal for Cancer Research). All of these help identify association and causation.

One critical area where GIS still requires improvement is data integration and interoperability. Effective public health responses depend on data from diverse sources, including hospitals, laboratories, and government agencies. However, these datasets often differ in format, standards, and resolution. Ensuring seamless integration is essential for expanding the use and effectiveness of GIS in public health (CDC 2024).

Further Reading

Centers for Disease Control and Prevention (CDC). 2024. "About Public Health Data Interoperability." *CDC*. https://www.cdc.gov/data-interoperability/php/about/index.htm.
Centers for Disease Control and Prevention (CDC). "GIS and Public Health at CDC." https://www.restoredcdc.org/www.cdc.gov/gis/php/index.html.
Centers for Disease Control and Prevention (CDC). "Travelers' Health." https://wwwnc.cdc.gov/travel/page/yellowbook-home.
D'Arcy, Beth. 2023. "14 Ways Health Departments Can Use GIS in 2023." *GovPilot.com*. https://www.govpilot.com/blog/health-department-gis-map.
Gibson, Meredith. 2020. "The Role of GIS in Public Health." *Govloop.com*. https://www.govloop.com/community/blog/the-role-of-gis-in-public-health/.
National Cancer Institute—GIS Portal for Cancer Research. 2025. "Cancer Map Stories: Rural-Urban Disparities in Cancer." https://gis.cancer.gov/mapstory/rural-urban/index.html. Accessed September 7, 2024.
Shaw, Nicola, and Suzanne McGuire. 2017. "Understanding the Use of Geographical Information System (GISs) in Health Informatics Research: A Review." *Journal of innovation in health informatics*, 24(2): 940. doi: https://doi.org/10.14236/jhi.v24i2.940.
Wang, Fahui. 2020. "Why Public Health Needs GIS: A Methodological Overview." Annals of GIS, 26(1): 1–12. doi:10.1080/19475683.2019.1702099.
World Health Organization (WHO). "WHO GIS Centre for Health." https://www.who.int/data/GIS.

How China and the United States Used Spatial Technology to Fight the Covid-19 Pandemic

After Covid-19 broke out in the city of Wuhan in December 2019, the Chinese government placed the city under strict quarantine. Residents were confined to their homes for a total of seventy-six days. As infections spread nationwide, this strategy evolved into the broader "Zero-COVID" policy. A key tool in enforcing the prolonged lockdown was GIS technology, which was used to monitor population movements, track outbreaks in real time, enforce antigen testing, and manage medical and logistical resources efficiently.

By integrating spatial technology, authorities were able to swiftly enforce lockdowns, implement quarantines, and ensure public compliance with routine antigen testing. During the pandemic, more than forty cities, each with millions of residents, underwent lockdowns, with spatial technology playing a vital role in their implementation.

The outcome was notable: as of March 2023, China reported 101,056 Covid-19-related deaths, less than 10 percent of the U.S. death toll during the same period, according to the Johns Hopkins Coronavirus Resource Center.

To control the spread of the infection, the Chinese government implemented two key measures: travel restrictions and social distancing. Individuals were required to install a dedicated mobile app called the "health QR code." This app enabled authorities to monitor users and alert them to potential exposure. It was also used to verify compliance with mandatory antigen testing and functioned as a digital pass for accessing public facilities, entering public spaces, and purchasing train or plane tickets.

The health QR system, co-developed by China's National Health Commission, China Electronics Technology Group Corporation, and tech companies like Alibaba. It was backed by government-controlled big data, including public transport information, such as flights and train booking, which required ID for booking, and medical data. The QR codes were color-coded: green indicated a healthy or negative status, red signaled a confirmed infection, and yellow denoted potential exposure requiring further observation and confirmation (Schneider 2020).

As a contact tracing tool, the health QR system notified users if they had been within close range of someone confirmed or suspected of infection within the past two weeks. Integrated with three of China's most popular mobile apps—Alipay, WeChat, and QQ—the system could identify whether an individual had worked with, shared a classroom with, lived in the same building as, or traveled on the same train (in the same carriage) or plane (within three rows) as an infected person. The health QR system also provided warnings and instructions on actions to take based on users' recent movements (Boulos et al. 2020).

In community settings, individual QR codes functioned as electronic keys for entering and exiting residential compounds. If individuals failed to complete the required swab tests by the specified deadlines—testing is typically conducted at street corner booths—their QR code status would change from green to yellow. This change would restrict their mobility at checkpoints until they met the testing requirements.

In general, the mobility restrictions defined by the tricolor health codes were applied consistently across China, though local variations were allowed. For example, under Hunan provincial government's regulations, an individual with a "red" code is required to isolate in government-designated facilities and remain under medical surveillance. However, with approval from a county-level

Covid Control Center, the individual may be permitted to quarantine at home. An individual with a "yellow" code, indicating potential infection, is subject to a more complex set of rules, including the following:

> Monitor your health at home and undergo regular nucleic acid tests. If you or a cohabitant exhibits symptoms related to COVID-19, such as fever or cough, you must immediately report to the community. In principle, you are not allowed to go out until the risk of infection is ruled out. If travel is necessary, a negative nucleic acid test result within 48 hours is required. However, you are not allowed to participate in gatherings such as dining, conferences, tourism, or training, nor are you allowed to enter schools, nursing homes, welfare institutions, agricultural wholesale markets, farmers' markets, supermarkets, libraries, museums, art galleries, exhibition halls, gyms, or other indoor venues. Additionally, you cannot enter cinemas, karaoke bars, bathhouses, internet cafes, or other enclosed spaces, and you are prohibited from using taxis, ride-hailing services, buses, subways, trains, or other public transportation. You may not enter medical institutions unless it is for your own medical treatment. When it is necessary to go out, such as to collect living supplies, deliveries, or participate in non-gathering activities, you must take personal protective measures. (Translated from Hunan Provincial People's Government Net 2022)

Beyond its role in Covid-19 control, the health QR code was reportedly combined with facial recognition and other technologies to monitor blogs on media platforms, raising significant privacy concerns (Huang 2020).

Similar contact tracing systems were adopted in countries such as the United States, Japan, Singapore, Poland, Israel, and South Korea. However, their use was often limited due to strong public concerns over privacy. A major apprehension was the potential misuse of individuals' biometric data, such as pulse rate, blood pressure, and other health parameters, for monitoring mental and physical well-being in ways that could infringe on personal privacy and autonomy (Chaturvedi 2020).

For instance, in India, the Aarogya Setu app faced criticism over privacy issues, with fears that the data collected could be used beyond its intended purpose of contact tracing (Clarance 2020). In Norway, the Smittestopp app was suspended after the Norwegian Data Protection Authority deemed it a disproportionate intrusion into users' privacy (Kelion 2020).

During the pandemic, governments, businesses, and hospitals utilized drones to assist communities under quarantine. Drones were primarily deployed in three ways: disinfection, delivery of medical supplies, and delivery of consumer goods. Some drones, originally designed for spraying pesticides on crops, were repurposed to spray disinfectants during Covid-19 outbreaks. In China, beyond delivery functions, drones were also employed for traffic control, including monitoring unauthorized driving (Yang 2020; Chaturvedi 2020).

Experts believe that the implementation of the extensive Zero-Covid policy, along with the heavy use of spatial technologies for tracking, was driven by multiple factors, one of which was the need to prevent the collapse of China's fragile health care system. Reports indicate that China faced a severe shortage of hospital beds, with only 5.2 beds available per 1,000 people (possibly even fewer in reality), compared to 12.77 in South Korea and eight in Russia (Statista 2021). This fragility was further compounded by the absence of a robust primary care system. As a result, people often rushed to hospitals for even minor symptoms, which, during frequent Covid-19 outbreaks, could easily overwhelm medical resources.

In the United States, reviews of published studies underscore the wide-ranging role that spatial technology has played in combating the Covid-19 pandemic. For instance, Johns Hopkins University (JHU) developed the web-based Coronavirus Resource Center to track global infection trends, which became the must-go-to resource worldwide. The center also offered tools to visualize social and economic disparities in affected communities, report on unemployment and business recovery, and monitor environmental changes such as pollution levels. JHU concluded its data collection operations on March 10, 2023.

In January 2020, the WHO launched its ArcGIS Operations Dashboard for Covid-19, providing maps of cases and deaths by country. The dashboard also includes links to information on other health emergencies monitored by the WHO, such as dengue fever, Rift Valley fever, and West Nile fever. The Covid-19 dashboard is updated automatically using ArcGIS GeoEvent Server, which pushes updates multiple times daily. This ensures strong map performance and optimization by leveraging content updates delivered through the Content Delivery Network operated by the Environmental Systems Research Institute (Esri) (Boulos et al. 2020).

The experiences of the United States and China demonstrate that spatial technology played a pivotal role in controlling the spread of Covid-19. These tools strengthened global response by enabling data-driven and location-specific strategies. At the same time, the Covid-19 pandemic served as a critical stress test for spatial technologies, showcasing their strengths and paving the way for broader deployment in public health.

Further Reading

Ahasan, Rakibul, Shaharier Alam, Torit Chakraborty, and Md Mahbub Hossain. 2022. "Applications of GIS and Geospatial Analyses in COVID-19 Research: A Systematic Review" (version 2). https://doi.org/10.12688/f1000research.27544.2 doi: 10.12688/f1000research.27544.2.

Boulos, Maged N. Kamel, and Estella M. Geraghty. 2020. "Geographical Tracking and Mapping of Coronavirus Disease COVID-19/Severe Acute Respiratory Syndrome Coronavirus 2 (SARS-Cov-2) Epidemic and Associated Events around the World: How 21st Century GIS Technologies Are Supporting the Global Fight against Outbreaks and Epidemics." *International Journal of Health Geographics, 19*(1): 8. doi: 10.1186/s12942-020-00202-8.

Chaturvedi, Aditya. Nov 5 2020. "The China Way: Use of Technology to Combat Covid-19." *Geospatial World*. https://www.geospatialworld.net/prime/technology-and-innovation/the-sino-approach-use-of-technology-to-combat-covid-19/.

Clarance, Andrew. 2020. "Aarogya Setu: Why India's Covid-19 Contact Tracing App Is Controversial." *BBC*. https://www.bbc.com/news/world-asia-india-52659520.

HealthMap. Healthmap.com. https://www.healthmap.org/en/.

Huang, Joyce. 2020. "China's Virus Tracking Technology Sparks Privacy Concerns." *VOANews.com*. https://www.voanews.com/a/covid-19-pandemic_chinas-virus-tracking-technology-sparks-privacy-concerns/6191538.html.

Hunan Provincial Government Net. 2022. "What Preventive Measures Should Individuals with 'Red' Or 'Yellow' Codes Follow? Answers to Frequently Asked Questions about the Health Code and Travel Code." April 29. www.hunan.gov.cn. Accessed September.

Johns Hopkins University Coronavirus Resource Center. https://coronavirus.jhu.edu/.

Kelion, Leo. 2020. "Coronavirus: Contact-Tracing Apps Face Further Hitches." *BBC*. https://www.bbc.com/news/technology-53051783.

Schneiger, Jordan. 2020. "How China Created Its Health QR Codes." *ChinaTalk*. https://www.chinatalk.media/p/how-china-created-its-health-qr-codes.

Statista. 2021. "Number of Hospital Beds in Select Countries as of 2021." https://www.statista.com/statistics/283273/oecd-countries-hospital-bed-density/.

The World Health Organization Covid-19 Dashboard. https://data.who.int/dashboards/covid19/cases?n=c.

Yang, Junwei. 2020. "3 Ways China Is Using Drones to Fight Coronavirus." *Webforum.org*. https://www.weforum.org/agenda/2020/03/three-ways-china-is-using-drones-to-fight-coronavirus/.

How Spatial Tools Empower Global Health Organizations

The World Health Organization (WHO), Food and Agriculture Organization (FAO), and World Organization for Animal Health (WOAH, formerly OIE) are key United Nations (UN) agencies tasked with safeguarding public health, food security, and animal health, respectively. During the Covid-19 pandemic, they confronted a shared challenge: mitigating the spread of the virus while ensuring critical supplies to affected communities. Spatial technologies played a pivotal role in enabling these organizations to achieve their missions while fostering collaboration during this global health crisis.

Infectious disease transmission is inherently spatial, closely tied to population mobility and community structures. According to the Centers for Disease Control and Prevention (CDC), technologies such as Geographic Information Systems (GIS), spatial statistics, and location-based data from Global Navigation Satellite Systems (GNSS) like GPS, along with remotely sensed imagery, were indispensable during the pandemic. These tools helped analyze transmission patterns, forecast trends, and implement targeted responses. For instance, integrating geographic data into Covid-19 modeling revealed correlations between health disparities and social vulnerabilities across regions. Globally shared spatial data also guided resource distribution, optimizing the allocation of personal protective equipment (PPE), ventilators, and hospital beds in countries like the United States (Boulos et al. 2020).

WHO's Use of Spatial Technologies

Spatial technologies enabled the WHO during the pandemic to coordinate global efforts by tracing virus spread, visualizing outbreaks with real-time interactive maps, and guiding governments in implementing targeted interventions. GIS was particularly useful for the WHO in assessing health care infrastructure, such as hospital and ICU availability, allowing governments to make data-driven decisions on resource allocation.

The ArcGIS Operations Dashboard for Covid-19 was one of the WHO's standout initiatives during the pandemic. This tool provided real-time visualization of cases, fatalities, and recoveries, integrating laboratory-confirmed data with interactive maps and curves of spread. Optimized for mobile use, it made critical information accessible to health care workers, policymakers, and the public, supporting the WHO's mission to monitor outbreaks, coordinate global responses, and inform resource allocation (Boulos et al. 2020). Additionally, the

Spatial Technology and Wastewater-Based Epidemiology

Wastewater-based epidemiology (WBE) analyzes wastewater to detect and monitor infectious agents such as viruses and bacteria. Unlike traditional methods requiring individual testing, WBE provides a community-wide health view by capturing indicators directly from sewage systems. It enables early detection of pathogen trends, supporting timely interventions. During the Covid-19 pandemic, WBE identified SARS-CoV-2 in wastewater days before clinical cases surged, aiding public health officials in implementing targeted measures such as testing and lockdowns. Cost-efficient and reliant on existing sewage infrastructure, WBE monitors health trends without individual testing.

Integrating Geographic Information Systems (GIS) enhances WBE by mapping viral concentrations and identifying transmission hotspots. GIS combines data layers—such as pathogen levels, demographics, health care facilities, and socioeconomic factors—into detailed visualizations, offering a comprehensive view of community health. For example, GIS overlays data on viral presence with vaccination rates, socioeconomic conditions, and lockdown zones, helping officials pinpoint high-risk clusters and allocate resources effectively.

Through spatial and temporal modeling, GIS can predict infection spread, track outbreaks, and assess intervention impacts. For vulnerable populations, GIS-enhanced WBE highlights at-risk communities, promoting equitable health care resource distribution. Together, WBE and GIS form a cost-effective, powerful approach to tackling public health challenges and improving global preparedness.

Further Reading

Cuadros, Diego F., Xi Chen, Jingjing Li, Ryosuke Omori, and Godfrey Musuka. 2024. "Advancing Public Health Surveillance: Integrating Modeling and GIS in the Wastewater-Based Epidemiology of Viruses, a Narrative Review." *Pathogens.* doi: 10.3390/pathogens13080685.

Geraghty, Easte. 2022. "How GIS Brings Wastewater Surveillance to Life." *ESRI.com.* https://www.esri.com/en-us/industries/blog/articles/how-gis-brings-wastewater-surveillance-to-life/.

WHO launched its first GIS Centre in Somalia in 2023 to enhance public health responses in a region plagued by conflict and climate shocks. This initiative tracks population movements, assesses healthcare access, and strengthens resilience against emergencies like polio outbreaks (WHO News 2023).

FAO's Application of Spatial Tools

During the Covid-19 pandemic, FAO employed spatial technologies to monitor food supply disruptions caused by market closures. Real-time data enabled the organization to assess changes in crop yields and livestock production, offering timely guidance for global food management. FAO's open-access platform featured tools like hunger maps integrated with Covid-19 incidence data, food chain disruption analyses based on social media, and maps tracking food price variations (FAO 2020). Furthermore, in the 2024 Gaza War, FAO, in collaboration with United Nations Satellite Center (UNOSAT), surveyed cropland damage, finding that 57 percent of Gaza's cropland—41 percent of its total land area—was severely affected. This analysis informed emergency efforts to restart food production and alleviate food insecurity (Van Damme et al. 2024).

WOAH's Contributions to Animal Health

WOAH's World Animal Health Information System (OIE-WAHIS), launched in 2021, exemplifies the use of spatial technologies to ensure transparency in animal health. This global database facilitates data reporting on animal diseases, offering tools for data extraction, mapping, and interactive dashboards (OIE IZSLT 2021). Beyond official reports, OIE-WAHIS leverages non-official sources, such as Epidemic Intelligence from Open Source (EIOS), to track unreported events, enhancing disease surveillance and control measures (Thompson et al. 2024).

The One Health Framework

The Tripartite Agreement between WHO, FAO, and WOAH, under the One Health framework, emphasizes the interconnectedness of human, animal, and ecosystem health. By fostering collaboration across sectors, One Health enables early detection and control of zoonotic diseases, which account for approximately 60 percent of human infectious diseases. Advances in spatial technologies have significantly bolstered the detection, prevention, and management of these threats, ensuring coordinated global efforts (WHO, FAO, and OIE 2019).

Overall, in the field of global health, geospatial technologies, such as GIS, remote sensing, and GPS, play a crucial role in infectious disease surveillance and public health management. A review study indicates that these tools facilitate real-time tracking, outbreak monitoring, and resource allocation, while integrating epidemiological, demographic, and environmental data to enhance understanding of disease dynamics. Predictive modeling and clustering techniques applied through these digital tools allow identifying high-risk areas and informed targeting interventions. Citizen science and crowdsourcing expand data collection by engaging the public in reporting symptoms, exposure, and environmental conditions—offering insights that might otherwise be overlooked. Meanwhile, digital contact tracing apps have proven effective in interrupting transmission chains by rapidly identifying and notifying potential contacts, though their use continues to raise concerns about data privacy and surveillance (Saran et al. 2020).

Spatial technologies have transformed how the WHO, FAO, and WOAH address global health challenges. By enabling data-driven decision-making, fostering collaboration, and enhancing resource allocation, these tools have strengthened the response to pandemics and other crises. Through these innovations, the organizations continue to ensure a united and efficient effort in protecting global health.

Further Reading

Boulos, Maged N. Kamel and Estella M. Geraghy. 2020. "Geographical Tracking and Mapping of Coronavirus Disease COVID-19/Severe Acute Respiratory Syndrome Coronavirus 2 (SARS-Cov-2) Epidemic and Associated Events around the World: How 21st Century GIS Technologies Are Supporting the Global Fight against Outbreaks And Epidemics."

FAO, OIE, and WHO. 2019. "Taking a Multisectoral, One Health Approach: A Tripartite Guide to Addressing Zoonotic Diseases in Countries." https://iris.who.int/bitstream/handle/10665/325620/9789241514934-eng.pdf?sequence=1.

Food and Agriculture Organization of the United Nations (FAO). https://www.fao.org/home/en.

Food and Agriculture Organization of the United Nations (FAO). 2020. "FAO Launches Hand-in-Hand Geospatial Data Platform to Help Build Stronger Food and Agriculture Sectors Post COVID-19." https://www.fao.org/director-general/news/details/FAO-launches-Hand-in-Hand-geospatial-data-platform-to-help-build-stronger-food-and-agriculture-sectors-post-COVID-19/.

OIE IZSLT. 2021. "OIE—WAHIS: New World Animal Health Information System." https://www.izs.it/IZS/OIE_-_WAHIS_New_World_Animal_Health_Information_System. Accessed September 16, 2024.

Saran, Sameer, Priyanka Singh, Vishal Kumar, and Prakash Chauhan. 2020. "Review of Geospatial Technology for Infectious Disease Surveillance: Use Case on Covid-19." *Journal of Indian Society of Remote Sensing*, 48(8): 1121–38. doi: https://doi.org/10.1007/s12524-020-01140-5.

Smith, Charlotte D., and Jeremy Mennis. 2020. "Incorporating Geographic Information Science and Technology in Response to the COVID-19 Pandemic." *Preventing Chronic Disease, 17*: 200246. doi: http://dx.doi.org/10.5888/pcd17.200246.

Thompson, Lesa, Chaire Claire Cayol, Lina Awada, Sophie Muset, Dharmaveer Shetty, Jingwen Wang, and Paolo Tizzani. 2024. "Role of the World Organisation for Animal Health in Global Wildlife Disease Surveillance." *Sec. Zoological Medicine*. doi: https://doi.org/10.3389/fvets.2024.1269530.

Van Damme, Olivier, and Anne-Sophie Faivre le Cadre. 2024. "Substantial Increase in Damage to Gaza's Cropland amid Ongoing Conflict." *United Nations Institute for Training and Research*. June 13. https://unitar.org/about/news-stories/press/unosat-and-fao-reveal-substantial-increase-damage-gazas-cropland-amid-ongoing-conflict.

World Health Organization (WHO). https://www.who.int/.

World Health Organization (WHO), Food and Agriculture Organization of the United Nations (FAO) and World Organization for Animal Health (WOAH). 2019. "Taking a Multisectoral, One Health Approach: A Tripartite Guide to Addressing Zoonotic Diseases in Countries." https://www.woah.org/fileadmin/Home/eng/Media_Center/docs/EN_TripartiteZoonosesGuide_webversion.pdf.

World Health Organization News (WHO News). November 14, 2023. "Inauguration of First Geographic Information System Centre for Health in a WHO Country Office—A Privotal Step forward for Public Health Systems in Somalia." https://www.who.int/news/item/14-11-2023-inauguration-of-first-geographic-information-system-centre-for-health-in-a-who-country-office.

World Organization of Animal Health (WOAH). https://www.woah.org/en/home/.

Mapping the Future—How Spatial Technology Is Revolutionizing Chronic Disease Prevention and Management

Spatial technology encompasses tools and methods for capturing, analyzing, and visualizing data linked to specific geographic locations. In public health, technologies such as GIS, remote sensing, and GPS are not just used for mapping—they support critical functions like identifying disease hotspots, monitoring environmental risk factors, and guiding the allocation of health resources. By linking health data to place, spatial technologies enable more precise and effective responses to both infectious outbreaks and long-term chronic disease patterns (Sinton 2023).

Spatial tools have been employed to track outbreaks of malaria, HIV/AIDS, and Ebola by identifying high-risk areas, thus facilitating rapid public health responses. They were widely deployed during the Covid-19 pandemic. These technologies also play a vital role in early warning systems by monitoring environmental changes—such as rainfall patterns linked to increased mosquito breeding—which can help predict malaria outbreaks. Spatial tools are also used to study chronic diseases, which develop gradually and are often preventable or manageable through lifestyle changes and medical interventions. Common chronic diseases include diabetes, heart disease, hypertension, and obesity. These conditions are closely tied to the lived environment, encompassing both physical and social factors (Jia et al. 2019).

For example, an obesogenic environment is characterized by limited access to healthy foods, a lack of safe places for physical activity, and high exposure to unhealthy food marketing. These conditions are often worsened by socioeconomic disparities, as low-income communities frequently experience challenges such as food deserts, unsafe neighborhoods, and restricted access to health care. Similarly, the geographic clustering of comorbidities—where individuals suffer from multiple chronic diseases—is often tied to the same environmental and social determinants. Spatial technology can help address obesogenic environments by identifying at-risk areas through mapping food deserts, limited recreational spaces, and health disparities. It supports targeted interventions by guiding resource allocation, monitoring environmental and health trends over time, and enabling predictive modeling to anticipate future risks. Additionally, crowdsourcing tools empower communities to report local needs, making public health responses more responsive and equitable (Casper et al. 2019).

On the hand, spatial technology opens new research fields, one of which is spatial epidemiology. Many environmental and social factors have contributed to the emergence of spatial epidemiology, an interdisciplinary field that combines the study of disease patterns with spatial analysis. The primary goal of spatial epidemiology is to identify high-risk areas for diseases, track disease trends over time, and provide insights into reducing disease burdens. Methods used in spatial epidemiology include spatial clustering analysis, hotspot detection, and spatial regression models, which map and analyze the relationships between diseases and environmental variables (Cuadros et al. 2021).

By identifying geographic concentrations of chronic disease, spatial epidemiology can offer guidance for environmental improvements. More generally, improving access to healthy food and creating safe spaces for physical activity can mitigate chronic disease risks in low-income communities. Research has shown that areas of economic distress tend to have higher rates of chronic diseases, likely due to a combination of environmental, social, and lifestyle factors.

A study led by Bravo et al. (2019), for example, examined the relationship between racial segregation and hypertension in Durham, North Carolina. The researchers found that neighborhoods with higher levels of racial isolation, particularly among non-Hispanic Black populations, had significantly higher rates of hypertension. A 0.20-unit increase in racial isolation was associated with a 1.06 to1.11 times higher likelihood of developing hypertension. These findings suggest that racial isolation, coupled with social and environmental stressors contributes to the disproportionate rates of hypertension among Black individuals.

Spatial technology has been used in assessing walkability, access to exercise facilities, in conjunction with developing prevention and treatment strategies for chronic diseases. GIS, for instance, has been used to assess the availability of sidewalks, parks, and recreational centers, identifying gaps in infrastructure that prevent regular physical activity. Improving neighborhood walkability, as many health experts advocate, promotes healthier lifestyles, and thus helps prevent chronic diseases.

In a study on walkability in Northern New Jersey, Plascak et al. (2019) used Google Street View imagery and a statistical approximation method called "kriging" to assess sidewalk conditions and identify barriers to walking-based physical activity. The study evaluated sidewalk presence and condition across 11,282 locations, revealing that sidewalks were more common and better maintained in urban areas like Newark and Hoboken, while suburban areas had fewer or lower-quality sidewalks. Even in urban cores, sidewalks along major roads were often in poor condition. The findings imply that improving sidewalk infrastructure, particularly in underserved suburban and urban areas, could potentially promote physical activity, help residents reach the 150-minute/week walking goal, and ultimately reduce obesity and heart disease rates in the region.

Spatial and environmental analysis goes beyond simple data visualization, such as that used in survey maps; by revealing epidemiological correlations, it can help identify the underlying causes of diseases. In this regard, the Centers for Disease Control and Prevention's Division of Diabetes Translation offers a model program: A Deeper Dive into Diabetes Disparities. This spatial analysis platform presents disparities related to diabetes across multiple dimensions, including prevalence, incidence, and complication prevention. For example, it provides national diabetes trends from 2001 to 2017 (as of this writing), with data disaggregated by education level, race and ethnicity, gender, geographic location, and Social Vulnerability Index metrics. The platform delivers information down to the county level, making it a valuable resource for researchers, clinicians, policymakers, educators, and the general public.

Integrating spatial analysis with emerging technologies such as artificial intelligence is expected to enhance our understanding of the complex links between environment and health. These innovations will enable researchers to uncover new patterns and support more targeted public health interventions.

Further Reading

Bravo, Mercedes A., Bryan C. Batch, and Marie Lynn Miranda. 2019. "Residential Racial Isolation and Spatial Patterning of Hypertension in Durham, North Carolina." *Preventing Chronic Disease, 16*: E36 doi: https://doi.org/10.5888/pcd16.180445.

Casper, Michele, Michael R. Kramer, James M. Peacock, and Adam S. Vaughan. 2019. "Population Health, Place, and Space: Spatial Perspectives in Chronic Disease Research and Practice." *Preventing Chronic Disease, 16*: 190237. doi: 10.5888/pcd16.190237.

Centers for Disease Control and Prevention (CDC). "Estimates of the Percentage of Adults with Diagnosed Diabetes." https://www.cdc.gov/heart-disease-and-stroke-data/data-vis/diagnosed-diabetes.html.

Cuadros, Diego F. Jingjing Li, Godfrey Musuka, and Susanne F. Awad. 2021. "Spatial Epidemiology of Diabetes: Methods and Insights." *World Journal of Diabetes, 12*(7): 1042–56. doi: 10.4239/wjd.v12.i7.1042.

Jia, Peng, Hong Xue, Li Yin, Afred Stein, Mingqi Qang, and Youfa Wang. 2019. "Spatial Technologies in Obesity Research: Current Applications and Future Promise." *Trends in Endocrinology & Metabolism, 30*(3): 211–23. doi: https://doi.org/10.1016/j.tem.2018.12.003.

Plascak, Jesse J., Adana A. M. Llanos, Laxmi B. Chavali, et al. 2019. "Sidewalk Conditions in Northern New Jersey: Using Google Street View Imagery and Ordinary Kriging to Assess Infrastructure for Walking." *Prev Chronic Dis*. doi: https://doi.org/10.5888/pcd16.180480.

Sinton, Diana. 2023. "GIS, Geospatial Technology, and Spatial Thinking in Geography Education." *Oxford Bibliographies*. https://www.oxfordbibliographies.com/display/document/obo-9780199874002/obo-9780199874002-0276.xml#:~:text=Geospatial%20technologies%2C%20including%20the%20use,availability%20of%20online%20mapping%20technologies.

Index

A
ABCG2 155
Abe, Shinzo 131
abortion 29–31
acquired immunodeficiency syndrome.
    See HIV/AIDS
ACTs (Artemisinin Combination
    Therapies) 50
acupuncture 100, 102, 170, 173
Aedes aegypti mosquitoes 24–5, 29, 69–70
Africa
    disease burden in 117
    Ebola outbreak in xi, 272–5
    health care in 78, 124–7
    health education in 78, 117–19, 124
    HIV/AIDS in 231, 234
    louse-borne diseases in 236, 238
    malaria in 48, 50, 117
    mpox in 256–9
    polio eradication in 227–30
    yellow fever in 24–5
aging, global
    challenges of x, 77, 80, 88–91, 96–9
    cultural perspectives on 77, 80–3
    and dementia 83–5
    and disease 96–9
    and health care systems 4, 96
    and Parkinson's disease 92–5
AIDS. *See* HIV/AIDS
air pollution
    and cancer risk 35–6
    from oil sands 57
    and Parkinson's disease 94–5
    post-Katrina 38
Alberta, Canada ix, 7, 55–9
Alfonso XIII, King of Spain 240
Amabie (yōkai) 175, 200
American College Health Association 208
American Expeditionary Force (AEF) 242
American Plague (yellow fever) 25
anxiety 176, 207–10
APOE gene 90
Appalachian region
    cancer rates in 177
    depression rates in 144
    drug abuse in 226
    health care access in 45
Arab Spring 244
Artemisia annua 49, 173
artemisinin 49–50, 173
Artemisinin Combination Therapies
    (ACTs) 50
arts-based health education 78, 118–19
Assad regime 244

B
babesiosis ix, 8–10
"barefoot doctors" 120
bats 13–14, 17, 21, 272
Behring, Emil von 211
benzene 35, 37
Beveridge Model (health care) 133
biosafety 7, 22, 60–4, 75
bird flu. *See* H5N1 avian influenza
Bismarck Model (health care) 133
bitumen 55, 57
Black Death 109
Blumberg, Baruch 203–4
body louse (*Pediculus humanus humanus*)
    236–7
Bordetella pertussis 211–12
Borrelia burgdorferi 66–7
Bovine Spongiform Encephalopathy (BSE)
    260–2
BRCA1 and *BRCA2* genes 32, 91
Broad Street pump 279
BSE (Bovine Spongiform Encephalopathy)
    260–2
Butantan-Dengue Vaccine 70

C
Canada
    health care system in x, 78, 132,
        135–7
    Lyme disease in 68
    oil sands in ix, 7, 55–9

cancer
  and Cancer Alley, Louisiana 35–6
  causes of 32–3
  and Chernobyl/Fukushima ix, 7, 41
  from mining ix, 7, 41, 72–4
  from oil sands pollution ix, 7, 55–9
  and PFAS 56
  prostate 34–5, 48–9
  racial and ethnic disparities in 33, 35–6
cardiovascular disease (CVD) 96–7, 159, 166
carfentanil 224
Center for Epidemiological Studies Depression Scale (CES-D) 144
Centers for Disease Control and Prevention (CDC)
  and chronic diseases 296, 297
  and Covid-19 278
  and GIS 283
  and H5N1 264
  and mpox 256
  on polio 228
  on smallpox 190–1
  and syphilis 194
CEPS (Health Care Products Pricing Committee) 140–1
Cercopithecus aethiops (African green monkeys) 12
Chernobyl disaster ix, 7, 41–2
Chikungunya virus 27
China
  antibiotic use in 171
  Covid-19 in 1–2, 95, 178–82, 285–8
  CSE in 105–7
  fatty liver disease and gout in 153–6
  health care system in x, 78, 120–3
  hepatitis B control in 176, 204–6
  HIV/AIDS in 235
  Lyme disease in 66
  MAFLD in 154
  mental health in 142–7
  overwork in 169
  population aging in 80
  SARS in ix, 13, 19–23
  syphilis resurgence in 176, 192–6
  TCM in x, 79, 100–3, 170–3
  urbanization in 11
  yellow fever in 27
  Zero-Covid policy in x, 1–2, 95, 175, 178–82, 285
Chinese Exclusion Act of 1882 110

chloroquine 49
cholera
  in Haiti 44, 281
  and John Snow xi, 279–81
  after natural disasters 7, 44
Chronic Wasting Disease (CWD) 260–2
Church Rock Uranium Mill Spill 7, 72–3
civet cats 15, 21
climate change
  and bat behavior 13–14
  and disease spread ix, 4, 7–8, 13, 27, 68
  and food safety 222
  and H5N1 266
  and heatwaves 88–9
  and MERS 16
  and mosquito populations 24, 27
  and natech events 37
  and wildfires 4, 37
Clostridium tetani 211
Comprehensive Sexuality Education (CSE) 78, 104–8
Confucianism
  and aging 81
  and CSE 105, 107
consumption. See tuberculosis
contact tracing 179, 286–7
coronavirus. See Covid-19; MERS; SARS
Corynebacterium diphtheriae 211
Covid-19
  in China 1–2, 95, 178–82, 285–8
  economic impact of 179
  global response to xi, 277
  and health care disruption 269
  and mental health 143, 146, 209
  origin of 13, 63–4
  political divides and xi, 175–6, 186–8
  quarantine measures for 1, 178, 285–6
  spatial technology and xi, 1, 277–8, 285–8, 290
  spread of 269
  stigma and 78, 109–11
  in Ukraine 177, 247
  in United States 1–2, 95, 184–8
  vaccines for 1, 95, 180, 185
  Zero-Covid policy for x, 1–2, 95, 175, 178–82, 285
Creutzfeldt-Jakob Disease (CJD) xi, 260–2
CVD (cardiovascular disease) 96–7, 159, 166
cVDPV (circulating vaccine-derived poliovirus) 228–30

cyanide spill 38–9
cytokine storm 172, 240

D
DDT 49
deforestation
　and disease ix, 7, 13, 21
　and Lyme disease 66–8
dementia
　and aging 77, 80, 83–5, 96–7
　care for 83, 85–7, 100–1
　education and 84
　global prevalence of 77, 83
dengue fever ix, 7, 69–71
Dentsu 167
depression
　in China 142–7
　in college students 176, 207–10
diabetes 96, 153, 158, 173, 215
diphtheria 176, 211–13
disasters, natural
　and disease outbreaks ix, 7, 44–7
　natech events and 7, 37–40
drones 287–8
drug prices
　control of x, 138–41
　in Japan 130
　In United States 134, 138
Dugas, Gaëtan 232

E
E. coli (*Escherichia coli*) 44, 177, 218–23
Ebola Virus Disease (EVD)
　in Africa xi, 272–5
　transmission of 13, 15, 272–3
　vaccines for 272
e-cigarettes. *See* vaping
ecocide 57
Egyptian rousette bat (*Rousettus aegyptiacus*) 12, 14
El Niño 14
endemic diseases 24, 69, 193, 229, 238, 257
environmental factors
　and cancer ix, 7, 32–3, 35–6
　and disease ix, 3–4, 7, 143
　and health ix, 3–4, 55
　and lupus 52–3
　and Parkinson's disease 77, 92, 94–5
epidemiology
　spatial xi, 277, 282, 295
　wastewater-based 291
Eradication of Smallpox program 176, 189–92
EVALI (E-cigarette or Vaping Product Use-Associated Lung Injury) 151
EYE (Eliminate Yellow Fever Epidemics) strategy 25

F
familial hypercholesterolemia 90
fatty liver disease 153–6
fentanyl 177, 224–5
filial piety 82, 105
Finlay, Carlos 25
First Nations (Canada) 57–8
Flaviviridae/flaviviruses 24, 26, 28, 69
Food and Agriculture Organization (FAO) 278, 290, 292
food deserts 160
food insecurity 176, 214–17
foot-and-mouth disease (FMDV) 63
forced migration. *See* migration
Four Corners outbreak (hantavirus) 10
France
　drug prices in 140–1
　heatwave in 89
　louse-borne disease in 237
　Salmonella outbreak in 222–3
Fukushima Daiichi disaster ix, 7, 41–2

G
gain-of-function (GOF) research 60, 64
Geographic Information Systems (GIS) xi, 277–8, 282–5, 290–2, 294
geography of health 45
Germany
　drug prices in 140
　Marburg virus in 12
　Wismut Uranium Mining in 73–4
Gilbert, Herbert A. 149
GIS (Geographic Information Systems) xi, 277–8, 282–5, 290–2, 294
globalization
　and disease spread ix, xi, 27, 255, 268
　and drug prices 138
　and health care 127
　and influenza 264
　and public health xi, 255–6
　and TB 268–70

GLP-1 drugs 158–61
gout 153–6
Greece 77, 82
Guillain-Barré syndrome 28
gwarosa (death by overwork) 168–9

H

H1N1 influenza (swine flu) xi, 177, 240, 264–7
H5N1 avian influenza (bird flu) xi, 264–7
Haiti 44, 281
hantavirus ix, 8, 10
HBsAg (hepatitis B surface antigen) 203–4
head louse (*Pediculus humanus capitis*) 236–7
health care systems
   in Africa 78, 124–7
   in Canada x, 78, 132, 135–7
   in China x, 78, 120–3
   comparative analysis of 78, 132–7
   financing of 121, 125, 129, 135–6
   in Japan x, 78, 129–31
   models of 133
   in United States x, 2, 79, 132, 134–7
health disparities. *See* socioeconomic disparities
health education
   in Africa 78, 117–19, 124
   arts-based 78, 118–19
   comprehensive sexuality education (CSE) 78, 104–8
   and nutrition (*Shokuiku*) 78, 112–16
health geography 45
health QR code 1, 278, 286–7
"Healthy Japan 21" program 163
heatwaves 88–9
hemolytic uremic syndrome (HUS) 220–1
hepatitis A 46, 245
hepatitis B (HBV) 176, 203–6
hepatitis E 46
herbal medicine 49, 100, 170
Hirayama, Takeshi 34
HIV/AIDS
   in Africa 117, 231, 234
   global prevalence of 231
   and migration 177, 231, 233–5
   origin of 231–2
   stigma of 110
   transmission of 233
   treatment for (ART) 233
   in Ukraine 177, 247
   in United States 231–2
Hon Lik 149
hospitals
   in China 121–2
   in Japan 129
Huanan Seafood Wholesale Market 63–4
Hurricane Katrina 38, 44
hypertension 96, 154, 215, 296

I

Incompatible Insect Technique (IIT) 51
India
   AIDS Amma and Corona Mata in 175, 200–1
   cholera in 200
   population of 80
   TB in 269
Indigenous communities
   cancer risks for ix, 7
   and oil sands 55, 57–9
   and uranium mining 72–3
influenza. *See* H1N1 influenza; H5N1 avian influenza; 1918 flu
in-situ extraction 57
Institute for Clinical and Economic Review (ICER) 139
International Atomic Energy Agency (IAEA) 43
International Organization for Migration (IOM) 233
Ixodes scapularis (deer ticks) 9, 66

J

Jack in the Box outbreak 219, 222
Japan
   aging population in x, 77, 80–1, 85
   CSE in 107
   dementia care in 77, 83, 85–7
   diet in 162–5
   health care system in x, 78, 129–31
   life expectancy in 162
   overwork in 166–7
   Shokuiku in 78, 112–16
Jenner, Edward 176, 189, 191
Johns Hopkins Coronavirus Resource Center 2, 180, 278, 286
JYNNEOS vaccine 259

K

karoshi (death by overwork) 166–7
Koch, Robert 268, 280
Korea. *See* South Korea
kyūshoku (Japanese school lunch) 164–5

L

lab leaks
    anthrax 61–2
    foot-and-mouth disease 63
    overview of ix, 7, 19, 59–64
    SARS 19, 21, 62–3
    SARS-CoV-2 (Covid-19) 63–4
Lancet, The 2, 182
Laveran, Charles Louis Alphonse 49
leptospirosis 46
lifestyle
    and disease x, 4, 79, 142
    and mental health 142–7
    and obesity 153, 158
    overwork and 166–9
    and *Shokuiku* 112, 163
Lik, Hon 149
lockdowns 1, 178–9, 182, 285
louse-borne diseases 177, 236–9
lupus (SLE) ix, 52–4
Lyme disease ix, 7, 66–8

M

MAFLD (metabolic associated fatty liver disease) 154–6
malaria
    in Africa 48, 50, 117
    control of ix, 48–51
    genetic biocontrol for 51
    after natural disasters 7, 44
    treatment for 49, 173
    vaccines for 50
malnutrition 176, 214–17
Marburg Virus Disease (MVD) ix, 12–15
measles 47, 245, 248
MDR-TB (multidrug-resistant TB) 270
Medicaid 134
Medicare 134
meningitis 47, 67
mental health
    in China 142–7
    in college students 176, 207–10
    and Covid-19 143, 146, 209
    and overwork 166

MERS (Middle East Respiratory Syndrome) ix, 13, 16–20
methamphetamine 177, 224–6
miasma theory 279–80
microcephaly 28–9
migration
    and disease spread xi, 177, 231, 233, 238, 268, 270, 274
    drivers of 251
    health needs of migrants 250–3
    and HIV/AIDS 177, 231, 233–5
    and louse-borne diseases 177, 236–9
    rural-to-urban 176, 195
    Syrian refugee crisis x, 177, 244–6
    and tuberculosis xi, 177, 268–70
mining
    and cancer 72
    and Marburg virus 13–14
    oil sands 55–9
    radioactive contamination from 7, 72–4
mirror bacteria 60
MMR vaccine 47, 246
Moderna vaccine 180, 185
monkeypox. *See* mpox
mortality rates
    from 1918 flu 240
    from cancer 34
    from Covid-19 2, 180
    from diphtheria 212
    from Ebola 272
    from H1N1/H5N1 264, 266
    from louse-borne diseases 238
    from malaria 48
    from Marburg virus 13
    from MERS 16
    from polio 228
    from smallpox 20, 190
    from syphilis 194
    from TB 269
mpox 256–9
mRNA vaccines 180, 185
Müller, Paul Hermann 49
MVD (Marburg Virus Disease) ix, 12–15

N

NAFLD (non-alcoholic fatty liver disease) 153–4

Natech (natural-hazard-triggered-technological) events ix, 7, 37–40
National Health Insurance (NHI) (Japan) 129–30
National Health Insurance Model (health care) 133
Native Americans
   and aging 82
   and uranium mining 72–3
New Safe Confinement (NSC) 41
Nicolle, Charles Jules Henri 237
non-communicable diseases (NCDs) 215–16, 245, 248
norovirus 44
nuclear accidents
   Chernobyl ix, 7, 41–2
   Fukushima Daiichi ix, 7, 41–2
nutrition education (*Shokuiku*) 78, 112–16, 163–4

O
obesity
   causes of 158–9, 215
   and GLP-1 drugs 158–61
   global rates of 159
   and malnutrition 215
   as a risk factor 155, 159, 215
   socioeconomic factors in 159–60, 215
O'Connor, John 58
oil sands ix, 7, 55–9
Okinawan diet 162–3
Ola Bibi (goddess) 175, 200–1
Omicron variant 2, 175, 178, 180, 182
One Health approach xi, 45, 256, 266, 277, 292
opioids 177, 224–6
oral polio vaccine (OPV) 228–9
osteoarthritis (OA) 96, 98
Out-of-Pocket Model (health care) 133
overwork 166–9

P
pandemics
   1918 flu x, 177, 240–3
   Covid-19 1–2, 178–88
   H1N1 (2009) xi, 264
Parkinson's disease (PD) 77, 92–5, 107
passive smoking 34
Patient Health Questionnaire (PHQ-9) 144
Patient Zero myth 232
PCR testing 178–9
Pediculus humanus humanus (body louse) 236–7
penicillin 171, 193
pertussis (whooping cough) 176, 211–13
PFAS (Per- and Polyfluoroalkyl Substances) 56
Pfizer-BioNTech vaccine 180
plague 109, 193
Plasmodium parasites 46, 48–9
polio
   eradication in Africa 177, 227–30
   in Ukraine 248
   vaccines for 228–9
pollution. See air pollution; water pollution
population aging. See aging, global
poverty
   and disease xi, 125, 215
   and drug abuse 226
   and food insecurity 214–15
   and health care access 125–6
   and malnutrition 215
   and TB 269
"Poverty Belt" (U.S.) 176, 215
prion diseases xi, 260–3
PRNP 261
prostate cancer 34–5, 48–9
Pthirus pubis (pubic louse) 236
public policies
   and Covid-19 x, 175, 178–82, 184–8
   and CSE 104–8
   and drug prices 138–41
   and health care 120–3, 129–37
   impact on health 3, 175–7
   and overwork 167–9
pubic louse (*Pthirus pubis*) 236

Q
qinghao. See *Artemisia annua*
quarantine
   for Covid-19 1, 178, 285–6
   for typhus 110
quinine 49

R
racism 4, 33, 35–6, 110
radioactive contamination
   from mining 7, 72–4

from nuclear accidents ix, 7, 41–3
Ranger Uranium Mine 73–4
Reed, Walter 25–6
refugees. *See* migration
relapsing fever, louse-borne (LBRF) 236, 238–9
Rickettsia prowazekii 237–8
Romania 38–9
Ross, Ronald 49
RTS,S/AS01 vaccine 50
Russia
   anthrax leak in 61–2
   invasion of Ukraine 42, 47, 177, 247–9
   nuclear power in 41
Rwanda 13

S
Sabin, Albert B. 228
Saint Roch 201–2
Saint Sebastian 201
Salk, Jonas E. 228
Salmonella 44, 177, 218–23
sanitation 3, 44, 126, 245, 279–81
SARS (Severe Acute Respiratory Syndrome)
   lab leaks of 19, 21, 62–3
   origin of ix, 13, 19, 21
   transmission of 13, 19, 21
SARS-CoV-2. *See* Covid-19
Saudi Arabia 16–17
schistosomiasis 120
school lunches
   in Japan (*kyūshoku*) 114–15, 164–5
   in United States 115, 165
sex education. *See* Comprehensive Sexuality Education (CSE)
sexually transmitted diseases (STDs). *See* HIV/AIDS; syphilis
Shokuiku (nutrition education) 78, 112–16, 163–4
single-payer system 79, 135
SLE (systemic lupus erythematosus). *See* lupus
smallpox
   eradication of x, 176, 189–92
   transmission of 190
   vaccine for 189, 191
Snow, John xi, 277, 279–81, 282
social determinants of health x, 3, 175–7. *See also* poverty; socioeconomic disparities

socioeconomic disparities
   and cancer 33, 35–6
   and chronic disease 96–7, 215–16
   and Covid-19 187
   and disease 3, 176
   and health x, 3, 90, 176
   and health care access 3
   and lupus ix, 54
   and mental health 144–5
   and obesity 159–60
Soul City (TV series) 118
South Korea
   CSE in 108
   health care system in 133
   overwork in 79, 168–9
Soviet Union
   anthrax leak in 61–2
   Chernobyl disaster in 41
   Wismut Uranium Mining and 73
Spanish Flu. *See* 1918 flu pandemic
spatial technology
   and chronic disease 294–7
   and Covid-19 xi, 1, 277–8, 285–8, 290
   in public health xi, 277–8, 282–5
   use by global health organizations 290–3
   wastewater-based epidemiology and 291
   See also Geographic Information Systems (GIS)
Spikevax vaccine 185
stroke 96, 216
Structural Adjustment Programs (SAPs) 127
Sverdlovsk anthrax leak 61–2
swine flu. *See* H1N1 influenza
Switzerland 139
syphilis
   congenital 194
   eradication and resurgence in China x, 176, 192–6
   prevalence 194
   symptoms of 193–4
Syrian refugee crisis x, 177, 244–6

T
Takahashi, Matsuri 167
TCM. *See* Traditional Chinese Medicine
tetanus 176, 211–13
Theiler, Max 25–6

tick-borne diseases. *See* babesiosis; Lyme disease
Traditional Chinese Medicine (TCM)
   decline and revival of x, 79, 100–3
   philosophy of 100, 170
   vs. Western medicine 170–3
trench fever 236–8
Tu Youyou 50
tuberculosis (TB)
   and Covid-19 269
   global burden of 269
   history of 268
   and migration xi, 177, 268–70
   transmission of 269
   in Ukraine 177, 247
   in United Kingdom 270–1
typhus, epidemic 237–8

U

Ukraine
   health crisis in x, 177, 247–9
   Russia's invasion of 42, 47, 177, 247
United Kingdom
   BSE in 261–2
   drug prices in 138
   foot-and-mouth disease in 63
   health care in 133
   TB in 270–1
United Nations (UN) 45, 125, 214, 277, 290
United States
   aging in x, 80–1, 85, 96
   cancer in 33–6
   Covid-19 in 1–2, 95, 184–8
   dementia care in 77, 83, 85–7, 100–2
   drug abuse in 177, 224–6
   drug prices in x, 134, 138–9
   E. coli/Salmonella outbreaks in 44, 219–20, 222
   health care system in x, 2, 79, 132–7
   hepatitis B in 203, 205
   HIV/AIDS in 231–2
   life expectancy in 162
   louse-borne disease in 237
   Lyme disease in 66
   malnutrition in 176, 214–17
   mental health in 143, 207–10
   mpox in 257–8
   obesity in 158–9
   polio in 228–9
   smallpox in 20, 190–1
   spatial technology use in 277–8, 288
   yellow fever in 25
uranium mining 7, 72–4
urbanization
   and dengue fever ix, 69
   and disease spread 3
   and health 155, 266, 270

V

vaccination/vaccines
   for Covid-19 1, 95, 180, 185
   for dengue 70
   for diphtheria/tetanus/pertussis (DTP) 212
   for Ebola 272
   for hepatitis B 176, 204–5
   for influenza 264
   for malaria 50
   for mpox 259
   for polio 228–9
   for smallpox 176, 189, 191
   for yellow fever 24–5
vaping (e-cigarettes) 149–52
variant Creutzfeldt-Jakob Disease (vCJD) xi, 261–2
VDPV (vaccine-derived poliovirus) 227, 230
Vibrio cholerae 44, 279
Vietnam War 50

W

war
   1918 flu and x, 177, 240–3
   and disease x, 3, 47, 177
   Syrian conflict x, 177, 244–6
   Ukraine conflict x, 42, 47, 177, 247–9
wastewater-based epidemiology (WBE) 291
water pollution
   and cancer 35
   from mining 72, 74
   from natech events 37–8
   from oil sands 57
   and refugee crises 245–6
Western medicine 100–2, 170–3
white-footed mouse (*Peromyscus leucopus*) 8, 10, 67
whooping cough. *See* pertussis
wildlife trade ix, 13, 15, 59, 257
Wismut Uranium Mining 73–4

WOAH (World Organization for Animal Health) 278, 290, 292
work-life balance 79, 169
World Health Organization (WHO)
  and Covid-19 22, 179, 278, 288
  and disease eradication 176, 189, 227
  and GIS 283, 290–2
  and hepatitis B 203, 205
  and mpox 256, 258
  and overwork 166
  on polio 228–9
  on social determinants of health 3
  on TB 269
  on yellow fever 24–5
World War I 177, 240–1
World War II 49, 130, 211, 236, 238
Worobey, Michael 63, 232

Wuhan, China
  Covid-19 origin in 1, 63, 178, 184, 285
  lockdown of 1, 179

X
xenophobia x, 4, 78, 109, 250
Xipe Totec (Aztec god) 175, 202

Y
yellow fever ix, 24–7
Yeltsin, Boris 62
yōkai. *See* Amabie

Z
Zaki, Ali Mohamed 18
Zero-Covid policy x, 1–2, 95, 175, 178–82, 285
Zika virus ix, 28–31

About the Author

Jing Luo is a professor in the Department of Languages, Literatures, and Writing at Commonwealth University of Pennsylvania. He earned his BA and MA from Peking University and his PhD from The Pennsylvania State University. In addition to teaching Chinese, French, and Linguistics, his research focuses on environmental issues, public health, and cultural topics. His recent publication, *Cities around the World: Struggles and Solutions to Urban Life* (2019), examines urban challenges and responses.

www.ingramcontent.com/pod-product-compliance
Ingram Content Group UK Ltd.
Pitfield, Milton Keynes, MK11 3LW, UK
UKHW022152230426
12049UKWH00003BA/61